The
Womanly Art
of
Breastfeeding

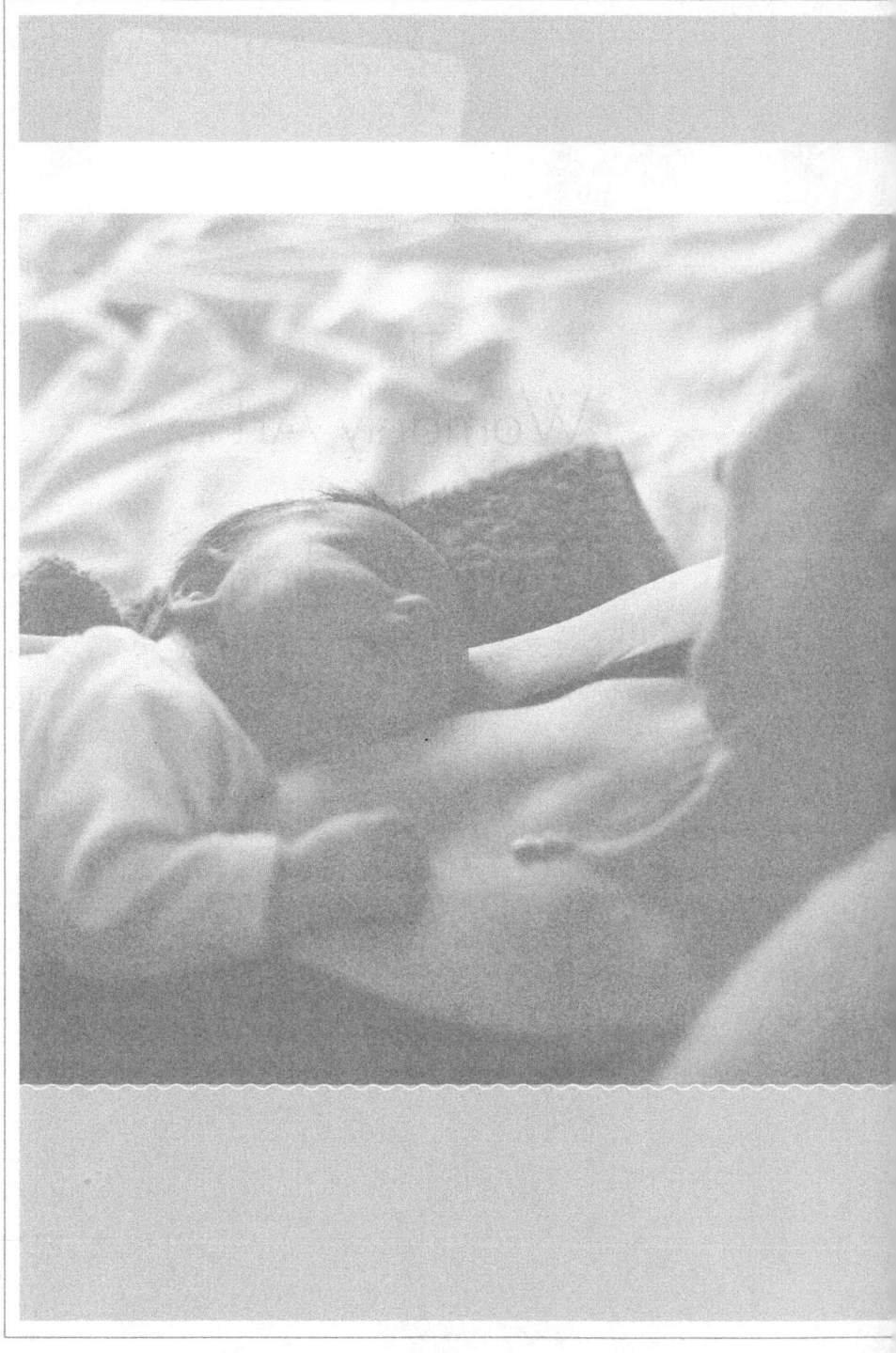

LA LECHE LEAGUE INTERNATIONAL

The
Womanly Art
of
Breastfeeding

8TH EDITION

Diane Wiessinger, Diana West,
and Teresa Pitman

BALLANTINE BOOKS | NEW YORK

Published in the United States by Ballantine Books,
an imprint of The Random House Publishing Group,
a division of Random House, Inc., New York.

BALLANTINE and colophon are registered trademarks
of Random House, Inc.

This work was originally published in 1958 by
La Leche League International.
Revised editions of the work were published in
1963, 1981, 1987, 1991, 1992, and 2004.

LIBRARY OF CONGRESS CATALOGING-IN-PUBLICATION DATA
Wiessinger, Diane.
The womanly art of breastfeeding.—8th ed. / Diane Wiessinger,
Diana West, and Teresa Pitman.
p. cm.
At head of title: La Leche League International.
Includes bibliographical references and index.
ISBN 978-0-345-51844-6 (pbk. : alk. paper)
1. Breastfeeding. I. West, Diana. II. Pitman,
Teresa. III. La Leche League International. IV. Title.
RJ216.W72 2010
649'.33—dc22   2010014031

Printed in the United States of America

www.ballantinebooks.com

4   6   8   9   7   5   3

EIGHTH EDITION

Book design by Cassandra J. Pappas

This book is dedicated to mothers and babies everywhere.
May you find your own way, with confidence and pride,
as you experience the womanly art of breastfeeding.

Contents

PART II Ages and Stages

PART III The Big Questions

PART IV La Leche League Resources

Welcome!

BEFORE THERE WAS *The Womanly Art of Breastfeeding,* there was what I've always thought of as "The Story of Breastfeeding." That Story wasn't written down; it was the breastfeeding wisdom passed down from one generation to the next, mother to mother. Unexpectedly, beginning in the first part of the twentieth century in the most developed parts of the world, the transfer of "The Story" practically ceased. But not entirely. The remembrance of "The Story of Breastfeeding" nourished the writing of the first edition of *The Womanly Art,* published in 1958, cradling it and sustaining its promise.

What never disappeared was the instinctive desire held by many mothers who longed to breastfeed their babies despite the highly touted advances of bottle-feeding (only later correctly labeled *artificial infant feeding*). For many of these hopeful mothers, the desire to breastfeed was thwarted early on due to misinformation or the plain lack of information.

I was one of those mothers with my Elizabeth, my first baby. Advised by the doctor that I didn't have enough milk, I began supplementing with formula. It was the beginning of the end of breastfeeding for us at three months, a regret I carry to this day.

A move to Franklin Park, Illinois, brought our family in touch with Dr. Gregory White, who was alternately referred to as totally out of step with the times or a prophetic maverick. My husband, Chuck, and I were delighted to learn he believed in "old-fashioned natural childbirth and breastfeeding." (Early in our parenting career, Chuck simply went along with my "offbeat ideas," but later he became a strong advocate of them.)

With the birth of our second child, Timothy, in 1952 and with Dr. White's steady guidance, we were on the right track. A protégé of Dr. Herbert Ratner, an early advocate of the wisdom of nature, Dr. White gave me the best mothering advice I ever received: "A baby's wants are a baby's needs." Gone were the confusion and worries about spoiling my baby, holding him too much or too little, following the clock, or nursing on demand. It was wonderful, blessed freedom!

Around the same time, I discovered other young mothers who were also breastfeeding their babies, an underground of "anti-establishment mothering," picking their babies up rather than letting them cry and taking them with them when going out. One of these mothers lived around the corner from me, Betty Wagner; her family was somewhat older than mine.

As we walked our babies on summer evenings, Betty shared her breastfeeding experience, little tips that made nursing the baby and caring for a growing family less stressful, more enjoyable. Various strands of "The Story" were coming together for me—caring, like-minded women companions, a supportive family, knowledgeable medical professionals.

In 1956, the most memorable instance of the revitalization of "The Story of Breastfeeding" came about when seven women in the Franklin Park area, all by then experienced breastfeeding mothers, chose the name "La Leche League" and committed themselves to reaching out to help other mothers who also longed to breastfeed their babies. The core group, hereafter known as the seven founders of La Leche League, consisted of Mary Ann Cahill, Edwina Froehlich, Mary Ann Kerwin, Viola Lennon, Marian Tompson, Betty Wagner, and Mary White. Both Dr. White and Dr. Ratner remained lifelong champions of breastfeeding and La Leche League, which spread rapidly, like a smoldering fire newly reignited.

And so the final element fell into place for the continuation of "The Story of Breastfeeding." A forum and process were put in place for mothers to come together, observe a loving and natural way of mothering, exchange information, and find support and companionship.

This new edition of *The Womanly Art of Breastfeeding,* the eighth, furthers this effort, opening new worlds of breastfeeding information, from pertinent findings from the scientific literature to the homey and highly prized experiences of ordinary mothers and babies. A totally new rewrite, it is a tribute to its three writers. Yet in the background, arrayed like a Greek chorus, stand the many mothers who have come before us.

Dear Reader, turn the pages, begin the story, and discover the beauty and power of breastfeeding. Step into history. There is a place for you in what will always be your own highly personal experience and enduring memories but also an act of great consequence to you, your child, and your family. To all of society. To the world. Thank you!

Mary Ann Cahill, La Leche League International co-founder

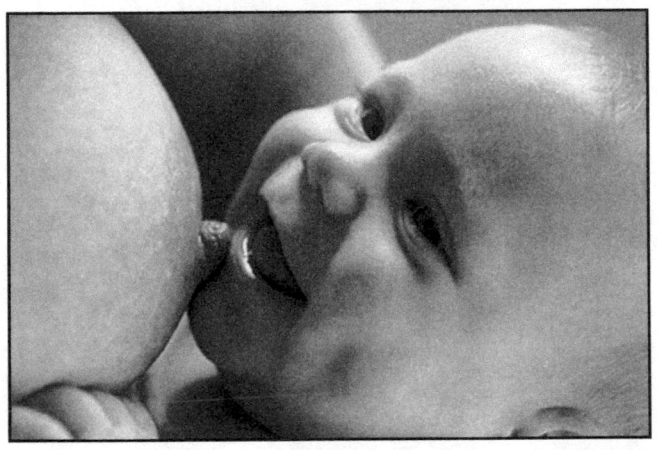

Introduction

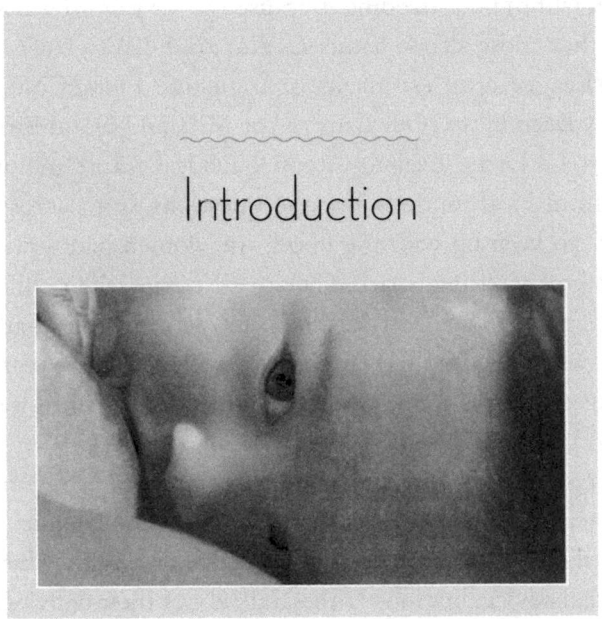

WELCOME TO THE newest edition of *The Womanly Art of Breastfeeding*! This is a book for you, wherever you are in your mothering journey. It's a book about developing a breastfeeding relationship with your baby, with strategies that help combine breastfeeding with your already busy life, and ideas for meeting any challenges along the way. There's some science, for sure, but we hope to bring to life the "art" part, the fun part, the way you and your baby figure out your own dance and make this work for you.

Does our title sound old-fashioned? That's because it's been around for more than half a century, dating back to 1956, when almost all TV shows were black and white and many countries' breastfeeding rates were at an all-time low. *The Womanly Art of Breastfeeding* was the first book about breast-feeding *for* mothers that was written *by* mothers—seven of them, in fact.

These mothers didn't start out to write a book. They were enjoying breastfeeding their babies—many of them had bottle-fed earlier children and breastfed later children—and they had all figured out, as mothers always have, that breastfeeding is much easier when we talk about it with friends. So they began holding monthly get-togethers in their homes for other women interested in (shhh) breastfeeding. Because the very word was shocking in those days, they chose a code name: *La Leche* (lah LAY-chay—Spanish for "the milk") League, after a shrine in St. Augustine, Florida, Nuestra Señora de la Leche y Buen Parto (Our Lady of the Milk and Good Birth).

That first La Leche League Group quickly became multiple groups. Questions from local mothers became questions from across the country. By 1958, to keep up with the flood, the women had written a simple overview of breastfeeding basics. They made copies, their children helped collate the pages, and the first *Womanly Art of Breastfeeding*—all thirty-one pages of it—was mailed from their homes. In 1963, just five years later, they wrote a longer version, found a company to print it, and ultimately sold over a million copies.

And so it grew. Today, from Bolivia to Bulgaria, South Africa to Singapore, breastfeeding mothers get together at La Leche League (LLL) gatherings to celebrate, laugh, cry, and learn from one another. They may share some technical advice, but mostly they talk about their daily breastfeeding experiences—life with a new baby, how to get a reasonable night's sleep, what solids to offer a breastfeeding toddler, what to say to doubting relatives. It's that sharing of experiences, mother to mother, that has been the heart of every LLL gathering and every edition of the *Womanly Art of Breastfeeding* from 1958 through today.

We hope this edition will be like a La Leche League meeting: just enough science to light your path and smooth any rough spots in the road, but mostly practical tips and stories from mothers who have been there. As you read it, we hope you'll think of yourself as being surrounded by all the pregnant women and mothers who are reading it at this same moment, as well as the mothers from the generations before you who have contributed to it. By breastfeeding your baby, you're joining a sisterhood of mothers that reaches back to our earliest ancestors and forward to future generations.

What Makes This Book Different from Other Breastfeeding Books?

What if you had to choose? You can either bottle-feed your baby with scheduled feedings and little body contact, but with your milk in the bottle. Or you can breastfeed your baby, responding to his cues, but only formula comes out of your breasts.

Which would you choose? You'd be choosing between the *product* of human milk and the *process* of breastfeeding…and you couldn't have both.

Some mothers would choose the milk, for all its protective and health-giving factors. Others would choose breastfeeding because they value the closeness and connection—they just couldn't imagine raising their child any other way.

There's no right answer, but in today's world, many women would automatically choose the product over the process because human milk gets all the glory. Studies of human milk are straightforward; relationships are hard to study. We have tons of research on the importance of a precious fluid that just happens to be delivered from your breast. But this book also celebrates the relationship—the *heart* of breastfeeding—not just the fluid. Breastfeeding is a connection as well as a food source, a baby's first human relationship, designed to gentle him into the world with far more than just immune factors and good nutrition. It's a way of *mothering* your baby— a relationship that develops feeding by feeding, building trust, closeness, knowledge of each other, and a deeply connected attachment that lasts long after weaning.

Every language has its own word to describe the infant at his mother's breast. North American English has two: *breastfeeding* and *nursing*. *Nursing* in other English-speaking countries tends to mean cuddling or caring for a baby. Maybe *nursing* began to mean *breastfeeding* in North America because it allowed the speaker to avoid the word *breast*, but we like it because it doesn't imply that it's just a feeding method. So in addition to talking about *breastfeeding*, we'll deliberately be using the word *nursing* because to us it means a connection that's more than just the milk.

What's Different in This Edition?

This edition is for you, the twenty-first-century mother. This new century has new attitudes, new expectations, new trends...and new babies built on a very, very old design. Today's babies have the same reflexes, the same instincts, the same needs that babies had thousands of years ago. We'll offer perspectives on how the age-old behaviors of babies affect breastfeeding today, what our babies need from us, and what we need from motherhood. And we'll help you find ways to adjust when your life and biology don't match.

The world you're living in also has more varied family structures. So we use the word *partner* in this edition to mean the person who shares your home, your life, and the care of your baby, whether that's a husband, wife, boyfriend, girlfriend, or significant other. Or you may have parents, friends, family members, or roommates whose presence is important to you and your child.

You have access to an almost infinite amount of information about breastfeeding online, but there's plenty of *mis*information out there as well, and it can be hard to know what to trust. So the concepts in this book are backed by the best practices in modern lactation science and solid research, with websites mentioned throughout the book and references in the back in case you want to learn more. They're also backed by decades and decades—maybe millennia—of "mother wisdom." Breastfeeding has always been something that women learn from one another, not from experts, so you'll read about other mothers' experiences throughout. Because our support networks are so vital to breastfeeding successfully, we've added a whole chapter just on this topic.

There's also a lot of information on birth in this edition, because while you can find plenty of books about *either* birth *or* breastfeeding, there is a vital connection between the two that isn't usually discussed. This is even more important today, when most women have medical interventions (such as induced labor, epidurals, or C-sections) during labor and birth. These interventions can have unexpected effects on both babies and mothers who are trying to get their breastfeeding relationship under way. To help get things back on track, we've added a chapter just about latching to explain approaches that tap into your and your baby's built-in reflexes and instincts. We've added a section of chronological chapters, with much more information about the practicalities of living with a breastfed baby at each stage of development, including the joys and journeys of breastfeeding a child beyond the first year.

We've delved deeper into ways to get enough sleep, start solids, and wean. If you're going back to work, we've added an expanded chapter to help you continue breastfeeding successfully, minimize your and your baby's stress, and reconnect with each other after your time apart. We've added more information about ongoing challenges like exclusive pumping, premies, multiples, milk supply issues, breastfeeding with a chronic illness, and babies with special needs. We've added a "Tech Support" chapter with to-the-point information on shorter-term problems such as engorgement, jaundice, breast infections, medications, and surgery. We have a chapter all about La Leche League—how we started and what we're all about. Finally, we've added a Tear-Sheet Toolkit of pages that you might want to keep handy or share with others.

Because sharing our stories is the way we women connect to one another most deeply, you'll find a story at the beginning of each chapter, written by a mother from the past or present, sharing her experience from across time and space. It's remarkable how much wisdom there is in the stories of mothers from many years ago; although the world has changed, much about breastfeeding is timeless.

This Edition's Authors

We are three La Leche League Leaders—accredited LLL counselors. We've breastfed our own babies (nine of them among the three of us) for a combined total of nearly thirty years (yes, they've all weaned!)—experiences that drew us to work with, write for, and speak about breastfeeding mothers and babies.

For each of us, breastfeeding was a transformational experience, central to the way we learned to parent our children. It wasn't always perfect or easy—we've struggled through mastitis, plugged ducts, thrush, and sore nipples. We've had babies who came early and babies who came late, babies who wanted to nurse constantly and babies who refused the breast altogether. We've had too much milk and not enough milk. We've worked in the home and outside. And when breastfeeding didn't work out, there was still a heart full of love and a parenting style that was as close to human biology as we could make it.

Diana's interest in helping mothers grew out of low supply with her first baby and her desire to find solutions. Diane wandered into it when she realized she was beginning to give as much help as she got at LLL meetings. Teresa figured from the start that if her horses, cats, and dogs could give birth and feed their babies, she could, too, and she became a Leader to help others find their own paths. But there also have been hundreds of contributors to this book—new mothers, older mothers, and great-grandmothers whose experiences have helped countless mothers over time. This is their book, and...

This Is YOUR Book!

We hope that this edition of *The Womanly Art of Breastfeeding* will help you settle comfortably into a breastfeeding style that fits *you, your* baby, and *your* corner of the world. We think that learning about other mothers and your own and your baby's natural tendencies will make finding your own style easier and more satisfying. As you'll hear at almost any La Leche League meeting anywhere in the world, take a look around, choose only what feels best for you and your family, and leave the rest behind. Whether you get ideas and information from our book, from research, or from talking to other mothers, you know yourself, your baby, and your family better than anyone else. Just as mothers always have.

We want to hear from you! Please visit the forums at llli.org and share your experiences. Tell other mothers how things are going for you and ask any questions that come up as you read this book. In every era, mothering skills have spread like the ripples of a pond, mother to mother to mother. Someone's ripple touches your life, you learn, and you send out ripples of your own. It's a method of sharing as old as humankind, and as soon as you share that first pregnancy hint with another woman, you've become one of the ripple-makers. So keep in touch! Your ideas and experiences might be just what the next mother needs to hear.

PART I

New Beginnings

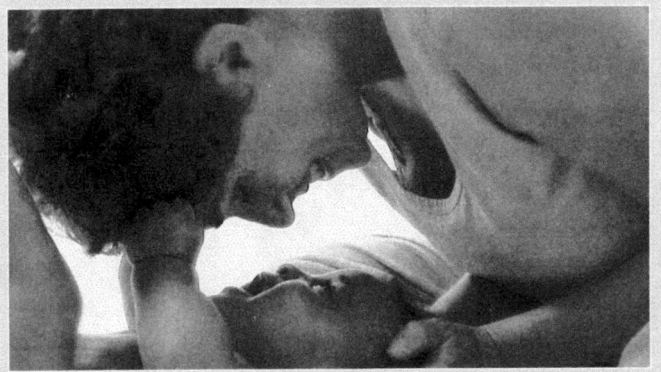

ONE

~~~~~~

Nesting

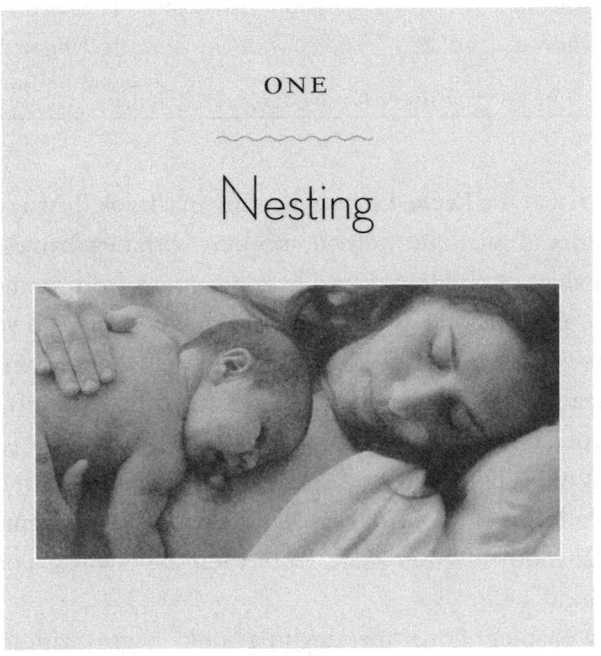

"When I was two, my mother came home from the hospital cradling two mysterious bundles wrapped in soft blue blankets. One was my new baby brother. She handed me the other. Underneath the folds of that soft blanket was a beautiful doll, which my mother explained would be my special baby. My father followed her with a red wooden rocking chair that he placed near my mother's rocking chair. I vividly recall watching my mother breastfeed my brother, and I followed her every move to be sure that I was feeding my own baby properly, even though my breasts looked nothing like hers. My mother and baby brother gazed at each other adoringly during the feeding. I looked down at my own doll, whose eyes closed when she lay on her back. I wanted that lifeless doll to be real. I told myself, "I can't WAIT to grow up so I can feed my own baby!"

"Twenty-five years later I gave birth to my first child. The day I came *home, I sat in our wooden rocking chair, and as I held my son close and nursed him, he opened his eyes to gaze at me. At once, an overpowering recollection of that early childhood memory returned, and tears began to flow as I realized, 'THIS is what I have waited my whole life to do!'"*   —Cathy, remembering 1981

WELCOME TO OUR "La Leche League meeting in a book"! At a real meeting, you'd see a mix of pregnant women, mothers with new babies, and moms with older babies or children. You'd hear questions from women at different stages of motherhood. Some of it would sound right to you, some of it would answer questions you didn't know you had, and some of it you'd shrug and leave behind. We hope you'll do the same with this book.

The cornerstone of La Leche League (LLL) meetings is addressing questions. While a book can never match sitting around with other mothers, we can address some of the typical questions at different stages, and tell you what mothers often share from their experience, along with the research behind it all.

This first chapter of our "meeting in a book" begins with the questions pregnant mothers often have about breastfeeding. Even if you've already had your baby, the answers to these questions should make you feel good about what you're doing and tell you more about why breastfeeding is such a great thing to do.

> *"The newborn baby has only three demands. They are warmth in the arms of [his] mother, food from her breasts, and security in the knowledge of her presence. Breastfeeding satisfies all three."*
> —Grantly Dick-Read, MD, from *Childbirth Without Fear*, 1955

Is Breastfeeding Right for Me?

The closer you are to meeting your new baby, the more you're probably thinking about what comes after birth. You're "nesting"—gathering the things your baby will need and making a place for him in your home. Those outfits are so cute! That changing table is precious! But while you're out shopping, your body is quietly preparing the real "nest" your baby will need—your breasts. They'll be all he really needs at first—his go-to place for warmth, security, comfort, love, and, yes, food. As cute as the outfits and décor are, what your baby will care most about is the way you and your body protect and nurture him.

Breastfeeding is far more than just a way to feed your baby. It's the way you're naturally designed to begin your mothering experience. So why doesn't it always come naturally? Some of your friends may have told you all about their tough experiences. Maybe your mother couldn't breastfeed and you wonder if you'll have trouble, too. The great news is that we've learned a lot since your mother tried. We've learned more about understanding and respecting the instincts that you and your baby both have. We've learned that the fewer interventions you have during birth, the easier these instincts will be to tap into. And La Leche League is always here to help you work through any issues that come up.

Maybe you want to breastfeed because you know it's best; science keeps finding new ways breastfeeding helps babies reach their potential and protect their mothers' health. Maybe you want to because it just feels right; every mother finds for herself all the little ways that breastfeeding brings her close to her children. Whether the urge comes from your head or your heart, breastfeeding *is* right for you. And it's *definitely* right for your baby.

How Important Is Breastfeeding, Really?

Extremely! There is almost nothing you can do for your child in his whole life that will affect him both emotionally and physically as profoundly as breastfeeding.

Breastfeeding is also important to our own bodies. We can't think of an aspect of your baby's health that isn't affected by breastfeeding, and it affects a surprising number of your own health issues as well. This would be a *much* longer book if we described all the ways that breastfeeding is valuable for you, your baby, and your family, but here are a few highlights.

Your Milk Is Your Baby's Normal Food

There's no formula that comes even close to the milk your body creates. Your milk has every vitamin, mineral, and other nutritional element that your baby's body needs, including many that haven't been discovered or named yet, and it changes subtly through the meal, day, and year, to match subtle changes in his requirements. Living cells that are unique to your milk inhibit the growth of harmful bacteria and viruses in his still-maturing system. And it's more than just living cells. For instance, interferon and interleukins are powerful anti-infectives. If you could buy them, they'd cost the moon. Your milk throws them in, free of charge. A squirt of your milk can even treat eye infections and speed the healing of skin problems!

Without his normal food, a baby is at higher risk of ear infections, intestinal upsets, and respiratory problems. Allergies and dental problems are more common. Vision, nerves, and intestines don't develop fully. Because of all these differences (and many others not listed here), a formula-fed baby has a different metabolism and a different development, and gains weight differently during his first year. His kidneys and liver work harder to process the waste products from formula. He needs more of any medication to get the same effect. His immune system's response to vaccinations is less effective. The risk of SIDS (sudden infant death syndrome or crib death) and infant death from many other causes is higher if a baby isn't breastfed.

As an older child or adult, he is at a greater risk of Crohn's disease, ulcerative colitis, type 1 diabetes, heart disease, and certain cancers. He responds to stress more negatively and has higher blood pressure, both as an infant and in later life. There's a higher risk of obesity, type 2 diabetes, heart disease, and osteoporosis in later years. There are numerous IQ studies showing deficits in children who didn't breastfeed, or who didn't breastfeed for long.

Colostrum, the milk you produce in small amounts in the first couple of days after your baby is born (and which you started producing during your pregnancy), has concentrated immunological properties that are your baby's first protection against all the germs he is suddenly exposed to. This "first milk" contains high concentrations of *secretory immunoglobulin A,* or sIgA, an anti-infective agent that coats his intestines to protect against the passage of germs and foreign proteins that could create allergic sensitivities. Scientists have also recently discovered a new ingredient in human milk called *pancreatic secretory trypsin inhibitor* (PSTI), which protects and repairs the infant intestine. It's present in all human milk, but it's seven times higher in colostrum, providing extra protection to that delicate and vulnerable newborn intestine. Think of colostrum as a complex paint designed to seal those brand-new intestinal walls (which were, of course, designed to receive it).

Colostrum has an acid level that encourages a baby's intestines to welcome just the right mix of beneficial bacteria. And colostrum is a laxative that gets his intestines up and running and helps clean out all the tar-like stool called *meconium* that built up in his system before birth.

Mature milk, which phases in during the first two weeks, has a still-unknown number of ingredients that contribute to lifelong health. Along with the interferon, interleukins, white blood cells, and SIgA, the breastfed baby gains an immune system nearly as sturdy as his mother's. Human growth factor continues to develop those intestines, bones, and other organs. Insulin for digestion, long-chain fatty acids for a healthy heart, lactose for brain development—it's all there. And just as important, it's there in forms that are available to a baby. Iron is added to formulas in forms that the baby can't readily use and which can actually be harmful since it increases the risk of intestinal infection, intestinal bleeding, and anemia.

The mechanics of breastfeeding are important, too. When your baby breastfeeds, the muscles in his jaws are exercised and massaged in a way that causes the bones in his face and jaw to develop more fully. The jaw that results from bottle-feeding and pacifiers is narrower, with a higher palate that's more likely to restrict nose breathing. Babies who use pacifiers, instead of soothing themselves at the breast, are more likely to need speech therapy later. The child who breastfeeds for less than a year is much more likely to need orthodontia later on. Snoring and related breathing problems are more common as well.

Your baby can design his own meal to suit his needs. If he's thirsty, he nurses for a shorter amount of time and gets a lower fat milk. Still thirsty? He asks to switch sides sooner and gets another thirst-quencher from the other side. Extra hungry? He stays longer on the first side or nurses more vigorously, to pull down more higher-calorie fat globules. Going through a growth spurt? If your baby takes more milk than usual, he'll have more milk available the very next time he nurses. If he drinks less than usual, your milk production scales back. Is he moving into toddlerhood and nursing less often? There will be more immune factors in your milk to keep him covered. Did he pick up some germs from the grocery cart handle? He communicates those germs to your breast at his next nursing, and it starts cranking out specialized antibodies. In a whole lot of different ways, your breast is Health Central for your baby.

Breastfeeding Helps Keep You Healthy, Too

Breastfeeding is the natural next step in the reproduction sequence: pregnancy → birth → lactation. When your newborn takes your breast soon after delivery, your uterus contracts and bleeding slows. Hemorrhage is a greater risk with formula-feeding, and your belly stays larger longer.

If you breastfeed exclusively (without giving water, solids, or formula) and your baby nurses often, including at least once during the night, then your periods most likely won't come back for *at least* six months. Your chances of getting pregnant again will be extremely low during that time, too (see Chapter 8 for details).

Breastfeeding helps many (not all) women lose weight readily. Nature gave you some of that pregnancy weight just for the purpose of making milk in the first few months. The natural design is for it to melt away by the time your baby is well started on solids.

Women who haven't breastfed are at greater risk for metabolic syndrome, a cluster of risk factors that makes heart disease and diabetes more likely. If you already have insulin-dependent diabetes, you're likely to need less insulin while you're a nursing mother.

Breastfeeding is also an insurance policy against breast, uterine, and cervical cancer. (It may be that the lower estrogen level of lactation provides the protection; the longer you breastfeed, the stronger your insurance.) This doesn't mean it's impossible for you to get these cancers if you breastfeed, but you are less susceptible to them. Osteoporosis and fractures are also more common in women who didn't breastfeed.

A formula-feeding mother's blood pressure is likely to be higher, probably because her neurological and endocrine responses are more pronounced than those of a nursing mother. Her overall physical and mental health take a hit as well, and in later years she remains at an increased risk of developing such autoimmune diseases as rheumatoid arthritis.

> "I didn't realize what immeasurable joy breastfeeding could give ME. I thought it was supposed to be about giving to the baby, not to the mother. Those hormones just poured into me and I was in a blissed-out, euphoric state when I was breastfeeding. And, I have to say, it gave this very un-confident mom something I could finally feel confident and proud of myself for."
> —Samantha

How Reliable Is Breastfeeding Research?

You've probably heard that breastfeeding reduces the risk of infection and a bunch of childhood and adult illnesses and diseases, that it reduces the risk of allergy, and that it even raises IQ. But (are you sitting down?) *none of it is true*!

Here's why: Let's say we're testing a new drug. We focus on the people who get the drug, with a group of ordinary people to compare them with. That's how we know what the drug did. It made things better or worse than normal. Accurate science focuses on the experiment, not the normal thing. Now think about most of the research on breastfeeding. Exactly—*it's research on breastfeeding!* And that means that virtually all our recent research was done backward, evaluating what's normal (breastfeeding) instead of evaluating the experiment (formula). It makes the high rates of formula-fed illness seem like normal baby health and breastfeeding seem like bonus points.

Breastfeeding doesn't *reduce* the risk of infection, illness, and disease. It doesn't *add* IQ points. Breastfeeding results in normal good health and normal IQ. When babies *aren't* breastfed—and this is using the same information from the same studies, just shifting the focus to the true experimental group—they are at *increased* risk for all those short-term and long-term illnesses and diseases.

Researchers have inadvertently hidden formula problems from us by focusing on the apparently fabulous "benefits" of human milk and breastfeeding, almost as if breastfeeding is a nice but unnecessary "extra." That's starting to change. More and more research articles are using the normal breastfed baby as the starting point, as good science requires, and are looking at what happens to babies when their normal system is altered. It can be a scary way for the public to look at infant feeding—to see a list of risks instead of a list of "benefits." But it's a more honest, accurate approach, and it's the one we've used.

Breastfeeding doesn't give you brownie points. It's simply the normal way to raise a baby.

> *"Breastfeeding is a 'safety net' against the worst effects of poverty.... Exclusive breastfeeding goes a long way toward canceling out the health differences between being born into poverty and being born into affluence. Unless the mother is in extremely poor nutritional health, the breast milk of a mother in an African village is as good as the breast milk of a mother in a Manhattan apartment."*
> —James P. Grant, former executive director of UNICEF

Breastfeeding Deepens Your Attachment to Each Other

Before you even picked up this book, you probably heard plenty about the nutrition and immunities in human milk. But if you talk to most experienced breastfeeding mothers, they're more likely to focus on the way breastfeeding helps you and your baby feel connected and attached to each other, weaving an emotional cord to replace the umbilical cord.

It's all part of the way Nature encourages us to take care of our babies and transition from birth. There's a surge of hormones in your body every single time you breastfeed that makes you feel loving and nurturing. These hormones, *prolactin* (pro-LAK-tin) and *oxytocin* (ox-ih-TOE-sin), not only foster a connection with your baby, they also help you recover from the emotional and physical stress of birth. Without these hormones, mothers tend to talk to their babies less, interact less, touch less.

As for your baby, breastfeeding is what he's born to expect. His nursing relationship with you becomes the foundation of the way he will think of himself and others. One mother pointed out that it's as if bottles fill his stomach, but breastfeeding fills his soul.

Many bottle-feeding mothers wish they had breastfed, yet very, very few breastfeeding mothers wish they had bottle-fed. This isn't to say that mothers who are bottle-feeding don't love and value their babies. But there's a difference. When a formula-feeding mother hears her baby fuss or cry, she responds using her mind. When a breastfeeding mother hears her baby make the little sounds that mean he wants to nurse, her whole body chemistry responds.

There is a difference in the intimacy of the feeding, too, that a baby can feel. When a mother bottle-feeds, she holds the baby loosely or off to the side so her breasts don't get in the way. The baby feels her clothes against his face and hands. As the baby gets older and more curious about the world, the mother may find it's easier if he faces away from her, or if the baby holds the bottle himself. When a mother breastfeeds, her body *is* the feeding, with the baby's cheeks on the mother's skin, and the whole nursing is a full-body hug.

The emotional connection created by those repeated full-body hugs is a strong one. After only a short time, you'll probably find that being away from each other, especially in the early months, can be just as difficult for you emotionally as it is for your milk supply. This is a good thing for your relationship, now and for the future.

The breastfeeding experience can also help heal many emotional wounds, from a difficult or traumatic birth to an abusive past. "Baby blues" are more common in societies such as ours where mother and baby are not able to stay together, nursing, from birth.

> "When my kids were teenagers, people were often surprised by our still-close relationship, our long, late-night conversations about everything from their girlfriends or boyfriends and school issues to politics and the future of the world. Other parents would ask me what I did to have this kind of relationship and it was hard to tell them—because I'd have to start out with 'Well, first you breastfeed until they wean themselves…'"
>
> —Ann

Breastfeeding Helps Teach You How to Be a Mother

Breastfeeding eases you into your identity as a mother. You're your baby's food source and you're the one who can comfort him best, so you're the one he turns to. Your body responds instinctively—you don't have to think through what to do once you get the hang of it. With all this intimate time together, you get to know his body and his personality better than anyone else. You know how to interpret his cries sooner than your partner. You know what makes him happy and what he doesn't like. Day by day, breastfeeding builds your confidence and mothering skills.

Many women are surprised by the passion they come to feel about breastfeeding. If you meet another breastfeeding woman anywhere in the world, you feel a connection, no matter how different her culture is, and no matter how long ago you or she breastfed your babies. Not many of us felt this passionately about breastfeeding until we did it ourselves, and many of us remember it as one of the best things we do in our lives. The experience is just that powerful.

> *"I live near a community of Old Order Mennonites. While we shop at many of the same stores, usually all we do is nod and smile. But when I showed up with my baby and sat on a bench near the river to breast-feed him, three other mothers wearing long dresses and bonnets and carrying babies of their own came over and sat by me. They asked how old my son was, admired his big blue eyes, and showed off their own infants. As we sat together breastfeeding our babies, our different ways of life seemed unimportant—we were breastfeeding mothers and that was all that mattered."*
>
> —Teresa
>
> ———
>
> *"What is established in the breastfeeding relationship constitutes the foundation for the development of all human social relationships, and the communications the infant receives through the warmth of the mother's skin constitute the first of the socializing experiences of life."*
>
> —Ashley Montagu, in *Touching*, 1971

And Then There Are the Practical Reasons

After the early weeks when you've learned the ropes and breastfeeding becomes second nature, you'll find you can gentle your baby out of almost anything—hunger, tiredness, overstimulation, fear, pain—with a little nursing. Breastfeeding stops being a feeding device and becomes an all-purpose mothering tool. It's these little social at-breast exchanges, in fact, that keep your milk supply in good shape and your baby growing well. Scheduling nursings, like scheduling kisses, would just make life harder for both of you.

In fact, one of the nicest things about breastfeeding is that it lets *you* take little breaks throughout your busy day. Nursing becomes efficient and easy. Your life may seem to speed up faster and faster, but when you're breast-feeding, you'll have to take time to gather him in your arms and be still for a few minutes. A few deep breaths later, and life seems simple again.

Some mothers say they don't want to breastfeed because they don't want to be tied down, but most breastfeeding mothers will tell you that breast-feeding actually frees them up! No cans of formula or bottles, no washing, sterilizing, or storing. No measuring, spilling, or heating. No planning, left-overs, or spoilage. Most likely a lot fewer trips to the doctor. Your milk is always available, always the right temperature, and never spoiled, no matter how hot or cold it is outside. The money that you don't spend on formula in a year could pay for a high-end appliance. And—this is a big one—in an emergency of any kind, from a minor problem to a natural disaster that means shortages of formula and clean water to prepare it, breastfeeding your baby is one way to ensure you'll always have a way to feed him.

> *"I was once on a plane with my two-year-old nursling, Quinn. There were thunderstorms and we circled the airport for two hours because we couldn't land safely. Eventually we were diverted to another airport two hours away for fuel. We sat on the tarmac for three hours more before we got clearance to take off for the original destination two hours away. None of the passengers were allowed off the plane, and no food or drinks were served (not even water). Quinn and I were per-fectly happy, nursing and playing to keep each other company. But a formula-fed baby and his mother were nearly hysterical because she had run out of formula after about the first two hours of our unexpected nine-hour delay."* —Diana

Will My Breasts Work?

There's a wide range of normal: big breasts to small, low breasts to high, soft breasts to firm, long nipples to short, flat nipples to round to multi-lobed, and more. We're all built differently, and most of us don't look like the women in the breastfeeding videos. Your baby will love your shape, what-ever it is.

Breast size doesn't matter. How much milk you make isn't related to how big your breasts are. There are a few breast shapes and breasts that have had surgery that have trouble making enough milk, and some women do need to breastfeed more often than others to keep a good supply flowing, but there are many ways to help any breast-related problems.

Nipple size doesn't matter. Most babies can give you a hickey or bruise by just sucking on your neck; they don't usually need an ideal nipple in order to latch, just a little matching of parts. If the nipple is too big or wide for the baby to latch, the baby just needs to grow until he has a bit bigger mouth, and then he'll do fine. Some otherwise prominent nipples become temporarily flat right after birth if too many intravenous (IV) fluids during birth caused the breasts to swell. Some nipples are tucked inside the breast (inverted) instead of sticking out, but there are ways to help them "untuck."

So it doesn't matter what size your nipples and breasts are. Sure, there are some breast or nipple types that require extra effort, especially at first, but breastfeeding can almost always work. You'll find tips for breastfeeding with all kinds of different nipples and breasts in Chapter 18.

Will My Baby Latch?

Your baby is born expecting to breastfeed. He has many innate reflexes designed to help him do it well, even if his birth is tough or problems come up. Babies are designed to deal with difficult births, cold, hunger, separation, and germs and still breastfeed well. It's how babies have survived difficult environments throughout history.

Maybe you've seen some of the videos of newborns, placed on their mothers' bodies right after birth, who wriggle their way to the breast and latch without help from anyone. Your baby will have those same instincts *and* he'll have you to help him along. It's not all on your shoulders to make breastfeeding work. Your baby is built for this, with all the reflexes he needs. You provide the access and support.

Your own breastfeeding instincts will guide you to providing the support your baby needs. Most mothers, without even thinking about it, pick up a crying baby and hold him vertically, so that the baby's chest and tummy are against her shoulder and chest. Why is this a good position? Well, it not only calms the baby but also puts him in a good spot to head toward the breast if he's hungry. Calming, access, and support. And we do it without a thought!

It's true, though, that today we see more babies who "can't get their act together" for a while. This is usually because their systems are overwhelmed with birth medications and interventions. Chapter 3 will help you understand and avoid or at least minimize, the possibility of this happening. If your baby does have difficulty latching, there's helpful information in Chapter 18.

Will Breastfeeding Hurt?

When a mother cat feeds her kittens, she's not thinking about how much milk each kitty is getting or what the latch looks like. She just lies there (usually purring) and lets them nurse. If it hurts, though—if one kitten gets on at a bad angle or gets too aggressive—Mother Cat reacts. She moves her body a little, nudges the kitten with her nose, or, if it's uncomfortable enough, gets up, shakes the kittens off, and starts over.

Same for humans. Nipple sensitivity is common in the early days. But if breastfeeding actually hurts, that's your body's signal to change something. As Christina Smillie, a physician specializing in breastfeeding, says, "Pain is the body's way of guiding us to find a more comfortable position. If you get a pebble in your sandal, you don't keep walking on the pebble. You'll stop to do something, maybe shake your foot, to get the pebble out. If that doesn't work, you'll intuitively do something else so you can walk comfortably." Most nipple pain is that simple, solved with a few simple changes that we'll explain in Chapter 4.

Nipple pain and damage are not *normal.* Not for cats, and not for humans.

Will I Have Enough Milk?

It's natural to worry about it, especially if a lot of your friends didn't seem to have enough. But most mothers are able to make plenty of milk. The chances are really good that you will be able to as well.

Some women do have difficulties with milk production, but most of the reasons are fixable. Sometimes the mother was given wrong information about breastfeeding, and sometimes it's because the baby had a problem removing milk effectively. Medicalized births can make it difficult to get breastfeeding off to a good start. Sometimes the mother has a hormonal problem that affects her ability to make milk, and occasionally women have anatomical problems that make breastfeeding difficult, such as previous breast surgery or a breast or nipple problem. So, yes, there are mothers who face challenges in making a generous milk supply. *But there are lots of ways to increase your milk supply* that we'll explain in later chapters. And LLL Leaders are ready to help you at any time.

If you suspect that you may have temporary supply problems for any reason, consider hand-expressing some colostrum to freeze ahead of time (see Chapter 15 for a hand expression technique). Not only can it give you a small "just in case" supply of colostrum, but there's some evidence that it may also boost your future supply.

If, despite all the best information and help, you aren't able to make a full milk supply, *you can still breastfeed successfully.* There are many mothers who nurse very satisfactorily with a partial milk supply. They supplement to make up for the amount of milk they can't make, but their main focus is on the milk they *can* make. They look at the breast as "half full" rather than "half empty"—it's all in how you think about it. One mother with an unusual condition could produce only about 1 teaspoon (5 ml) of milk each day. She thought of the milk as *medicine* for her baby, which she very proudly gave him each day.

Every single drop of your milk that your baby gets is wonderfully beneficial, containing all the immunities of a full milk supply and many, many elements that are completely absent from formula.

How Long Will I Be Doing This?

The short answer is "as long as you and your baby want." You may have an idea now about when you want to stop. Once things are going smoothly, you may decide to keep going longer than you'd originally intended. Unfortunately, many women end up weaning sooner than they had planned, because they ran into challenges and didn't know how to get help. (That's not likely to happen to you, of course, because you have this book and access to the resources of LLL, including the support of other mothers you'll find at LLL meetings.)

What do the experts recommend? Based on research, the World Health Organization and many national pediatric associations around the world advise exclusive breastfeeding (no other drinks or solid foods) for about six months, with solid foods gradually added and breastfeeding continuing for *at least* two years.

Can't imagine nursing a two-year-old? Not many of us can when we have a new baby. For that matter, it's hard to imagine what it's like *caring* for a two-year-old when you've never done it. For now, focus on feeding your new baby and getting help if you need it. Then, when breastfeeding is going smoothly, you'll be able to make decisions about when you want to stop from a position of strength, instead of stopping because you had no choice. When you're ready to think about weaning, we have an in-depth discussion in Chapter 16.

What "Stuff" Do I Need for Breastfeeding?

There are lots of products sold for breastfeeding mothers, but a breastfeeding baby really doesn't need much. Here are our thoughts on the most common products you'll hear about.

Nursing Clothes? Not Really

Clothes made especially for nursing with hidden flaps and access to the breasts are nice but certainly not necessary; most mothers just wear a top that's loose enough to pull up from the hem. Your shirt can droop over the baby and hide any bare skin. Or you can wear a shirt that buttons in front and unbutton it from the bottom. You can also wear a loose jacket or overshirt with a T-shirt or tank top underneath to cover a bit more.

Nursing Bras? Not Necessarily

Bras are never a health necessity; if you're happy bra-less, stay bra-less. If you like wearing one, figure that whatever you wore in your last trimester will probably fit after your baby's born, though your cup size may run somewhat bigger for the first couple of months. You'll probably want two or three. A regular bra that's loose enough and flexible enough that you can pull the cup down or up to breastfeed works well for many mothers. It's a good idea to avoid underwires, at least at first. They can cut across milk-making tissue and increase the risk of milk plugs or infections. Avoid any bra that's tight enough to leave marks on your skin.

Some mothers find that bras made for nursing are handy because they have flaps that open for easy access without having to remove the bra for each feeding. They come in many different styles and fabrics, but cotton is usually the most comfortable. Better-quality nursing bras stand up better to a lot of wear and tear. You'll find good ones at specialty breastfeeding and maternity stores in your area and online. La Leche League carries a line of good-quality nursing bras online at llliclothes.com and in select stores at llliclothes.com/locations.html.

A really good place to ask about bras is at a La Leche League meeting, where women are happy to share what they've learned.

Breast (or Nursing) Pads? It Depends

Some women find breast pads helpful to soak up leaking milk, but some breasts never leak at all. (Leaking has nothing to do with milk supply.) Both disposable and washable brands are available. Or you can make your own washable pads from layers of soft cotton circles sewn together. Many women leave a cloth diaper here and there around the house to catch any drips while they're nursing, and don't need pads in between.

Breast Pump? Not Always

If you won't be separated regularly, you probably don't need a pump at all. Many breastfeeding mothers never need to pump or express their milk. If you want to have one for unexpected separations or the occasional night out with your partner, hand expression or a good-quality manual pump may be all you need. Manual pumps are relatively inexpensive and may remove milk better than the mid-priced electric pumps available at discount stores and drugstores. Hand expression works fine, too, and doesn't cost a thing! See Chapter 15 for an explanation of how to hand-express your milk.

If you're going to go back to work while your baby is still small, this is a good time to investigate pumps—see Chapter 15.

Nursing Footstool? Not Necessarily

Mothers who nurse sitting up and have short legs may find that a low stool raises their lap to support their baby and relaxes their lower back. But mothers who lean back slightly when they nurse, or who simply cross one knee over the other, may have no need for a nursing stool at all. If you use one, it doesn't have to be a commercial product—a thick book, diaper bag, or coffee table crossbar works, too. As you become more practiced, you'll find other creative ways to get comfortable. Try raising just one foot, so your baby's feet are lower than his head.

Soft Carrier? Almost Always!

One of the most helpful tools of motherhood is a cloth carrier, sling, or wrap, so you can "wear" your baby while you go about your day, inside or out. Babies get heavy fast, and it's much easier on your back and arms to have your baby secured to you in fabric that holds him against your body You can use a carrier from birth until he is about 35–40 pounds (16–18 kg)—much heavier than you'd be able to manage with a car seat. Mothers in all cultures have used slings to make life easier. Many a baby who cried the first time will get excited when he sees his sling a few months later.

Having your hands free is great. But baby wearing is even more important to your baby. Research shows that babies who aren't "worn" by adults for much of the day fuss more than those who are.

We're not just talking mothers here. Diana's husband, Brad, used to carry their sons in slings when he'd take them with him to run errands. Teresa's grown son, Matthew, carries his baby in a sling with fabric featuring the logo of his favorite hockey team.

Carriers come in all kinds of fabrics, from mesh to cotton to luxurious washable silk, and in all kinds of colors and patterns. There are many different designs, from ones that tie in a criss-cross pattern to the basic kind that is secured with two large rings. They're not only baby carriers, they're also a clean surface for diaper changing (in a pinch) and a blanket to cover a sleeping baby. Most people won't be able to tell when you nurse your baby in a sling. Some even have pockets for your cell phone and keys. And there are sizes to fit all body types.

Patterns for sewing your own custom sling or carrier are available from several companies online. Sewing can be as simple as two straight seams, and many are just a length of fabric, no sewing needed. Simple styles often work best.

Wearing a carrier does take a bit of practice, and how you use it—even which one you use—may change as your baby grows. Be sure it's cinched firmly so your baby is secure and fairly upright against your chest, not flopping loosely in a hammock, and avoid positions that have the baby with his head tucked toward his chest. Google "sling instructions," check with other mothers at LLL meetings, take a look at Chapter 6, or just keep experimenting until you find what works for you and your baby.

> *"Nursing is the best thing I've ever done (besides having Leah!)."*
> —Kate, a mother whose baby didn't latch for two weeks,
> who had sore nipples for two months, who never had a
> full milk supply...and who ultimately breastfed
> with joy and fulfillment into toddlerhood

What Do I Need to Do to Prepare My Body?

Not much! All the heavy-duty preparation is automatic.

Before Your Very First Period

Some of your earliest milk-carrying ducts were formed at this time, looking something like a cluster of sapling trunks and small branches. Separate "trunks" (ducts) began forming behind your nipple, from which the smaller "branches" grew.

Before Each Period Pre-Pregnancy

Your ducts added more and more branches, the branches themselves began to sprout buds, and milk-making tissue grew, causing the breast tenderness you may have felt just before your period.

During the First Three Months of Pregnancy

Growth accelerates at this time, and more buds are added. Your breasts are probably more tender now than before your periods, and all that internal growth will probably cause visibly larger breasts in the coming months. Each bud grows into a tiny cluster of milk-making cells called an *alveolus* (al-VEE-oh-lus). These *alveoli* (al-VEE-oh-lie) are hollow, surrounded by microscopic bands of muscle. Milk will collect in the hollow center of each alveolus, will be squeezed out by those tiny muscles, and will follow the ductal branches and trunks toward your nipple. Some of the ducts will join along the way, so that you will probably have between four and eighteen nipple pores where the milk flows out.

Now take a look at the outside of your breasts. They might begin to have visible blue veins, and your *areolae* (ah-REE-oh-lee, or one *areola*, ah-REE-oh-luh), the dark area around your nipples, may be getting darker and possibly larger. You may notice small bumps begin to form on your areolae—*Montgomery glands,* which secrete a small amount of oil and maybe milk after the baby comes, and which may help to keep your nipples clean and moisturized.

If you've always felt that your breasts looked "different," or if you're not experiencing any tenderness or changes, consider talking to a breastfeeding-savvy health care provider, and take a look at Chapter 18 to get breastfeeding off to the best possible start.

During the Middle Three Months of Pregnancy

Breast growth continues, inside and out, during the second trimester. "Lifting and shifting" your breasts (see below) will give you a better sense of their changing weight and contour and increase your comfort with a part of your body that you may never have handled before.

MOVING YOUR BREASTS

Here's an idea worth pondering. Cheryl Chapman is a nurse, massage therapist, and author of *The Happy Breast Book,* who suggests that all women, especially pregnant and nursing mothers, move their breasts at least twice a day. She believes that this has many benefits, including improved lymph drainage to remove toxins and improve the immune system, reduce breast tenderness during pregnancy, and improve a woman's awareness of changes in her breasts. Bend at the waist, cup your hands under each breast, and gently move your hands in an up-and-down motion, as if fluffing a pillow. It will give your breasts a chance to shift and move a bit.

During the Last Three Months of Pregnancy

In the last trimester many mothers can express, or even leak, drops of colostrum, the thick, yellowish (or other-colored) early milk that is your baby's first food. It's a mixture of carbohydrates (sugars), proteins, lipids (fats), and immune factors. If you express colostrum, you'll make more to replace it; there isn't a finite amount. And if a pregnancy ends at any time from this point on, almost all mothers will automatically begin full milk production within a few days.

These last three months are a great time to learn hand expression. Even though it's usually just drops (or less), learning how to hand-express is a skill that may come in handy in the months to come. See Chapter 15 for a description of how to do it.

After Birth

The hormonal "wall" that held back milk production comes down when your placenta is delivered. In the first few days, the alveoli continue to secrete colostrum. The sugar and fat content rise dramatically on about the third or fourth day, pulling additional water (and many other elements) into the alveoli, so your milk is now whiter and increased in volume. Mothers often say this is their milk "coming in." But the basics were there from the start, though in smaller amounts and with different concentrations.

During the first two weeks, the extra sugar, water, and fats keep increasing the volume. All of this will happen whether or not milk is removed. Even if you do nothing at all—even if you don't *want* to breastfeed—your body's going to do everything it can to feed your baby.

Your gradual increase in milk gives your baby time to practice everything from breathing to digesting. By about ten days, you're near full production, and your supply won't increase much from about one month on. Your baby may have growth spurts, when he nurses a lot and increases your supply for a few days...but then he'll slow down and your production will return to its usual level.

Shortly After Your Baby Is Born

Your milk production will start to work on a "supply and demand" system, meaning that the amount of new milk *created* depends on how much has been *taken out*. The resulting milk-making process can continue for years once it starts, but only as long as milk keeps being removed from the breasts.

Milk removal is especially important during the first two to three weeks because that's when your milk production capability is established. It's like "calibrating" your milk supply, and it happens all over again with each new baby. Each breast is calibrated independently. The more milk you remove during the early weeks, the more milk you'll be able to make for this baby. If you don't remove much milk in the first few weeks, it will be harder (but not impossible) to make more milk later on. The system is built to work, even with a rough start, but getting started well helps a lot.

Once you start, milk is *always* being made. It's made more rapidly when the breast is less full. The fuller the breast, the more slowly milk is made. This is why your milk production slows down if you wait to feed your baby until your breasts "fill up." It's also why your breasts are never truly empty.

When your baby nurses, nerves in the nipple and areola send a signal to the pituitary to release a hormone called oxytocin. Oxytocin causes those little muscles around the alveoli to squeeze, building milk pressure inside the breast and creating a *milk release* (or *milk ejection reflex* or *let-down*). The tiny ducts yawn open as milk spurts down them. You might feel a tingling in your breasts or shoulder blades, you might feel thirsty or sleepy...or you might feel nothing at all. In the early weeks, a milk release may be triggered just by thinking about nursing or by hearing a baby (any baby!) cry. Your body wants to breastfeed!

What Do I Need to Do to Prepare My Head?

Talk to friends and relatives who've enjoyed breastfeeding. If you know anyone who's currently breastfeeding, hang out with her. Do some reading. If you can, check out a La Leche League meeting (pregnant women are always welcome—no pressure, no commitment). Even watching casually, you'll pick up a lot of little tips and tricks that will help a lot. This will all help you picture yourself happily feeding your baby at your breast.

Most important, decide this is something you are GOING to do, not something you are going to TRY to do. That can make all the difference. Most women who "can't" breastfeed simply don't have enough information or support. With this book in your hands, you have a lot of both. Now all it takes to become a breastfeeding mother is the realization that *you already are one.*

BREASTFEEDING RESOURCES

Some Other Good Breastfeeding Books
The Breastfeeding Café, by Barbara Behrmann
Breastfeeding Made Simple, by Nancy Mohrbacher and Kathleen Kendall-Tackett
So That's What They're For, by Janet Tamaro
The Ultimate Breastfeeding Book of Answers, by Jack Newman and Teresa Pitman

Some Good Breastfeeding Videos
Baby-Led Breastfeeding... The Mother-Baby Dance, by Christina Smillie
Biological Nurturing: Laid-Back Breastfeeding, by Suzanne Colson
Follow Me Mum: The Key to Successful Breastfeeding, by Rebecca Glover

Breastfeeding: A Guide for Success, by the Northwest Georgia Breastfeeding Coalition

Some Good Breastfeeding Websites
llli.org—La Leche League International
ilca.org—International Lactation Consultant Association
usbreastfeeding.org—U.S. Breastfeeding Committee
lowmilksupply.org—Diana West and Lisa Marasco's website
normalfed.com—Diane Wiessinger's website
kellymom.com—Kelly Bonyata's website

Who Will Help Me?

Everyone will want to help you breastfeed your baby. Formula companies, furniture companies, pump companies, baby food companies, ointment and cream companies, relatives, friends, websites, and, um, authors—they'll all tell you how helpful they can be. And they all have different styles and levels of expertise. Almost all have good intentions and want to help you breastfeed successfully (with the notable exception of those funded by formula companies, who have a different agenda altogether). But commercial companies put their own bottom line first, friends think their own experiences are how it always works, not all "experts" *are,* and not all websites or books will suit your style. Here are some helpers that you may get to pick from, in the order in which you're likely to meet them, with some pros and cons:

Who is she (or he)?	How can she (or he) help with breastfeeding?	Points to remember
La Leche League Leader	In-person and phone help, leading meetings, finding information and resources	Is an experienced nursing mother; not usually medically trained; can direct you to medical and other resources in your community

Who is she (or he)?	How can she (or he) help with breastfeeding?	Points to remember
Obstetrician	Minimizing interventions and keeping you and your baby together	May have little or no breastfeeding training
Midwife	Facilitating normal birth and keeping you and your baby together	May have little or no training in breastfeeding
Doula	Help with a smoother birth and early breastfeeding	Usually trained in basic breastfeeding help; some postpartum doulas have had extra training
Hospital nurse	Keeping mother and baby together	May have little or no training in breastfeeding
Pediatrician	Keeping mother and baby together	May have little or no training in breastfeeding
Lactation consultant, lactation counselor, lactation educator, peer counselor, breastfeeding specialist	May be able to help with basic breastfeeding problems	Titles have no standardized or legal meaning; individuals may have very little or no experience helping mothers
International Board Certified Lactation Consultant (IBCLC)	Experienced and legally certified to give breastfeeding help in special situations	May not have breastfed own children

At La Leche League and in this "meeting in a book," we're sharing information based on research and on the experience of generations of mothers. But at the end of the day, we can't go home with you and our lives won't be affected by the decisions you make. You need to do what's right for you and your family. When it comes to breastfeeding, the decisions are always up to you. Listen to your heart and trust that you know—or will know—your baby better than anyone else. Because you are your baby's *mother.*

TWO

Building Your Network

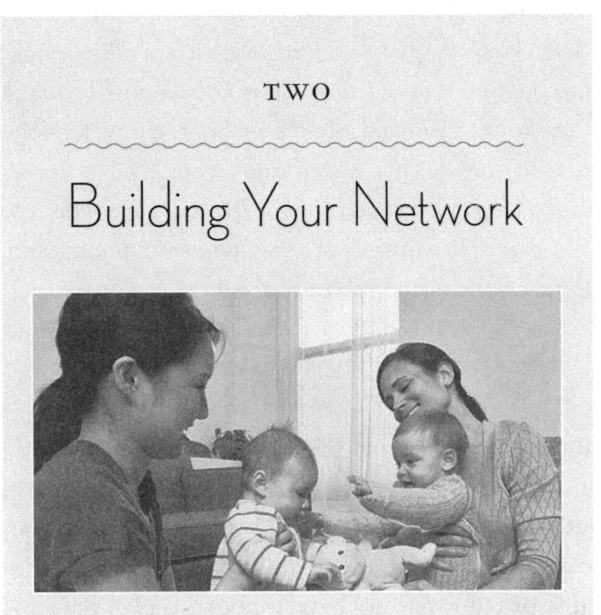

"*I never questioned how I would feed my own babies—babies nursed; this was just the way my world worked. And this, I thought, was normal.*

"*Then I had a child of my own, and the questions and comments started. I quickly realized: to most of America, the way I had been raised was anything but normal. I had grown up in a bubble without realizing it, and now I had moved outside the bubble. It was hard to face the criticism, stated and implied, but everything I knew—from science, from my faith, from my upbringing, and from my own experience with my daughter—told me that no other way of parenting could provide what my child and my family needed.*

"*Thanks to my mother, I had plenty of support and information only a phone call away. But surrounded by startling evidence of the 'abnormality' of what I was doing, I started to long for, and found, local support—other women with young children to whom I could talk without feeling weird. Now I have friends with whom I can freely discuss the joys and challenges of toddler nursing—a small version of my childhood bubble where I know that I am normal, that my child is normal, and that what we are doing is right. Secure in this knowledge, I can take a little bit of that confidence with me into the rest of the world, and surprise a few people with how well my 'weird' ideas work.*

"And, just as my mother did for me, I'll nurse my children as long as they need to, even if this raises eyebrows when we go out. And they will be taught that all this is normal—because it is."

—Newt, remembering 2002

IF YOU'RE READING this book from beginning to end, instead of just dipping into it for the information you want, you may wonder why this section is near the front of the book. Why aren't we starting with the how-tos of initiating breastfeeding? Why are we talking about building a network of support when your baby may not even be born yet?

Here's why: Being part of a supportive community is more important than you might think in succeeding at breastfeeding and smoothing the road to parenthood. It really is part of the basic how-to.

The statistics tell the story. Today, the majority of new mothers in almost every country in the world opt for breastfeeding. As a new breastfeeding mother, you're in good company! But the statistics also tell us that, in many places, most of those mothers stop breastfeeding within a few weeks or months, usually earlier than they had wanted to. What goes wrong?

There's no one answer—every mother's story is unique. Often, though, those many individual challenges that led to weaning can be boiled down to one thing: not having the support network they needed.

You'll sometimes hear at La Leche League meetings that people are more important than things. It's true once you have your baby, but it's also true when you are getting ready. In the last chapter, we talked about "nesting" being more about preparing your mind, getting to know your breasts, and arranging to keep your baby close than it is about buying baby equipment. Nesting is *also* about gathering the people you'll need around you.

What kind of practical help will you want? What kind of emotional support? Who do you want to be in touch with to share stories, concerns, and those moments of pure joy? That's the foundation of your community, your village, your extended family, your network.

We're Designed to Have Networks

Different types of mammals live in different ways. Some are almost always found in groups or herds or packs, like dolphins, horses, and elephants. Others are more solitary, like tigers and bears. Force an elephant to live alone and you'll have a very unhappy elephant who won't be able to care for her babies well.

So what about people? How do humans normally live? If you look at our ancestors and at people in the developing world, you'll see people in tribes and villages: small communities, often of people who are related to one another in some way, where everyone pretty much knows everyone else. We're not like bears, happy to live alone in our caves; we're a lot more like elephants, who crave the company of other elephants.

Traditional tribes are usually made up of people from several generations: great-grandparents, grandparents, parents, and children. When a baby comes along there are plenty of experienced relatives to help and support the new family. In fact, new parents probably don't need much advice and information. In traditional tribes, where babies are part of everyday life, the new mom and dad have been watching other parents since they were babies themselves, and they've absorbed most of the skills they need without even trying. They've had plenty of chances to practice, too, because they've been carrying and soothing and entertaining babies—their own siblings and cousins and neighbors—for many years.

So the new mother in this traditional village is pretty confident about breastfeeding. She's watched everyone else around her do it, she's seen the variations, and she knows that sometimes people have challenges—their nipples get sore, or they get plugged ducts or mastitis—but she's also seen people solve those problems, so she knows they can be fixed. She's watched mothers breastfeeding in every imaginable position, including walking around to see what their toddlers are up to, and she has a mental image of the way that breastfeeding looks when it's working well. So does her partner.

Babies operate on pure instinct at first—who would they have watched and learned from ahead of time?—but they have to be in the right place at the right time to make it work. That's the mother's job, and that's partly learned. Even elephants struggle to feed their babies if they haven't learned it by observation.

So it can be hard for a new mother today. Your mother might not have breastfed at all, or only for a short time. The images that you carry around in your brain of babies being fed might feature bottles than breasts.

And support can be hard to find. One mother commented that before she had her baby her childless friends all promised to visit and help out. "Maybe they would have helped, but we were in a new-baby fog and didn't call. *They* didn't call because they didn't want to intrude. 'We'll be glad to help out' ended up being one dinner a month later. The support we'd counted on from casual friends really wasn't there."

Every situation is different, and you may have a family around you that understands and supports breastfeeding, or a ready-made circle of friends who are experienced nursing mothers. Or you may be trying to build your support network from scratch. One great place to start is La Leche League.

La Leche League

When those seven mothers created La Leche League in the 1950s, they were just thinking of providing information to other mothers. But for many women, their local LLL Group became a kind of community or extended family—exactly the kind they needed, a place where breastfeeding is *normal*. At La Leche League, because breastfeeding is recognized as the normal way of feeding a baby, difficulties are just something to resolve in order to keep a normal process going.

That's not always the case with mothers' groups. Go to some of them and ask a question like, "My baby wakes up a lot at night and I'm really tired. What can I do?" The responses often zero in on breastfeeding as the probable cause of the problem, with suggestions that your baby shouldn't be eating that often, that you don't have enough milk, that formula would help, or that your partner should take the night shift, bottle in hand. Breastfeeding itself isn't the problem in this situation, and formula isn't the answer. But breastfed babies are still unusual in many communities, so people figure that any problems are probably related to it, even when the mother hasn't really asked about feeding.

You'll hear some different answers at La Leche League meetings. We know that many baby behaviors, including wanting to be held, needing to nurse "again," and waking at night, are perfectly normal, and we can help you figure out ways to meet your baby's needs and your own without sacrificing breastfeeding. Whatever question you have, whatever concerns are worrying you, at La Leche League meetings we'll try to help you in a way that keeps the "normalness" of breastfeeding in mind.

So La Leche League can be one cornerstone of your network. Who else?

Other than Mother

Most new mothers have a life partner: a husband, wife, boyfriend, girlfriend, significant other, or whatever name you give your relationship. It may also be a non-parent, such as a grandmother, other relative, or close friend. Your partner is another cornerstone of your tribe, and his or her support can make a huge difference to your breastfeeding experience. But this person can also be at a huge disadvantage when it comes to supporting you. He or she may be enthusiastic about breastfeeding and knowledgeable about all the reasons it's important, but when problems crop up that person may feel helpless. If you're crying because your nipples hurt and the baby never seems satisfied, your partner has a big dilemma: tell you to keep trying (or even try to repeat some of the suggestions the midwife made at her last home visit) and risk being labeled insensitive to your pain and struggles, or pop out to the store to pick up some formula and risk being told it undermines breastfeeding.

There is a happy medium! Partners don't need to know how to solve breastfeeding problems; *they just need to help you link up with the support and information you need.* Sometimes it's the partner who makes the first call to a

LLL Leader or finds the date and location of the meeting on the website (llli .org). Or maybe your partner searches through the folder you were given by the midwife or hospital nurse with contact information about breastfeeding clinics or lactation consultants and makes an appointment for you.

Partners want to connect with their babies, too, and when they see the closeness and intimacy of the breastfeeding relationship, feeding the baby themselves looks like the obvious way to do it. But there are a gazillion ways to bond with a baby without bottle-feeding—in fact, partners have the key role of teaching the baby that love sometimes comes without food. Some partners take over bath time. Your partner might like to let the baby have daily "tummy time" by leaning back on the couch, baby on chest, or by wearing the baby in a wrap or sling (tummy time doesn't have to be horizontal!).

Partners can be wonderful comforters. Babies like different voices, from low and rumbly to soft and motherly. Most partners soon figure out their own repertoire of baby-soothing tricks. They will be different from the birth mother's. But "different" can help!

Partners can often help by doing *everything but* feeding. They can take charge of diaper changes (most babies' favorite non-nursing activity after the early weeks), bring you a drink or snack (or both), and take baby off for a relaxing walk or in-arms snooze when the feeding ends. Nursing itself isn't especially tiring—after the first few days or weeks the baby can usually latch just fine even if you're half asleep, so this kind of everything-else help can make a huge difference, with no need to involve bottles.

Why not just give a few bottles? Some babies seem to be able to adapt easily to the different kind of sucking involved: But even with these babies, mothers often find that they end up with feeding problems over time if there are too many bottles. The baby can learn to like the fast, steady flow from the bottle and get frustrated at the breast because the milk flows more slowly at first. There's also an effect on your milk production. If the baby is getting bottles and you don't pump or express your milk, your breasts will make less milk.

One of the most helpful things a partner can do is to be a buffer between you and other relatives and friends who may be uninformed or even opposed to breastfeeding. If your mother or mother-in-law didn't breastfeed, or tried to breastfeed for a short time but ended up weaning early, she might feel that your decision to nurse your baby is a subtle way of criticizing her choices and decisions. If breastfeeding was difficult for her, she may want to protect you from the pain and struggles she went through. Or she may feel that a longer breastfeeding relationship than hers is not only long but wrong.

Don't have a partner at all? That's a tougher road, for sure, but many, many single mothers have successfully breastfed and built their own unique community of support. There are sources of paid support, such as doulas and nannies. But there are no-cost possibilities, too—enlisting friends to help with meals, entertaining your older children, and conversation when you need it. You may have friends or family eager to help out who just need some suggestions on what to do. (You'll find a suggestion list for them ready to fill in and tear out in Chapter 20.) If you don't have an already-built support network, you can begin building one today, whether or not your baby is here. You can ask your caregiver about support groups available in your community, ask at your LLL meeting if anyone would like to get together informally, or check with local religious and community centers to see if they offer groups for new parents.

You may have heard "it takes a village to raise a child." That can be interpreted to mean that the other "villagers" play a direct role in teaching and encouraging the child. But there's another way to look at it. The role of the village can be to support the new mother and her family, so that she can put her time and energy into mothering her baby and the child that her baby becomes.

TEN WAYS A PARTNER CAN HELP

1. Before the baby's born, help stock the freezer with meals that can be eaten with one hand.
2. Find a good phone number for help and *call it as needed*. (La Leche League's website, llli.org, and U.S.-based phone line, 877-4-LA LECHE (877-452-5324), can both lead you to your closest local group, and that's a fast route to anything else you might need.)
3. Buy the grocery basics, and keep easy, healthy snacks on hand.
4. Get dinner—*any* dinner!

5. Nights can be tough at first. Be flexible about where and when everyone sleeps. Going to bed early helps!

6. Do more than your share. You may be what keeps the household running for a while.

7. Everything won't get done. Talk about what's most important *to her*—a clean kitchen? a cleared desk?—and do that first.

8. Get home on time. You're like a breath of fresh air for mother and baby both.

9. Helping out means helping emotionally, too. Remind her how much you love her, how wonderful she looks, and what a great job she's doing. There she is, holding your child. She really is beautiful, isn't she?

10. Remind her that this part is temporary. Most women feel it takes at least six weeks to start to have a handle on this motherhood thing. Life will settle down. But it takes a while.

Online Support

In the villages and networks we've been talking about, new parents get face-to-face support: someone to demonstrate when you want to see how to hand-express a little milk, someone to wash the dishes, and someone to give you a hug when it's been a long day. But many mothers today find they can get an important layer of support from e-mail, texting, instant messaging, or online forums.

Where do you find this kind of network? Your local LLL Group may offer an e-mail list that you can join, or your prenatal class may create one that allows you to stay connected after your babies are born. You may find it especially helpful to communicate electronically with people you can also get together with in person.

Or you might be able to connect with mothers around the world. Many websites, such as llli.org, offer forums where mothers ask and respond to questions. Some are more active than others and some are more breastfeeding-friendly than others. So pick carefully, and be aware of the limits to Internet support. A few people take advantage of the anonymity that e-mail and forum usernames provide to post "flames"—unkind, rude, and insulting messages that no new mother needs. You also don't know whether a website or poster's qualifications are valid, so weigh any information gathered this way against what you get from known, reliable sources.

Those limitations aside, though, forums and e-mail lists can be a great way to connect with other mothers. Sometimes it's easier to tell strangers about your struggles with thrush or the hurtful comment your mother-in-law made. If you have an unusual challenge—maybe you've given birth to triplets, or your baby has an uncommon problem, for example—you may be able to find a list for that specific issue. A huge help for those days when you're feeling alone in the world! And what faster way to connect with other wakeful friends at two in the morning?

Paid and Professional Support

After Lorna's baby Morgan was born, her mother came to stay with her for six weeks to look after the older children, take care of the house, and prepare all the meals—including stocking up Lorna's freezer with extra food she could pull out for weeks to come. Sadly, the techniques for cloning Lorna's mom haven't been perfected.

If it fits into your budget, though, you can hire support. Postpartum doulas, for example, are available in many communities. They will come into your home for several hours a day (depending on your situation and needs) to help with housework and basic baby care (other than feeding the baby, of course). Many have some experience in helping breastfeeding mothers. You can also hire a nanny, cleaning service, personal chef, and so on if your budget will stretch this far. One mother of breastfeeding twins hired a personal chef who came to her house, discussed the foods she liked and didn't like, then spent another day in her kitchen preparing, packaging, and freezing meals she could thaw and eat over the next month or so. Money well spent, she felt, and certainly less expensive than eating out in restaurants or buying formula for two babies.

TEN THINGS NOT TO SAY TO A NEW BREASTFEEDING MOTHER

1. Is he eating *again*?
2. He's just using you for a pacifier.

3. Here, I'll feed the baby a bottle and you can go get some house-work done.
4. Maybe your milk isn't good enough.
5. We've never made enough milk in our family.
6. Can breasts that size really make enough milk?
7. If you're going back to work, shouldn't he get used to having some of his feedings from other people?
8. You look like a cow attached to that pump.
9. I feel like your breasts really belong to me, not the baby.
10. Don't let him fall asleep at the breast—he'll get into bad sleep habits.

A Diverse Network

It's tempting to build your entire community around people who "get" exactly what you are going through. But there's value in diversity. Many of us were surprised, as new mothers, to discover the important role played by those who don't agree with us! Maybe you don't *want* to be like your mother or your friend, and her model of what *not* to be helps to guide you. Maybe you rise to challenges better than you respond to encouragement, and sometimes having someone disagree with you helps you solidify the reasons for your choices. There will always be people who have a different point of view, and it's not always a bad thing. This was part of the value of having multiple generations of relatives in those early villages. If you include some more experienced moms, even grandmothers, you get a longer-term perspective that can really help. What you need is a community of people who care about you and who won't try to coerce you into following their ideas. Your community doesn't have to speak with the same voice. It just has to love you.

Having a Positive Health Care Provider

Negative voices have their place, but not in your health care provider. Most doctors these days say—and believe—that they're supportive of breastfeeding. But if there are formula cans visible in the office, if suggestions are made to breastfeed less or to use formula as the first approach to a problem, if what you hear just doesn't feel right to you, you can always shop around. You'll probably hear some names more than others, but remember that part of what makes for a good relationship with your doctor is just plain personality combinations. This conversation took place between two mothers at a La Leche League meeting: "I'm so pleased with our doctor. He's flexible, he listens to us, and he really seems to care." "You're lucky. Ours is incredibly rigid. I don't get the sense that he's really listening to me at all." It turns out they were talking about the same doctor!

Networks Can Start Small

Many women breastfeed their children with a very small network behind them at first—just one or two friends or relatives who breastfed. When things are going well, that's all you need. But oh, the pleasure of a playgroup, a knowledgeable and enthusiastic doctor, an experienced mom who can share her insights, a teenage girl who can play with the baby sometimes as you take a shower, the friend to go on walks with, the La Leche League Leader who's just a phone call away....More than one woman who never, ever called La Leche League found her path easier just knowing that she could if she needed to. Tailor your network to your needs, and keep an "outside line" open in case you decide to expand.

Your Baby as a Member of Your Network

Diane felt much of her new-motherhood stress lift when she stopped trying to get away from her newborn. It was a realization that finally hit at about six weeks. Your baby is *part* of your support system, not just the reason you need support. Yes, he gives you an excuse to leave parties or end phone conversations whenever you choose. But it goes much deeper than that. You may discover that you begin to feel lost when your baby isn't with you. Babies and breastfeeding can give us a confidence we never had, an ability to cut through the nonsense and make solid decisions, to know for sure what's right for us and our families. Babies turn us into mothers, and motherhood is astoundingly powerful. Yes, we all need to find our network, but don't forget that your baby is part of it, too, with his smiles, his warm body against yours, his bright eyes focused on you when you say his name. Someday soon this amazing little person, who led you to need a network in the first place, will be its most important member.

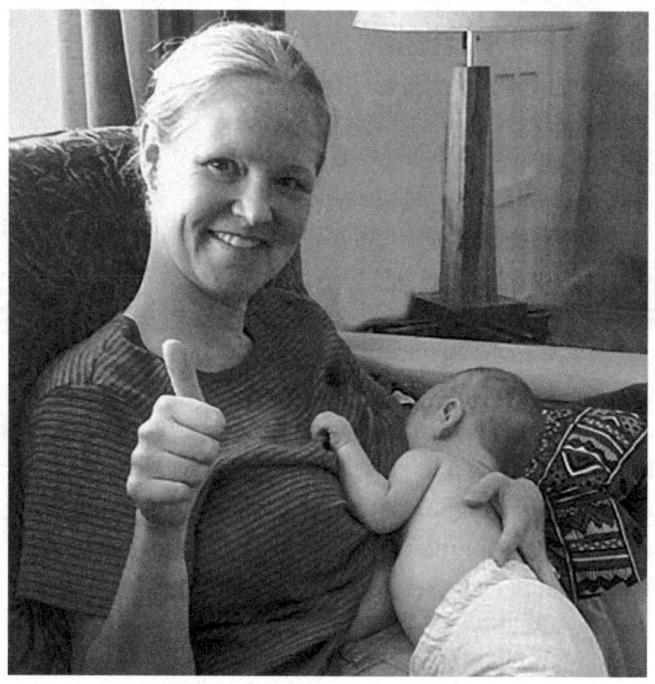

THREE

Birth!

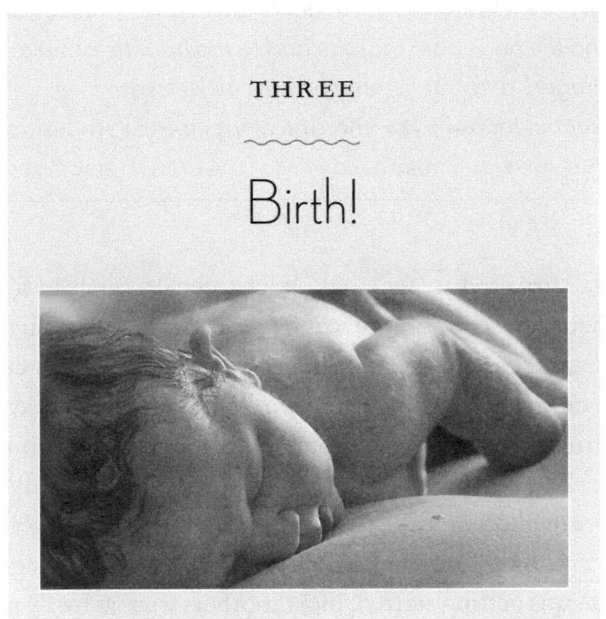

"When I had my second baby—no medications or interventions—babies were test-weighed before and after every feeding. If the baby wasn't 'getting enough,' you were supposed to top up with formula. My daughter nursed for thirty minutes or so in the delivery room. After she had her second time at the breast, the nurse came back to tell me that my baby was getting 'too much'! I asked how that was possible. She said that I must be nursing her for too long and I'd end up with sore nipples. I ignored that and we soon checked out of the hospital. My daughter was four ounces over birth weight by the time she was a week old.

"My roommate during that short hospital stay had a lot more difficulty. I remember her curled up on the bed, looking miserable. I asked what was wrong and she said the pain meds were wearing off. She'd had her labor induced, had six hours of an epidural, and ended up *with an episiotomy for a forceps delivery. When the nurse brought in her baby to feed, she struggled to find a comfortable position and the baby didn't seem to know what to do. I tried to give her tips, but it didn't go well and the nurse said that she had to top up with formula. She was so discouraged, and commented on how lucky I was.*

"We kept in touch for a while. She stopped trying to breastfeed by the time her son was a month old."   —Krissy, remembering 1978

YOU MIGHT BE surprised to see a whole chapter on birth in a breastfeeding book; there's a trend today away from learning about birth or taking childbirth classes, trusting instead to an obstetrician and an epidural. But becoming a mother isn't just getting the baby out. A complex hormonal sequence during labor sets us and our babies up to take on our new roles with confidence and enthusiasm, and if that sequence is disrupted too much, both early motherhood and breastfeeding can be harder.

We've been down this road before. A full half century ago, when La Leche League was getting started, most mothers were actually unconscious during the birth. Mothers woke up from anesthesia to be handed a freshly washed and dressed baby that they had to assume was their own. It wasn't thrilling, but they were certain it was better than the pain of an unmedicated childbirth.

The women who started La Leche League were interested instead in the unmedicated, partner-attended, often at-home births that the new natural childbirth movement promoted. They discovered that birth can be exhilarating. They also discovered that breastfeeding was a whole lot simpler and, well, *natural* after a simpler, more natural birth.

But somewhere along the line, we found ourselves back on that "medicated birth road." Mothers are usually conscious for birth today, but the majority have some medications—such as an epidural anesthetic—that prevent them from feeling labor and birth. Unfortunately, medicalized birth tends to disrupt a mother's sense of motherhood and impede a baby's ability to breastfeed easily, just as it did in the 1950s. You can improve your odds for a smooth start to breastfeeding by planning for a birth with as few interventions as possible.

Breastfeeding is likely to begin more smoothly if you *read* at least one book that promotes normal birth, *take* a childbirth class that gives lots of non-medical ways to handle all kinds of labors, and *find* a birth helper who is experienced in helping to keep births normal. A La Leche League meeting can be a terrific place to start. Coming *before* your baby is born connects you immediately with other mothers and mothers-to-be. All you have to do is ask, "Do you know any good birth resources around here?" You'll learn in minutes what's available in your area and what other mothers' experiences with those resources have been. A downloadable list of questions to ask and think about when choosing a caregiver and birthing location is available at motherfriendly.org/downloads.php.

SOME COMPREHENSIVE BIRTH BOOKS

The styles of these books vary; find one whose tone makes you want to keep reading.

The Birth Book: Everything You Need to Know to Have a Safe and Satisfying Birth, by William Sears and Martha Sears

Gentle Birth, Gentle Mothering: The Wisdom and Science of Gentle Choices in Pregnancy, Birth, and Parenting, by Sarah J. Buckley

Ina May's Guide to Childbirth, by Ina May Gaskin

The Official Lamaze Guide: Giving Birth with Confidence, by Judith Lothian and Charlotte DeVries

Pregnancy and Birth, by Teresa Pitman and Joyce Barrett

Pregnancy, Childbirth, and the Newborn: The Complete Guide, by Penny Simkin, Janet Whalley, and Ann Keppler

The Thinking Woman's Guide to a Better Birth, by Henci Goer

Natural Childbirth the Bradley Way, revised edition, by Susan McCutcheon-Rosegg, Erick Ingraham, and Robert A. Bradley

SOME THOROUGH CHILDBIRTH PROGRAMS

Independent classes—not taught by your local hospital or clinic—are more likely to present a full range of information and options. If you have a midwife or doula, she may recommend specific classes.

Lamaze (lamaze.org)

Bradley Method (bradleybirth.com)

International Childbirth Education Association (icea.org)
Hypnobirthing (hypnobirthing.com)

About Labor

Let's cut to the chase: LABOR. The right word for the hard physical work of opening your body for a baby to squeeze through. If you've ever helped move a mattress up a flight of stairs, worked up a better-than-usual sweat at the gym, or ridden a bike up one last hill, then you've already "labored." You didn't always get a break when you wanted to, but you *did* get periodic rests. And if you didn't, your muscles gave out and made you stop. Muscles just can't work beyond their own ability. Same with labor. Natural contractions *always stop within your ability to cope,* because it's your own unmedicated muscles that are doing the work. You get a break after every surge of work. And you relax from each surge almost instantly, just as you do at the gym. It's very different from an injury-based pain. Labor is an effort-based pain, nothing more.

Birth is like putting on a snug turtleneck sweater: before you can get your head through the neck, you have to gather up the body of the sweater (labor) and use your hands to fold down the neck part and pull it open. *Then* you push your head through (birth). Think of your uterus as a sweater that doesn't bunch quickly. It's spent nine months repelling all attempts to dislodge this baby, and now it has to change tactics. Most of labor is simply changing from "holding safe" to "opening up."

Em and Abe

Television births are edited for drama, with hospital equipment and screaming and helplessness and the doctor sailing in to take control. Forget that. Let's follow Em (for Everyday Mother) through the birth of her baby, Abe (for Average Baby). Could be yesterday, could be thousands of years ago.

How Labor Starts

Abe is Em's first baby. She's been pregnant for about forty weeks, but Abe isn't quite ready yet—not surprising, since the average first labor starts at forty-one weeks or so.

Until your baby is ready, your uterus does *everything it can* to keep the baby safely inside. That's why attempts to induce labor with Pitocin (artificial oxytocin, the hormone that causes contractions) often "fail." (A "failed induction"? You could just as well call it a successful defense against premature birth.) Attempts to induce labor in the face of a determinedly protective uterus can be long and painful and are more likely to end in a C-section. If the induction requires many hours of IV fluids, often with synthetic oxytocin, the added fluids may increase breast engorgement in the mother and weight loss in the baby. And a baby who was not quite ready to be born—even if just by a few days—may have more difficulty breathing and coordinating sucking and swallowing when he tries to breastfeed.

Eating and Drinking During Labor

At first, Em just feels the same old Braxton-Hicks contractions—those "warm-up exercises" that her uterus has been doing for months. Gradually, she notices that they're a little stronger or lower than usual, a little harder to ignore. Her cervix begins to change shape, stretching a little wider, growing a little thinner, and finally breaking loose the mucous plug that helped protect Abe from outside germs. Em sees the bloody mucus and thinks maybe this is the day. But she eats and drinks as usual. She's about to become an athlete, and all athletes need a good supply of fuel and liquid to perform at their peak. This is no time for fasting!

Like an athlete, Em might change the kind *of food and drink she chooses, though, switching to lighter, easier-to-digest foods so that her muscles get energy faster. As labor progresses, she's likely to stop eating altogether, although she'll probably still want to drink.*

In the past, mothers were often told not to eat once labor starts, to reduce problems from "aspiration"—inhaling stomach contents while unconscious if general anesthesia was needed. But newer research has overturned that recommendation. Eating and drinking as much as you want to in labor gives you more energy to manage your contractions, the birth, and those amazing first hours after your baby arrives.

We Need to Feel Safe

Em's contractions grow stronger as the hours pass, and she goes for a walk, with pauses whenever she needs them. As contractions get stronger still, she heads for home. At this stage, if Em left home instead, or if unfamiliar people came in, she would probably release catecholamines—fight-or-flight hormones that could cause her labor to slow down or even stop. Our biology says we shouldn't labor in a risky place, and being with strangers or in a strange place can signal risk to the unconscious part of our brains that controls labor.

Hospital routines, feeling like a patient, bright lights, scary equipment, unaccustomed smells—they can all make us feel uneasy and make labor more difficult. Birth is easier, faster, and safer for both mother and baby when we *feel* completely safe, supported by familiar and caring people, and "at home." This is one of the reasons that bedroom-like birthing suites have become so popular.

Doulas

Em stays put, and relies on an experienced and familiar friend—a labor support person, sometimes called a doula—to keep her feeling secure. The doula focuses on Em's comfort—anything from fixing food to rubbing her back—and supports her partner as well. After all, Em's partner has probably never been at a birth, any more than Em has.

Research indicates that a doula—a trained labor support person—can provide as much physical comfort as, and far more emotional comfort than, any medication, whether or not your partner is also present. She can be your single best ally in creating a memorable, smooth, exhilarating experience. Without a doula, women who birth in a hospital are more likely to:

- Have an epidural or other pain medication
- Have an instrumental vaginal birth
- Have a Cesarean
- Have synthetic oxytocin during labor
- Have a baby with a low five-minute Apgar score
- Have a baby admitted to the special care nursery
- Rate their birth experience negatively
- Recall severe labor pain

Choose someone who makes you feel safe, although women who have *any* support person (in addition to their partner) during labor seem more likely to succeed in breastfeeding—even if the support person knows nothing at all about breastfeeding!

To find a certified doula in your area, visit dona.org, alace.org, and icea .org. Your local childbirth educators or LLL Leader may have names of other good doulas in your area.

Keep Moving

Em looks for ways to get comfortable. She holds on to something and sways her hips. She gets down on her knees and rests her head, rocking her hips back and forth. Moving into these positions as she tries to get comfortable helps to line her baby up for an easier birth. For many months now, hormones have worked to make the connections among her pelvic bones more relaxed, so that they'll allow the baby to ease through. Now their flexibility allows her changes of position to help work her baby lower and lower.

As labor progresses, Em may groan or moan during contractions. The sounds help with the work she's doing. Like any athlete, she's too focused to smile or chat. Her body releases endorphins, the same pain-relieving hormones that athletes' bodies release during a tough, satisfying workout. No one checks her cervix to see if it is "time to push." That's something Em will gradually sense for herself, just as any mammal would.

Having to lie still or lie on your back during labor has been shown to lengthen labor, increase the desire for medications, and make it more difficult to position the baby well for birth—all of which can interfere with breastfeeding.

Can an Epidural Affect the Baby?

Yes! An epidural keeps you from moving around, feeling, or finding good positions to direct the baby, and it often slows down labor, increasing the risk of interventions such as vacuum and forceps extractions and possibly C-sections. *All* medications, including those in epidurals, reach your baby through the placenta, affecting his ability to find the breast, latch, and suck effectively after he's born. Depending on how long the epidural was in place and the drugs used in it, these effects can last from a few days to a few weeks. Pain-relieving drugs reduce your own endorphins, which may increase your *baby's* discomfort, both before the birth and after the birth, when more endorphins are passed on through your milk. Your baby may cry more. Or, without your natural endorphins, you and baby may feel "flatter" emotionally, making it harder for you to respond to each other.

Epidurals can cause your temperature to rise, which raises your baby's temperature. He may be sent to the nursery for observation and antibiotics in case he has an infection. And if an epidural or induction included hours of IV fluids, your normal breast and nipple shape may be distorted, making latching difficult even with skilled help.

This can be hard information to read, but it's what the research very clearly shows. As childbirth educator Linda Smith, IBCLC, comments, "If your friend tells you how she 'loved her epidural,' ask her how her first month of motherhood went."

Em now reaches the "transition" stage, between the first stage of labor (gathering up the turtleneck sweater) and the second stage (pushing through the opening). Contractions are intense and close together. She might even throw up, just as some athletes do. She might feel panicky. This is when she needs the support and encouragement of her partner and doula the most—her baby is almost here.

At the end of transition, her cervix is fully opened, but she may not feel like pushing her baby out right away. Her contractions may subside or even stop as her uterus "takes up the slack" from her now-much-lower baby, preparing for a more efficient pushing stage. In response to the pressure, her cervix, vagina, and perineum (the tissues around the vaginal outlet) loosen up, becoming stretchier, ready for the baby to pass through. Waiting until her body wants to start pushing means Em has less risk of tearing or needing help to get the baby out, and that means a faster recovery. As the tissues slowly stretch, sensors in them respond by increasing her oxytocin levels, making this last job easier and her "openness to motherhood" greater. (Some mammal mothers won't know their babies belong to them if their "stretch receptors" have been numbed.)

Labor starts up again. Soon Em feels a mild urge to push, and pushes mildly. With her next contraction she finds herself in the grip of a powerful force: her face contorts and she grunts and strains. No one tells her how to breathe; she knows, just as you know how to breathe to move heavy furniture. She can feel Abe moving down the birth canal. He slips back just a little at the end of each contraction, then moves farther the next time. Sometimes she "holds the push" between contractions to keep him from sliding back; sometimes she doesn't. It's her show. She has a surge of catecholamines, which don't shut labor down at this stage; they act as cheerleaders to strengthen it. Before, if danger threatened, it was important to stop labor from going too far. Now, if danger threatens, it's important to get that baby out! Same hormone, different responses at different stages.

Em may be on hands and knees or squatting or lying on her side or supported under her arms. If she sat back on her tailbone, it would be like holding a gate shut, and it could be harder to work Abe through. And if she had to lie on her back, she'd be pushing him uphill, fighting gravity. Em finds the position that works best for her.

Because her body's comfort guides her, she's far less likely to tear, or to tear badly. No one makes a cut, or episiotomy, which increases the risk of more serious tears. There is a short period of burning when it seems that her skin must surely give way completely, but then Abe's head emerges facedown and automatically turns to the side, so that his shoulders can slip through on their own, first one and then the other. And then his body tumbles out in a gush of amniotic fluid.

Allowing the Cord to Stop Pulsing

Em reaches down and strokes Abe, as his full blood supply—only partial at the moment of birth—is pumped to him from the still-pulsing cord. She picks him up, looks him all over, and gathers him against her. He begins to squirm and takes his first bewildered breaths. Along with those first breaths, his movements against her belly cause her uterus to contract again, and the placenta separates from her uterus. Abe's skin color changes from purplish to rosy, and the umbilical cord that has been his lifeline stops pulsing. There's no rush to cut it.

Babies squeeze through the birth canal with only about two-thirds of their blood, which makes them a smaller package. The rest comes "on board" afterward through the cord. By waiting until the cord stops pulsing, the baby gets his full supply of blood. And that means his resulting iron stores are high—enough to last comfortably for six or nine or more months while he begins to add other food sources to his diet.

The Gaze

Em soaks in the first sight of Abe and feels a new rush of oxytocin. It helps to contract her uterus still more, reducing the risk of hemorrhage and sending a rush of loving feelings through her as she and Abe gaze at each other. That first deep gaze of his is part of what makes her fall in love. She says, "Hello, baby," in that wondering voice that mothers use when they greet their new babies. She bows her head to smell and rub her lips on the bare top of his head.

An alert newborn finds his mother's eyes and gazes at her, long and deeply, drinking her in and drawing her in. It's one more piece in the falling-in-love dance. If there are interventions, babies may be too disoriented to gaze, or someone else may end up getting the gaze that Nature intended for the mother—one more little complication in the mother-baby love affair.

> *When I was in transition with my second, third, and fourth babies, and coping with really intense contractions, I'd tell myself, "It won't be long until you have that feeling again." I was thinking about the overwhelming feeling of love and joy that came from looking into my newborn baby's eyes. It was all worth it, just to experience that.* —Jade

Drying Your Newborn

Em draws a warm blanket over herself and her newborn. The warmth helps reduce those now-unnecessary catecholamine levels, reducing her risk of hemorrhage. And in a ritual shared by virtually all mammal mothers, Em dries her baby.

The simple act of drying our babies probably contributes to our feelings of love; when mammal mothers are deprived of the chance to sniff and dry their still-wet babies, their bond with the baby is weakened. When the moisture has been dried off, you may see a white waxy coating called *vernix* (some babies have more than others). Rubbed in, it will help prevent much of the peeling skin that babies so often experience in the first week after birth. A water bath can happen anytime you like...or not at all.

Skin to Skin

After a few minutes of cleaning and cuddling, Em settles back comfortably in a semi-reclining position, with Abe on her chest and the blanket over the two of them. Because his bare skin is against her bare skin, Em warms Abe quickly and precisely.

The most elaborate hospital warmer can't warm a baby as quickly or as well as full-body skin contact with his mother—his *bare* chest and stomach against her *bare* chest and stomach. (There's no need to remove your shirt completely, just open it up.) In fact, if you have twins, the temperature on each breast rises and falls to warm or cool them independently! It's no surprise that stress hormones are much higher in babies who are kept away from their mothers in these critical first hours. Any exams or minor procedures can be performed while you hold your baby on your chest.

First Nursing

Abe begins to nuzzle Em's sloping chest. His head wobbles and bobs like a determined little woodpecker. He takes a short rest, his head falling against her and turning to the side. The feel of his cheek against her skin is exciting, and he lifts his head again, searching. His hands, still smelling of amniotic fluid, stretch and reach. When a hand finds her nipple, made erect by oxytocin, it leaves some of its scent behind, and helps him find his way. But he certainly doesn't work on this project alone. Em, as excited as her baby, moves him closer to her breast. Between the two of them, with experiments and blunders, exploration and near misses, his cheek lands next to her nipple. He lifts his head, opens wide…and contact! He begins to suck.

The feeling surprises Em—it's stronger than she expected but not unpleasant. And it causes yet another whoosh of oxytocin. Her uterus contracts again in response, and, because this oxytocin comes from within her own brain, another wave of affection washes over her. Her colostrum (early milk) moves through her breasts in a small gush, reinforcing Abe's sucking efforts. Thick and small in quantity, it's just the thing for practicing sucking, swallowing, and breathing. It provides a protective, anti-infective coating for his brand-new intestinal tract and stimulates his first bowel movements.

The oxytocin they produce during their first nursing makes both of them drowsy. Their eyes close, and, although Abe keeps nursing, they both semi-doze through the next hour or two. Em shifts him from one breast to the other as she chooses. She'll be hungry enough for a solid meal soon. For now, it's enough to soak in the sights and smells and sensations of this amazing new little person—this most wonderful of all babies, her beautiful son, Abe.

Too romantic and perfect? Normal births may be longer, shorter, harder, easier, earlier, or later, but Em and Abe's experience is the basic plan on which they're all built. Many of today's interventions have not been shown to improve outcomes as much as they've been shown to complicate the birth. Most women today *want* to breastfeed, but many are finding it hard, and the way we give birth today is a big part of the problem.

"THE MACHINE THAT GOES PING"

The Monty Python 1983 comedy movie *The Meaning of Life* included a parody of modern birth. Search online for "machine that goes ping" for a video of the scene.

The Birth-Breastfeeding Connection

Pick a mammal, any mammal, and imagine it giving birth the way we do. Let's say you take your laboring dog to a strange place with bright lights, lots of strangers, people who stick their fingers in her vagina repeatedly, tubes going in, tubes coming out, drugs, needles, belts around her belly, and a "machine that goes ping." Is she likely to have an easy time with motherhood? Our instinct is to give her a familiar place, quiet, dim lights, and privacy. Those are good instincts for humans, too.

Can you still breastfeed after any or even all of today's interventions? ABSOLUTELY! But it may take a while. See "Moving Forward After a Difficult Birth," below, for strategies.

Pregnancy Decisions: Who and Where?

You might be choosing between obstetricians, between a family doctor and a midwife, or between various midwifery practices. Your place of birth options may be home, birthing center, or hospital. It's well worth investigating C-section rates, other intervention rates, and whether the hospital or birth center is certified Baby-Friendly (see below). All your decisions will make a difference in how easily breastfeeding happens.

THE BABY-FRIENDLY HOSPITAL INITIATIVE

In 1991, the World Health Organization and UNICEF sought to improve breastfeeding outcomes by outlining Ten Steps to Successful Breastfeeding and urging all maternity facilities around the world to follow them and achieve Baby-Friendly certification. More than twenty thousand in 152 countries have become certified. Is your facility one of them? Check to see: unicef.org/programme/breastfeeding/assets/statusbfhi.pdf.

Choosing a Caregiver: Midwife, Family Doctor, Obstetrician?

Midwives' skills and limitations can vary with their setting, but they generally have the lowest rates of interventions. Most home births involve midwives. If yours is hospital-based, it will help to learn about the facility where you and she will be working together.

Family doctors sometimes include birth in their services. They are generally less likely than an obstetrician to reach for an intervention, and they can provide continuity of care for both mother and baby. They may not have the knowledge of a midwife who specializes in birth, but many provide excellent care for normal pregnancies and births. In some areas, they provide backup services for home births.

Obstetricians are experts in the complications of pregnancy and birth, though they may have little experience with unmedicated birth. An obstetrician will be on call at any hospital or birth center, and provides backup services for home births.

Doulas can be extremely helpful in any birth setting. Or have we said that already?

Choosing a Setting: Home, Hospital, Birthing Center?

It's been said that the first intervention in modern birth is leaving home. Research finds that home birth is just as safe as hospital birth for low-risk pregnancies, with a lower rate of interventions and higher rates of breastfeeding success and maternal satisfaction. Midwives are skilled in handling common problems, and the time it takes to transport you to a hospital in a true emergency is generally about the same as the wait for an operating room setup if you're already there. A hospital has more equipment for overcoming problems...but the hospital environment is what causes many of those problems in the first place.

It's worth investigating *all* the birth options available to you in your community. If possible, talk to some women who have given birth in more than one setting (easy to find at LLL meetings), and ask what differences they experienced in the birth, in their satisfaction, in breastfeeding, and in their relationships with those children. Whatever the setting, find out what breastfeeding help will be available, and on what days. See Chapter 1 for information on various types of breastfeeding helpers, and check the hospital section below for lots of ideas on keeping birth simple no matter where you give birth.

CHANGING YOUR MIND

Almost any birth decision can be changed, at just about any time. More than one woman has changed her planned birth place or caregiver in her last month of pregnancy. Trust your feelings. You don't owe people and places your loyalty; you owe yourself and your baby peace of mind and a smooth transition. Motherhood involves some very effective instincts. This may be your first one kicking in, and it may be really important to listen to it.

Birth at Home

At home, you get to decide who will be with you for the birth. Some women like to have supportive family and friends around, and feel safe and protected within a fairly large group. Others need more privacy and quiet in labor. You may not know which you want until labor. Maggie and her husband agreed beforehand that if she said, "I need more room," he would remove part of the crowd.

There are no institutional routines to separate mother and baby after a birth at home, but sometimes grandmothers, visitors, or even partners can end up taking over the baby. Right now, your baby just needs you. If you keep your baby's bare skin against your bare skin for the first few hours before passing him to others, you'll make sure he's thoroughly colonized with your "friendly" bacteria.

Birth Centers

Birth centers and birth clinics still mean leaving home, but they usually work hard to recapture the course of normal birth after that first intervention, and they generally have experience with a wide range of helping techniques. They can manage many types of complications, so they're a good option for those who want the comfort of a homey atmosphere within a medical setting. You can take a prenatal tour to see where your baby will be born, ask questions about whether options you're interested in—such as laboring in water—are available, and find out what help there is for getting breastfeeding under way.

Hospitals

Hospitals can also provide a positive experience and are essential in some higher-risk cases. The risk is that one seemingly minor intervention can lead to another, and then another. Here are some ideas hospital-birthing mothers have found helpful in reducing interventions:

- Protect your privacy and treat the room as your (temporary) home. Keep the door at least partly closed and have your labor support person "approve" anyone who comes in. Bring your favorite music. Put your own pictures up with poster adhesive. Wear your own clothes (with warm socks if the room is cool).
- As long as you're comfortable, stay on your feet. You're a competent person, not a patient. Walking and moving help line your baby up and keep labor going. Wander the halls or go outdoors, taking a helper with you.
- Cover the clock. When labor really gets under way, you won't care much about time, anyway.
- Avoid routine vaginal exams, which increase the risk of infection and cause stress. You'll know when you feel like pushing! (You can ask to have an exam to see how much your cervix has dilated, if *you* want, especially if that might help you make decisions about whether you want a particular intervention.)
- If the hospital requires an IV for all laboring women, even though it isn't supported by research and could waterlog both you and the baby and delay your milk coming in, consider asking for a *hep-lock* instead. It allows an IV to be plugged in instantly if needed, but doesn't interfere (much) otherwise.
- The bathroom can be a good place to labor. Try sitting backward on

the toilet, resting your head on your arms. We're used to relaxing and opening up on a toilet.

- A shower can help you relax deeply. Soaking up to your neck in a tub can be an amazing comfort. See waterbirth.org for more information.
- Remember that the staff are there to support you, so let them know what you need—like extra pillows, a darkened room, or a closed door.
- Avoid routine external fetal monitoring. Research indicates that its main result has been to increase the number of unnecessary Cesareans. Same with the internal monitor. Monitors hamper movement and make normal labor more difficult.
- Ask the medical staff not to offer you medication or an epidural. Instead, have your doula and midwife suggest other simple comfort measures.
- Gravity can help you, if you find a comfortable upright or side-lying position for pushing. Gravity works against you if you lie flat on your back. Your birth helper can adapt his or her position to whatever position you choose.
- Take off the baby hat. It's a holdover from the days when babies were taken away and were at risk of losing body heat. *Your* baby is lying on a furnace—you. Now you can smell the top of that delicious head without getting a noseful of synthetic fiber!
- *Keep the baby with you, on your body, bare skin against bare skin, at least until after he has that first nursing, which could continue off and on for several hours.* There's ample research to support the importance of skin-to-skin contact immediately after birth and during the hours that follow. It's important both for breastfeeding and for minimizing your baby's stress responses, which in turn will minimize a host of other large and small problems. Even after the first few hours, he'll be healthiest in your arms, next to your body, or on another adult's body, 24/7.
- If they want a first-day weight on a flat scale, you can request that he be weighed tummy down. He'll be calmer that way.
- Almost any measurements or procedure short of weighing and surgery can be done while he lies on you, even if the hospital staff are not used to doing it that way.
- The sooner you're home, the sooner you can do things your way.
- A one-on-one visit with a La Leche League Leader or other breastfeeding supporter at two or three days is often helpful.

Coping with Labor Interventions

This is the twenty-first century, and sometimes life happens fast. Here are some thoughts for coping with two common interventions.

Induction

An induction may be necessary in some situations. However, not all inductions are needed. You may have been told that your baby is getting too big, but prenatal size estimates are notoriously inaccurate. Or the date may have been chosen for your or your doctor's convenience, or you may be told that your facility routinely induces mothers at thirty-nine or even thirty-eight weeks. Research indicates that the "too-big," "convenience," and "new standard of care" reasons have not only increased the number of inductions, they've also increased the risk of prematurity and surgical delivery. The World Health Organization recommends limiting medical inductions to those that are truly necessary, fewer than 10 percent of all births. A baby who is born even a week or two early is at a higher risk of having breast-feeding difficulties and other health issues.

If an induction is recommended, here are some ideas that mothers have found helpful:

- 🔆 Ask some questions: What will happen if you don't induce labor? What are the odds of the "worst-case" scenario? How long can you wait? What is the doctor's plan if the induction doesn't work?
- 🔆 Find out about the medications involved. (*Medications and Mothers' Milk* by Thomas Hale can give you information on how the medication will affect your baby. Most LLL Leaders will have a copy. Learn more about it in the "Medications and Breastfeeding" section of Chapter 18.)
- 🔆 You may want to ask that misoprostol (Cytotec) *not* be used. It can result in very intense contractions, beyond what your body and your baby are designed to handle, and can result in serious complications, especially if you've had a previous C-section. Although it's inexpensive and easy to use, its safety as a cervical ripener is still controversial.
- 🔆 Consider asking that any artificial oxytocin used to jump-start your

labor be *given at intervals* instead of continuously. Once labor is under way, experiment with tapering off the Pitocin/Syntocinon. Your labor may continue without it. Research indicates that a lower, *slower* rate reduces the risk of emergency C-section.

- ☀ You may want to ask that your doctor or midwife *not* rupture your membranes (break your water) to help get labor going or speed up the induction process. It does very little to speed labor, and once your membranes have been ruptured, many caregivers limit how long labor can continue, with a C-section as the next step. If your labor doesn't get going *and your membranes are intact,* you can go home and try again later.

- ☀ Prepare yourself for how well a uterus protects a baby. Others may have decided that this is your baby's birthday, but your uterus may not have acquired those oxytocin receptors that allow the Pitocin to work.

"I had a very fast birth with my third baby, Quinn, and even though I didn't want to have any medications, at one point I started to panic and thought I couldn't stand the pain. Looking back, I was probably close to transition, but I didn't realize it at the time and I asked for a shot of Nubain to help me cope. The midwife reluctantly agreed to give me a half dose. But that may have been too much. I was loopy for the rest of the birth, and when Quinn was born I didn't really feel connected to him. He had very little interest in nursing, and he was very sleepy. I started pumping to get my milk supply going. By the end of the first day, we were getting worried and began finger-feeding him my pumped milk. Thankfully, he started waking up on the third day and started nursing eagerly. Everything went just fine after that and we were a happy nursing couple. But I sure learned how devastating even a little birth medication can be to the breastfeeding experience. I'm very thankful that we hung in there until Quinn was able to nurse—it would have been so easy to give up in those shaky first two days." —Diana

---

Cesarean Section

In many parts of today's world, one mother in three leaves the hospital with an abdominal incision; in some places the rates are even higher. This is way beyond the 10 to 15 percent that the World Health Organization finds reasonable, but it's still a reality that every pregnant woman needs to prepare for. The effects of medications and IV fluids, and the difficulty in finding comfortable positions for breastfeeding when your abdomen is tender from surgery, can make breastfeeding more difficult. And it's challenging to recover from major surgery and look after a new baby at the same time. *This doesn't mean that you can't breastfeed after a C-section—many, many women do*—but if you can reduce your risk of a C-section—and you can, in most cases—it's worthwhile. How can you normalize the experience if it happens to you?

- If possible, don't schedule a C-section; let labor begin on its own since even a little labor is good for both of you. *Your* body gets to go through labor's hormonal setup, and y*our baby's* body isn't taken without warning from his dark, safe world.
- If your only reason for having this C-section is a previous C-section, find out about vaginal birth after Cesarean (VBAC) options in your area.
- Be conscious, if possible. With a C-section using an epidural, your recovery and your baby's will be easier than if you had a general anesthetic. Sometimes, of course, general anesthesia *is* necessary, especially if speed is important.
- Even though you are having a surgical birth, you are still entitled to make decisions about your care, and to have your wishes and choices respected. If you're not quite ready and need a few more minutes (assuming there's no emergency), *say so*. If there's someone or something you want—or don't want—say so. If you want to have a good cry about the whole thing, that's okay, too. This is still your birth. Many mothers have found their second C-section to be a much better experience than their first, in part because they felt more in charge. It's when we feel helpless that we're most likely to feel bad about an experience.
- You may want to have someone describe the birth (not the surgery) to you—the moment that hair, then face, then body are visible, and the bringing forth of your baby into the world. You or your partner, *not the surgeon,* should have the privilege of announcing the baby's gender.
- Consider asking the surgeon to delay cutting the cord, and to hold the baby low until the cord stops pulsing. It won't take long. Once the cord is cut, ask that your baby be brought to you right away, for you to see and touch.

- ⚬ If the baby is to be taken to a nursery, or if your hands aren't free, you might want to have him touched to your cheek. *Nuzzle* him, smell him, take a mental photo of that little face. One mother of Cesarean-born twins found that she fell in love with the first, who had been touched to her cheek immediately, faster than with the second, whom she saw but didn't touch.

- ⚬ Put your baby skin-to-skin in the operating room if possible, while they finish the surgery. Your baby can be laid on your chest above the drape, where your helper can hold him and help position him near your breast. It's a memorable moment for both of you, no matter what your baby does. If he nurses, it's a wonderful extra. His smell and touch can go a long way toward emotional healing from the surgery. More and more hospitals are doing this because they recognize how much more smoothly breastfeeding goes when mother and baby are kept together. Some have even noted that the uterus clamps down more quickly and satisfactorily if the baby's sucking drives the process. Every hospital had to have a first time. Maybe you'll be the first for yours!

Getting Breastfeeding Started After a Cesarean

- ⚬ In the recovery room, you can ask for help with breastfeeding. Your baby can nurse in any of a number of positions: kneeling at your side, lying across your chest toward your opposite shoulder or below your opposite breast, cuddled in your armpit, even lying alongside your face with his feet toward the headboard. Any position that gives your baby access to your breast without being near your incision can work. After surgery, while the incision is still numb and temporarily comfortable, may be the simplest time for you and your helper to find a breastfeeding position that will work well for the next couple of days.

- ⚬ You might opt to have family or friends with you 24/7, or as close to that as you can manage, so that you can have your baby stay with you even though you're immobile or affected by medications.

- ⚬ Feel free to undress the baby if he comes to you all bundled up. A blanket will keep both of you warm, and your partner will probably be happy to take some shifts, leaning back in a chair to share skin time with your baby. Skin-to-skin contact is what your baby expects. The feeling of that warm little body against yours is pretty wonderful for *you,* too.

☀ You and your baby deserve good help with breastfeeding, and now's the time to get it. So make use of breastfeeding helpers—those on staff, or a friend, La Leche League Leader, or private-practice International Board Certified Lactation Consultant (IBCLC).

What if I'm High-Risk?

If you've been told that you are high-risk, your birth plans (and dreams) may have gone out the window, and your caregiver may already have given you a list of interventions you can expect. While some may be needed, you may be able to avoid others. Talk to your caregiver about what you can do to make your birth as normal and low-risk as possible, and about how you can help get breastfeeding off to a good start.

Most mothers and babies can breastfeed, even after the most severe birth complications. The more complicated the birth, the harder it may be to get started, however, so line up your birth resources, and know that there's plenty of good help out here.

Moving Forward After a Difficult Birth

If you feel that what happened during birth is getting in the way of your relationship with your baby, you're not alone. Most mammal mothers have difficulties if they didn't feel labor or birth, or if the experience was unusually traumatic, or if the baby is taken away from them. As Donna wrote in the early weeks after her unexpected C-section, "I still feel like something is missing, but I don't know what. I feel as though I adopted Edwin and he is not biologically mine. I feel like I only know he's mine because everyone tells me he's mine. I love him, but there really seems to be this big gap. I don't know what happened to the bump on my belly and I have no idea where this child came from. He's totally cute, though, and *he* seems to think I'm his mother. So I will go with that...I don't know if/how normal birth would have changed this feeling. But the more we nurse, the more I believe he's my kid."

But many babies won't latch after a difficult birth, and some mothers aren't sure they even want them to. This makes a lot of sense biologically—the birth didn't happen the way it "should" have, so neither of you received the sequence of motions and hormones that helps bonding happen immediately. You and your baby need to connect in a fundamental way. Here are some ideas to speed the process:

- It can help to keep your baby with you 24/7, *even if you don't feel like you want to be with him yet.* The familiarity that develops with being together will help your bodies to recognize each other on a primal level. He'll grow on you. Bit by bit, you'll find more about him to adore.
- Spend as much of this time as possible with your baby's bare skin against your bare skin. Smell him, feel him, caress him, savor him. One mother decided at three days to lick her baby, and told us, "I felt something melt as I did it. And I felt a whole lot better about the Cesarean." (See Chapter 4 for interesting thoughts about licking your baby.)
- You could take a warm bath together by candlelight, just the two of you and no one else. Stroke and massage him as you enjoy the soothing water. Admire his wonderful skin, nuzzle him, kiss his toes. Let him nurse while you soak if he can and wants to.
- Try holding your baby and watching his face while friends or family give you a relaxing massage—foot, scalp, shoulder, back—anywhere that feels good. Give yourself over to the sensation and open yourself up to the enjoyment. This releases oxytocin, the bonding hormone.
- Make some decisions about him—what he'll wear, how to hold him, how to comfort him. Taking responsibility for him helps you feel more nurturing toward him.
- If your baby won't latch, understand that it's just temporary, and try to be patient rather than panicked or frustrated. He'll get there in time.

"I missed something in the delivery room, something huge, and at nine months, the window was still open enough that I got it. I was sitting next to his wading pool looking at him. I reached over and touched his little arms and hands and shoulders and I felt a lightning bolt of joyful recognition and a gap filled in where I had been hurting so much. I think it

was very important that he was wet and without clothes. It was important that we were alone. I felt completely different after that. I held him differently. He was mine in a more fundamental, physical way."

—Laura

Owning Your Birth

If absolutely everything you didn't want happens to you, or even if your birth just isn't what you hoped, *this was still your story and nobody else's*. It's a story that you will probably want to tell in detail someday to a caring friend or maybe even to your child. At some point—even years later—it can help to write it down. The good parts and the bad parts, what you saw and did, and how you felt. Your story will become precious to you for exactly what it is—the beginning of your life with your child.

There really is life after birth, and it really will be wonderful (most days). No matter how the birth goes, most mothers and babies can go on to breastfeed. In the next chapter, we'll show you the basics of keeping your milk supply high, your baby well fed, and your breast a happy place while you and your baby recover from any birth issues and learn to breastfeed. There are good days ahead.

Em and Abe are drowsy again, but full of the knowledge that they belong to each other. "So this is who you are," she thinks. "Surely I've known you, my absolutely right baby, all my life." Their days together begin.

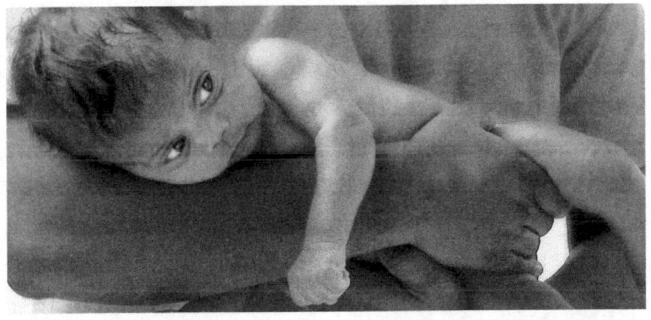

FOUR

Latching and Attaching

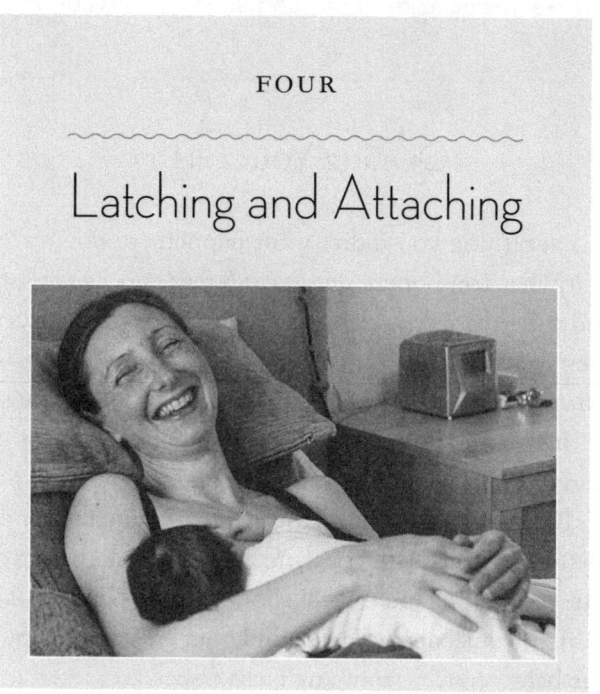

> *"When Shay was born, the nurses tried hard to get him to latch on and breastfeed, but he arched his back and didn't seem to know what to do. I couldn't get him to nurse at all. We went home when he was eight hours old, and the first thing I did was call the La Leche League Leader I met when I was pregnant. She suggested I get into bed with Shay and just let him lie on my chest, tummy to tummy and skin-to-skin. My husband, Chris, got into the bed with us, too. I kept dozing off, and after a couple of hours I woke up because Shay was nursing! He'd found the breast on his own."*
>
> *—Emma, remembering 2006*

YOUR BODY AND your baby have instincts and abilities not just for birth but for breastfeeding as well. Yes, it may seem a little awkward at first, especially if you haven't seen many breastfeeding babies, but even though this is *your* first time, it's a process that has worked *billions* of times before.

Laid-back Breastfeeding

When a baby is born, his instincts and reflexes help him crawl to the nipple and latch on, even if you don't help at all. But most of the time you'll want to help—and that's instinctive, too!

Here's an approach that takes advantage of the natural instincts you both have. Ideally, your baby will be in your arms moments after she's born. Ask for some pillows or adjust the bed so that you are not lying flat or sitting up straight—just reclining at an easy angle that's comfortable for every part of you. Your baby can lie on top of you, her front on your front, with a towel for you to dry her with and a blanket over the two of you for warmth if you need it. There! Now gravity will paste her entire front against yours, while your hands are free to rub and stroke her wherever you like. That's really all you need to do at first—just find a totally comfortable way to cuddle together so that you're completely supported—head, neck, shoulders, body—by whatever you're leaning back against, and she's completely supported by your body, or maybe also by the bedding around you.

Your baby might start searching for your breast almost immediately, or she might be a little shocked to find herself outside her warm, wet home of the past nine months. If the trip was a rough one, she may just cry at first. As one experienced helper said, "She needs to tell her story." And you can tell her yours! Soothe her, stroke her, talk to her, snuggle her. As she recovers from the journey from womb to world, she'll begin to think about sucking, usually sometime in that first hour. She may start by drooling, or making sucking movements with her lips or bringing her fist to her mouth or licking. After a while, she may lift her head (look how strong she is!) and bob her face on and off your skin. You can help her move closer to the breast or support her as she finds her way. She's doing all this by feel and by smell, not sight, and she welcomes having you share in her efforts. You don't need to be skilled; fumbling is a normal—even helpful—part of the process.

At some point, when her face is near your nipple, she'll lift her head, open her mouth wide, latch, and begin to suck. She's breastfeeding!

The feeling may surprise you. That's a strong little mouth, and it may tug and compress your nipple more than you thought. If it's downright pinchy or painful, try moving her body or yours around just a bit to see if it helps. It doesn't have to be a big adjustment to make things more comfortable.

Your baby can nurse as long as you both want. Most likely, after a while she'll either fall asleep with your nipple in her mouth or let go and fall asleep. Or you might decide to stop nursing because you need to shift your position or get up for a bit. If you're the one who ends the feeding, take your cue from the baby about whether to offer the other breast. If she's putting her fist in her mouth or fussing, she probably wants to nurse some more.

Until now, your baby was fed continuously through the umbilical cord, and she's designed to expect frequent feedings now. So she may nurse, let go, and doze for a bit, then wake and start looking for the nipple again. That's normal. It's how a good milk supply and a well-fed baby get started.

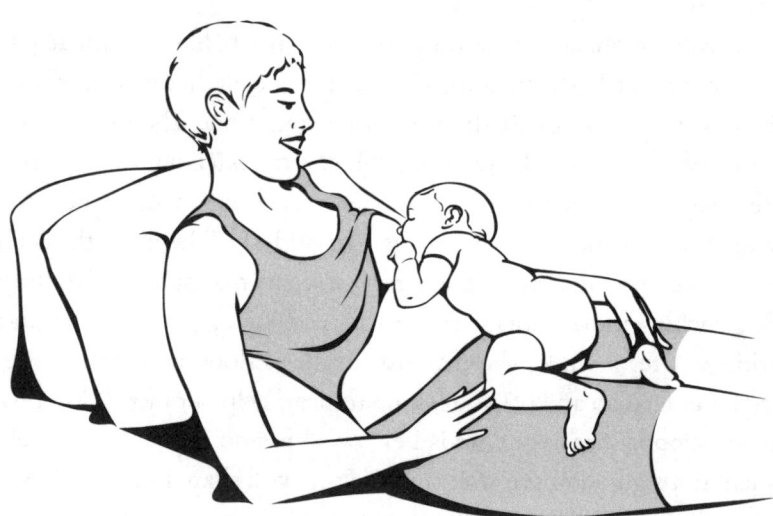

Laid-back breastfeeding: gravity does the work!

What's So Cool About Laid-back Breastfeeding?

Leaning back and letting gravity hold the baby is as old as humankind, but it was recently revived, analyzed, and named Biological Nurturing by British midwife Suzanne Colson, PhD. Here are some of its advantages over the long lists of instructions of the past quarter century:

- There *is* no long list of instructions!
- Gravity "sticks" your baby against you, so you don't have to worry about a precise hold.
- You get to decide on your position, your baby's position, how much each of you wears, whether or not to hold or move your breast, and whether or not to move the baby.
- Your torso "opens up" so that your baby can lie in any position on it, instead of having to lie across your lap because there's nowhere else to go. If you're "laid back," you *have* no lap, and the number of arrangements becomes limitless!
- Gravity gives your baby full, consistent, comforting support—no gaps or pressure points.
- Gravity brings your baby *toward* your breast as he bobs around, instead of pulling his head *away from* it as can happen when you sit up.
- Your baby's whole body touches yours, triggering more instinctive responses in both of you.
- Your baby isn't likely to flail his arms and get in his own way, because he feels secure against you.
- You can be totally relaxed—no tight shoulders or aching wrists.
- You have at least one hand free to stroke your baby or pick up that glass of water you're suddenly thirsty for.

Will you use laid-back breastfeeding forever? That's up to you. You can modify it, enjoy it for naps, or switch completely once you and your baby are more skilled. Consider it training wheels for all kinds of positions!

LAID-BACK BREASTFEEDING REVIEWS

From a breastfeeding helper in Ireland: *"I took a leap of faith this morning and tried Biological Nurturing with a mum and baby. Mum had sore nipples, very anxious and tense, but baby was great. It was pretty amazing—fabulous latch, the baby looked sooo comfortable and the mum couldn't believe there was no pain. I'm still smiling."*

From another in Mexico: *"I took that same leap of faith last week, with two different babies on house calls. Both babies did amazingly well and easily latched in the abdominal [whole front against the mother's front] position. What hit me smack in the face was the realization that in this position, with baby on his/her tummy on TOP of a slightly reclining mom, the earth's magical gravity does most of the work. When I have the mother sitting more straight up, the mother needs to help the baby much more. What a difference!"*

And from a mother in the United States: *"After our visit with an LLL Leader, I was using the laid-back technique, but I tweaked it by switching to basically the cross-cradle hold, which gave me better control of her head but wasn't painless. Yesterday she was rooting around on my chest and I just decided to try the laid-back approach again, and it was PAINLESS! Both in terms of the latch, and afterward. Since then, I have had thirteen out of fourteen PAINLESS nursing sessions!!! Even with the nipple wounds still not healed! I think the laid-back approach is easier now because I am basically not really trying to guide her that much; I just put the nipple in front of her mouth and she does the rest! So I think maybe previously I was trying too hard to control the latch.*

"I am just over the moon to have had so many painless sessions; it is like a different world. I am overwhelmingly relieved and thrilled beyond belief!!!"

Sitting Up, Baby Leading

If you or your baby prefer to breastfeed sitting up, try starting with your chest bare and no bra. You don't have to be topless—you can wear a button-down shirt, jacket, or robe and just open it up. Undress your baby down to his diaper. Lean back a little bit (not quite as much as with laid-back breastfeeding). Hold your baby vertically against your chest, facing you, with his head under your chin, and follow his lead. After he rests on your chest, if he's hungry and not sleepy from birth medications he'll begin bobbing his head and working his way down toward one breast or the other. Be prepared—he might move really quickly, like a lunge. Keep his body against yours, and help him, in any way that feels right, with what he's trying to do. When his cheek or nose is near your nipple, he will probably move his head, open wide, and gently take your breast.

Like laid-back breastfeeding, this approach lets your baby "make the trip to the kitchen" on his own, something all other mammal newborns do. Imagine shoving a puppy at his mother's nipple. You'd probably just confuse him! That's why the laid-back and baby-led approaches tend to work so well. Like any other baby mammal, your baby gets to organize himself, sense his landmarks, and choose his own moment.

Sitting Up, Shortcut

You can also start by choosing a breast for him and then holding him so his body angles across yours, his hip resting on or near your thigh, with his whole front against your front. Since babies latch by feel, he'll need his face or cheek or chin touching your breast, or your nipple resting above his top lip, to understand what to do. If he fusses, just bringing his lower face into contact with your breast may help him focus.

Baby held behind his back and shoulders, head resting on arm.

Try to avoid having any gaps between the two of you by holding him behind his back and shoulders. His head will rest on your wrist or forearm, and he can control it himself. If he fusses, calm him by holding him vertically for a minute or two, and maybe walking and talking to him, and try again. It may be tempting to push on his head. This almost *never* helps and can make him dislike being at the breast. It also pushes his chin toward his chest, making it hard for him to get a good mouthful if he does latch on.

If you hold him so that your nipple falls in the space between his upper lip and nose, he can tip his head back slightly to take it into his mouth. Or let his cheek come to rest just above your nipple and help him move to take it into his mouth. You may have seen him turning his head, mouth wide, to latch on to his own collar or shoulder, if it happened to brush his cheek. You're taking advantage of that same turn-and-open reflex when you let his cheek touch your breast or nipple.

What Babies Need to Breastfeed

Laid-back, sitting up but baby-led, and sitting up with a small shortcut all let the baby lead the way. Some babies, whether from birth medications or other issues, need a bit more help at first. We'll show you some more "mother-guided" approaches, all of which provide certain elements that babies need in order to figure out what to do. So let's look first at what babies need.

Babies Need to Be Calm

Your first job is to calm your baby. If he's upset, take time to soothe him. Bring him up higher on your chest, stroke him, talk to him in the voice that he already knows so well. You'll gradually learn what calms *your* baby. It also helps to begin when your baby gives *early* cues for wanting to eat—sucking on his hand, smacking his lips, turning his head toward you—rather than waiting until he's crying from hunger. If you feel he's agitated because he's hungry, a little colostrum expressed and fed to him with a dropper or spoon can calm him and help him focus.

Babies Need Good Support

Whether you're laid-back or sitting up, your baby will be most competent if he's well supported. If you're lying back, gravity does it for you. If you're sitting up, hold him behind his back and shoulders and remember "his front to my front." His shoulders, especially, should be tucked in closely to you. This helps keep him stable while he moves his head to search. Babies who don't feel stable may wave their arms around, which can make latching much more difficult.

Babies' Lower Jaws Need Room

Your baby's *lower* jaw needs to be deeply placed on your breast. His upper jaw isn't all that important for nursing. Rest your index finger under your nose like a mustache—on your upper jaw—and make exaggerated chewing motions. Your finger doesn't move, does it? Your baby is built the same way: his lower jaw is his moving jaw and it needs plenty of room to move. If your fingers are in the way of his lower jaw, that can't happen. You can shape your breast or lift it, if you want to, but do it from a respectful distance, so that his chin can sink into your breast, with his head tipped back a bit to bring his lower jaw forward. Be sure to keep your fingers totally away from where his chin and lower jaw need to be.

Babies Need a Big Mouthful

While there might be some milk in your nipple, the milk is mostly in the ducts in your breast. The baby who just chews on a nipple won't get much, and it'll hurt! When your baby has a good big mouthful of breast *beyond* your nipple, *that's* when it's comfortable. And *that's* where the milk is. So when it *feels* good, it *is* good. As Toronto pediatrician Jack Newman often says: "It's called breastfeeding, not nipple-feeding."

Babies Need a Big, Fat Sandwich

Some women like (or need) to hold their breast when they nurse. They flatten their breast as they would a big sandwich they were offering their baby, which helps the baby grasp more breast tissue. When you eat a big sandwich, you keep your thumbs way back on the sandwich so there's room for a big lower-jaw bite. You don't worry about the fingers closer to your upper jaw. In the same way, if you hold your breast, keep your "lower jaw fingers" *w-a-y* out of your baby's way.

Babies Need to Choose Their Own Timing

We used to be told to "latch the baby on" when her mouth was open wide. But mammal mothers never take that much control over a feeding, and babies don't expect it. Unless there's a specific need, your baby will probably do best if *he* picks the moment. Your job is just to see that that moment becomes possible, by having a well-supported baby in easy reach of the breast.

Babies Need to Reach Forward with Their Lower Jaw

The baby who has to tuck his chin to reach the nipple loses breast contact with his lower jaw. His jaw does much better if he lifts his chin so that his head tips back slightly, chin in firm contact with the breast, nose lifted free or nearly free of the breast. Tipping his head back a bit helps with swallowing, too; it's easier to swallow when our chin is lifted than when it's tucked.

Babies Need to Breathe

In most cases, babies get plenty of air if their heads are tilted back, which lifts their noses free or nearly free of the breast. Even if his nose is lightly touching, your baby can still breathe just fine. If he can't, of course he lets go! But what if his nose is buried? Try shifting him in a way that tips his head back a bit more, maybe by pulling his back and shoulders in closer.

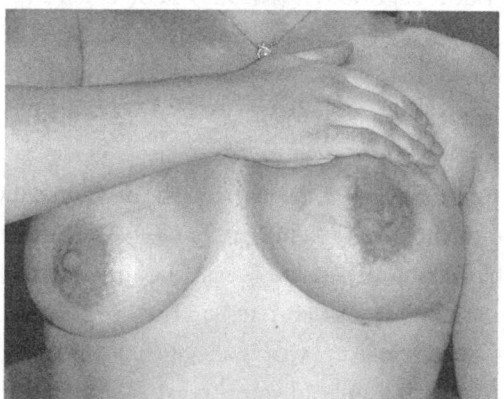

Raising breast with flat of hand.

You can also lift your breast slightly (try pressing your hand flat on your chest between breast and collarbone and lifting).

DO I HAVE TO LIFT OR HOLD MY BREAST THROUGHOUT THE FEEDING?

Not necessarily! First, try starting where Nature and Gravity (not your bra) have already put you. If you lift your breast for your baby, you'll probably have to hold it throughout the feeding. Some babies do have to have the breast stabilized for them, or need it lifted slightly to make breathing easier. But unless you're very long-breasted or wide-breasted, it will probably be easier to let your breast be wherever Nature puts it.

What About Those "Holds" and "Positions" I Hear About?

Over the years, breastfeeding helpers have tried to find ways to help mothers and babies get a good latch, especially those babies who may be dealing with the challenges of labor medications. One approach has been to have the mother hold the baby in certain ways. When all is going well, specific holds and positions don't really matter because you and your baby figure out your own system. But if you're having trouble getting things going in the beginning, it can help to have a "recipe" to follow until you know what works for you. So let's talk a bit about each of them.

The *cradle hold,* or some variation of it, is what most of us use

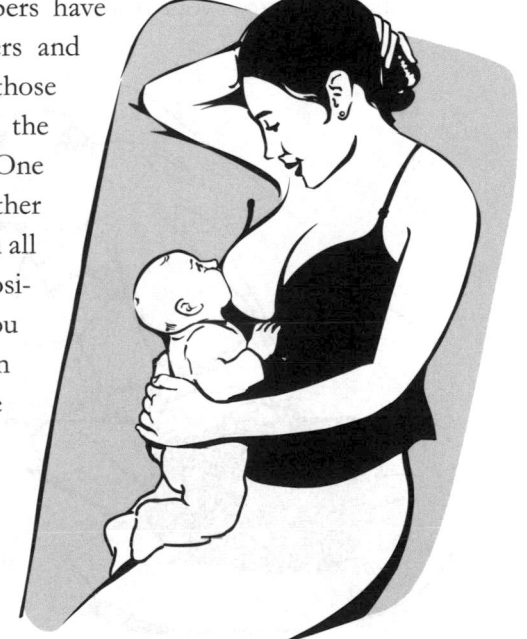

Side-lying.

when we're more comfortable with breastfeeding. To try it, hold your baby's front against yours by holding him behind his back and shoulders, his head resting on your forearm or wrist (not the crook of your elbow) and his hip resting on or near your thigh. His chest is snuggled into your breast, and your nipple is near his nose. As he opens to take your nipple in, gently snuggle him closer. If he seems confused, shift him so his cheek rests near your nipple, or use the nipple tilt described below.

The *across-the-chest hold*, or cross-cradle hold, works especially well with small babies and is often taught in hospitals. For this position, you hold the baby with the arm *opposite from* the breast he is going to latch onto. Hold him underneath your breasts, his hip near or resting on your thigh. Your hand supports his neck (not the back of his head) as your arm hugs him against you; his chest is snuggled against the mound of your breast. Your other hand is free to shape or stabilize your breast if you want to. As your baby opens to take your nipple, gently snuggle his chest in closer. Touching his cheek or using the nipple tilt described below may help.

The *clutch hold* is often suggested for mothers who have had C-sections, because the baby's weight is kept away from the incision. Instead of holding the baby across your front, position him next to you, his front against your side, your hand under his shoulders and neck and his body supported between your arm and the side of your body. He'll be a bit below your breast, which may work well if your breasts are fairly large; you may need to move him into a semi-sitting position if your breasts are smaller.

Side-lying can helpful to the baby who is having difficulty in other positions, and it is definitely helpful at night. Try laying your baby on her side facing you, and pulling her down so that your nipple is level with her nose or eye. It may *or may not* help to

Nursing from the top breast.

make a "sandwich" of your breast, aligned to match her mouth, fingers well out of the way, nipple rolling in last. As she latches, press on the middle of her back to bring her closer. She may be arched somewhat; bringing the middle of her back closer helps to keep her head tipped back. If you keep a small towel or receiving blanket rolled up nearby, you can tuck it behind her back to hold her there, and have that hand free to stroke and enjoy her.

Sometimes babies just do better if you *stand up*. You can sway or bounce gently to help calm your baby, and the lack of a lap can be helpful. As always, keep your baby nice and stable, let him lead the way, try angling his legs down instead of holding him horizontal, and see what happens.

Small-breasted Kim was curled up on the sofa, talking with another mother about her birth, her knees drawn up almost to her chin, her three-month-old resting on her thighs. "It was incredible!" she said, and her arms flew straight up over her head. "I have to ask," her friend said. "Are you nursing right now?" Kim, arms still high in the air, glanced down. "Oh. Yes," she said.

Large-breasted Anita came to a La Leche League meeting with her two-week-old because they were having a lot of trouble starting each nursing. Two months later she came again, sat cross-legged on the floor, started nursing, and passed around some handouts from

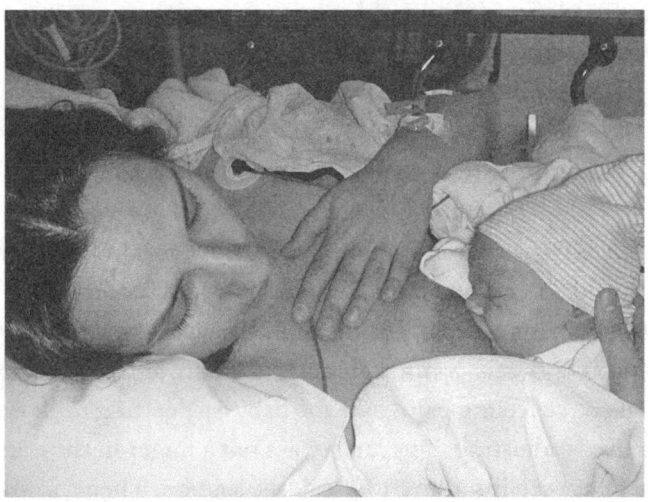

Latching after a C-section.

her spot on the floor. "Are you nursing while you're doing that?" we asked her. "You sure couldn't have done *that* two months ago." "Oh!" she said, surprised. "I guess I couldn't have. I'd forgotten!"

C-section and Episiotomy Adaptations

If you've had a large episiotomy or a C-section that makes it hard for you to get into a semi-reclining position, you can lie flat on your back and let the baby lie on your chest (avoiding your incision) or even kneel (with someone's help) at your side as he finds the nipple. Or you may be more comfortable using a clutch hold or sitting upright, with a pillow or two behind your back and a pillow on your lap to protect your incision.

Easing into the Feeding

If you used a "technique" to "get your baby latched on," *don't relax immediately* or he could lose your nipple. Instead, give your baby time to get everything arranged in his mouth and start sucking. *Then* you can slowly relax the hand on your breast, making sure to bring your baby in closer if relaxing your hand means your breast sags away from him. Rearrange yourself comfortably, and settle in. You'll find more about what to expect during your nursings in Chapters 5 and 6.

He's Latched, but It HURTS

Good breastfeeding has nothing to do with how good it *looks*, and everything to do with how good it feels and how well it works. Your baby is nursing well IF he is able to get the milk he needs without getting too tired AND you both feel comfortable. If *either* part of that description isn't working—if you're feeling pain, or if the baby isn't getting milk well—then something needs adjusting. You can always put a finger in the corner of his mouth, right between his gums, to break the suction. Then slip your nipple from his mouth and start again. Try not to do this too many times, though, because it can be frustrating for him. Instead, get some help finding a more comfortable approach. Here are some ideas you might try.

Tilting Your Nipple

Rebecca Glover, a midwife in Australia, suggests putting your thumb (or a finger) near the base of your nipple on the side where your baby's *upper* lip will be. Press or tug a little, and notice how your nipple tilts away from the baby. Now you're presenting your baby with a nice full bit of breast rather than presenting her with your nipple, and there are no fingers near her important lower jaw. You can use that bit of breast to "tease" her lower face. If she opens wide, reaching with her mouth for the nipple that's beyond her, snuggle her straight in (don't

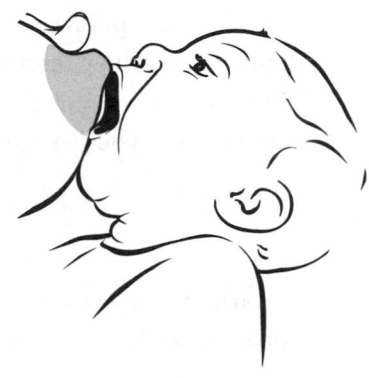

Tilting your nipple can give your baby more breast.

shift her to try to put the nipple in the center of her mouth). You can use your thumb or finger to help push or tuck the bit of breast into her mouth. Your nipple is the *last* part in, still tilting away from her and unrolling inside her mouth. It doesn't matter if your thumb or finger ends up under your baby's upper lip for a moment. You're just tucking in the last bit of the sandwich! Remember to keep your baby snug against your body, her chest against the mound of your breast, and let her control her head herself.

For pictures and additional description, go to Rebecca's website, rebeccaglover.com.au, and click on her various handouts to enlarge them.

Narrowing the Sandwich

You probably sometimes compress a really fat sandwich so you can get your mouth around it. Narrowing the "breast sandwich" to make it easier for your baby to get a deep mouthful will do the same thing. You can combine this with the nipple tilt. Remember to keep the "lower jaw fingers" well away from the nipple. The upper jaw finger, though, can be right next to the nipple.

Pillows

If your body supports your baby, there's no need for pillows. If you need support for your arm, a squishy pillow or two may help. Supporting your baby on a pillow can put extra space between his body and yours, and has caused more sore nipples than it has cured. However, there are some situations where a pillow can be a temporary help. You may do better with a flat-surfaced pillow than with a rounded one, especially with a small baby (they tend to roll into the crack). If using a pillow means you have to lift your breast to your baby, you probably don't need the pillow!

Footstools

If you're nursing sitting up and have short legs, a low footstool (or thick book, diaper bag, or coffee table crossbar) may raise your lap to support your arm and baby and relax your lower back. As you become more practiced, you'll find other creative ways to get comfortable. Cross your legs or try raising just one foot, so your baby's feet are lower than his head. Paintings from earlier centuries tend to show *one* foot on a stool, with the baby's body angled down somewhat.

None of This Is Working! My Baby Isn't Latching!

If you had medications, such as an epidural, or had other interventions, such as induction or forceps, your baby may not be able to respond in the way we've described. For some babies, the effects of the labor medications can last for days or weeks. Other babies may have physical or neurological difficulties. It can be incredibly upsetting and frustrating when you want nothing more than to get your baby happily nursing at your breast. You might also be feeling a lot of pressure from hospital staff and even friends and family to "make it happen NOW."

This is a temporary setback that many, many mothers have worked through before going on to breastfeed happily. Remember that a baby who *won't* breastfeed *can't* breastfeed, at least for the moment. If he acts frustrated or angry at your breast, maybe it's because that's a place where he can let his frustrations out, in a way he wouldn't do with a stranger. Or maybe he feels like the child in a candy shop who throws a tantrum not because he doesn't like candy but because he does.

But if we can get tigers to jump through hoops, which they're not built to do, then *of course* we can find ways to help your baby nurse.

The key in this situation is to be patient and to have good help. Your baby WILL get it, but it might take some time. A full-term, healthy baby does not need any food or liquids for at least twenty-four to thirty-six hours. Nature provides this buffer to give babies and mothers time to figure things out. Many babies wake up to nurse just fine the next day.

The "Three Keeps"

There are three things to take care of if breastfeeding isn't working. Take care of these "Three Keeps," and you'll be ready and able to breastfeed when your baby is.

1. Keep *Your Milk Flowing*

Your milk supply will start to increase automatically after the first couple of days, whether you remove milk or not. But these early days are when your breasts are planning for future milk production. The amount of milk you remove now tells them how much you'll be needing. If your baby isn't nursing yet, it will help if you start now to hand-express or pump, so that your breasts will be ready and waiting, with plenty of milk, when your baby is finally able to nurse.

In the first few days, colostrum is thick and easier to remove by hand expressing (see Chapter 15) than by pumping. Massage and breast compressions will also help. Most mothers can express more colostrum in the first hours post-birth than they get later—that's the large first meal your baby would normally get. You can ask for help expressing it if your baby isn't nursing. Afterward, you can take about a six-hour break (rest and enjoy being with your baby) and then begin expressing milk every two to three hours around the clock, or eight to ten times every twenty-four hours.

If your baby isn't nursing by Day Three (the third twenty-four-hour period), when your volume starts to increase, you can continue to hand-express (maybe into a pump flange attached to a collection bottle) or get a rental-grade pump (most hospitals have them readily available or contact your local Leader for sources). It's helpful to express for about fifteen minutes on each side every two to three hours, using breast massage to encourage more milk.

2. Keep *Your Baby Fed*

At first you may get only drops. No worries. His needs at first are very minimal. Even if he was nursing beautifully, he wouldn't be getting huge amounts at first. In fact, there's some evidence that giving lots of food at first may rev up his metabolism and cause him to require more. A little colostrum goes a long way.

You can hand-express into a plastic spoon and tip the drop(s) into your baby's mouth. If possible, have an assembly line, expressing into one spoon while another is being fed to the baby. If you find you have much more than drops, you can collect it from the spoon with an eyedropper or medicine dropper.

If you're hand-expressing into a pump funnel or pumping, you can wipe precious drops off the funnel part with your finger and let your baby suck them off, and collect the colostrum from the pump's bottle with an eyedropper.

Once your volume increases, or if you need to supplement, you can use any of several other breastfeeding-supportive feeding methods described in Chapter 18 to feed your baby away from the breast until he's ready to breastfeed.

3. Keep *Your Baby Close*

Your baby's bare skin against your own bare skin really helps encourage breastfeeding in a baby who's still getting himself organized. With a covering over the two of you that keeps *you* warm, your baby will be just as warm. He won't burn valuable calories trying to stay warm on his own (research shows the most expensive high-tech warmer or incubator in the world doesn't do as good a job as your own bare skin), he won't burn valuable calories trying to keep a steady heart rate and breathing (your own heart and breathing will pace and steady him, exactly as they always have; he's not supposed to have to take care of this on his own yet), and he'll have lunch close by, ready and waiting, whenever he decides he's ready.

You can let him doze on your chest or at your breast as much as you like, have your breast nearby when you feed him—little happy things that will remind him that your chest is still the most satisfying place in the world, even if it doesn't seem like a food source yet. This will encourage breastfeeding and also stabilize and comfort your baby.

The first step toward breastfeeding may be that the baby will mouth your nipple but won't suckle. Sometimes compressing your breast between your thumb and fingers so that a few drops gather on your nipple will encourage him to start sucking.

One out-of-the box idea is *licking* your baby. All mammals lick their babies after birth, not only to clean them but also to stimulate their breathing, digestion, and neural responses. Licking is also used to show affection and enhance the sense of smell. Human mothers don't typically think to do this, but some mothers have felt drawn to do it and their babies have responded surprisingly well.

If your baby hasn't nursed by several days of age, even with skilled help, you could try a nipple shield (see Chapter 18).

These feeding times should be relaxed, happy, and low-pressure. Play at breastfeeding when you both feel like it, instead of working at it because it's mealtime. Time, trust in the process, and a skilled helper are your best allies. Almost all babies begin nursing, though it may take some several weeks or more. Breastfeeding will come in its own good time, so long as you remember the Three Keeps—*Keep* your milk flowing, *Keep* your baby fed, and *Keep* your baby close.

Find and Keep a Good Breastfeeding Helper

We ought to add one more Keep: *Keep* in touch with someone who really understands breastfeeding, someone whose approach you respect and enjoy. You can get some general and helpful information from a book like this one, but for real help for individual challenges, and ongoing support, contact with a knowledgeable breastfeeding helper can make all the difference: it provides a pair of expert eyes, a mind that can pull from multiple resources and past experience, and a shoulder to cry on and lean on. The right person can shorten this extremely frustrating time and help you find not only answers but ways of streamlining your efforts.

Expect your helper to:

- Ask questions before giving ideas
- Be kind and respectful to both you and your baby
- Be endlessly patient
- Be fully supportive of your choices and goals
- Know other people and places to turn to for help
- Have books on how to help
- Keep up to date on research through conferences and other resources
- Adjust the information and ideas to your situation
- Be ready to change any suggestion that's not working for you
- Leave you feeling better than you did
- Leave you feeling stronger than you were
- Stick with you as long as you want to stick with her

The best way to find a local helper may be to start with La Leche League, if there is a Group or Leader in your community. Some breastfeeding difficulties may exceed her skills, but she'll know who to refer you to. You can also check ilca.org for a list of International Board Certified Lactation Consultants (IBCLCs) near you. And of course you don't have to stay local. Larger cities will often have more resources. Again, La Leche League is a great place to find your starting thread.

There's a reason your baby isn't breastfeeding, and a good helper will keep looking as long as you want her to...or until, as often happens, that magic "something" happens and your baby starts nursing. We've seen babies who suddenly "got it" at two weeks, four weeks, six weeks, three months, six months, and so on. When La Leche League Leaders work with mothers, we don't worry that the baby will never latch. We worry that the mother won't be able to "keep the faith" until it happens. It will work, and in the meantime there are ways to keep your milk supply strong. Babies *are* built to breastfeed. Early babies, small babies, sick babies—they're all designed to feed themselves at breast.

Practice Makes Perfect

It takes time for you and your baby to really get the hang of this new skill. Fortunately, you'll be breastfeeding very frequently and getting LOTS of opportunities to practice. Eventually you'll be able to nurse on this chair and that sofa, in a parked car and in the park, lying on your side in bed or sitting cross-legged on the floor, even getting up to answer the door. You might find that you like to cross one leg over the other, resting your supporting arm on your thigh and your baby's weight in your lap. Maybe you'll settle on a style wildly different from anything we mention—something tailored to your breast length, waist length, favorite postures, and baby's preferences. At that point, you'll be able to put all the breastfeeding books back on the shelf. Your baby will be a pro. And you will be, too.

OTHER GOOD RESOURCES FOR LATCHING APPROACHES

Breastfeeding Made Simple, by Nancy Mohrbacher and Kathleen Kendall-Tackett

The Latch, by Jack Newman and Teresa Pitman

Mother-Baby Experiences of Nurturing, by Suzanne Colson

Supporting Sucking Skills in Breastfeeding Infants, edited by Catherine Watson Genna (an excellent book for your breastfeeding helper but probably more technical than you want)

Baby-Led Breastfeeding, by Christina Smillie (DVD)

Biological Nurturing: Laid-back Breastfeeding, by Suzanne Colson (DVD)

Follow Me Mum, by Rebecca Glover (DVD)

PART II

Ages and Stages

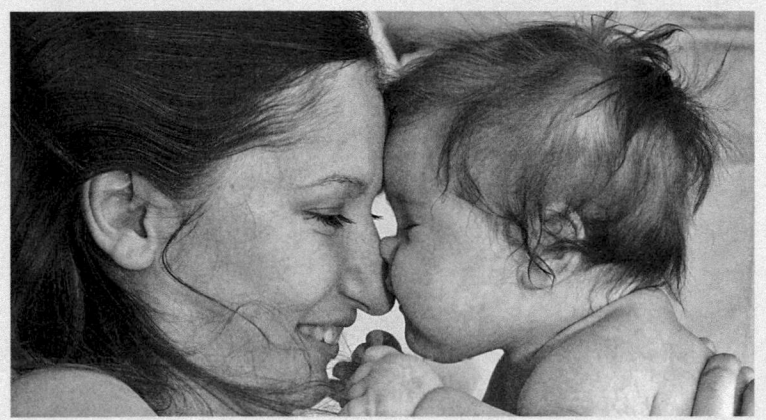

FIVE

The First Few Days: Hello, Baby...

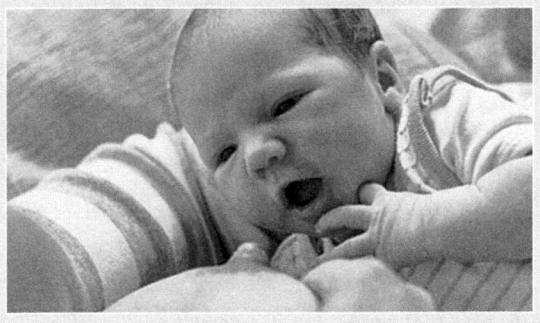

> "*We were home again and tucked into our own bed four hours after Melissa was born. She had begun breastfeeding just minutes after her birth, but the nurse at the hospital told me she'd probably sleep quite a bit for the next few days. Hah! That wasn't Melissa's plan. She surprised me by how alert she was much of the time. She'd lie in my arms and solemnly study my face as though she was trying to memorize what I looked like. Maybe she was! And she nursed a lot. She'd nurse for twenty minutes, doze in my arms for fifteen minutes, then nurse again. I spent most of those early days in bed with her, just gazing at my beautiful daughter.*" —Julie, remembering 1988

SO HERE YOU are—just you and your new baby (or maybe babies). Your emotions are probably all over the place, and your body doesn't feel anything like the one you had before you were pregnant. Having your baby in your arms is even better than you'd imagined, yet your whole world has tilted and you know there's a lot to learn.

Getting to Know Your Baby

Let's pick up where Em and Abe left off.

Em is tired after giving birth, but also euphoric. She wants to look at her son all the time, and when he opens his eyes and looks back at her, it's the best feeling in the world. She doesn't want him out of her sight, and of course there's no reason he should be. Within a day or two, the tiredness and soreness fade and she's surprised by how much energy she has.

Em is learning Abe's nursing signals, and she finds he nurses frequently, which is just fine with her. Her mother and a young cousin have come to stay and help out so Em can focus on Abe. When the weather is nice, Em puts Abe in a sling and they go for short walks. The fresh air and moving around feel good.

If Abe fusses, Em tries different things to soothe him. She always tries breastfeeding first, and most of the time that works, but if it doesn't she'll walk with him, talk or sing to him, do a bouncy little step that he sometimes likes, or go outside with him. Gradually she learns to identify what he needs—the way he makes little noises and holds his body still for a minute when he's about to pee, the way he squirms and rubs his fists against his face when he's tired and wants to sleep, the way he bobs his head against her chest when he wants to nurse again. Each time she settles him, Em feels a little more confident about being a mother.

Your own early days may not go as smoothly: you may be recovering from surgery, dealing with the after-effects of labor medications, or really struggling to get breastfeeding going. Fortunately, Nature has given both you and your baby the instincts and skills that can help you overcome any early challenges you might face. See "Moving Forward After a Difficult Birth" in Chapter 3 for further strategies.

SKIN-TO-SKIN

For at least the first two hours of your baby's life, the two of you deserve to be—*need* to be—together, with your bare or diaper-only baby on your bare skin, chest to chest. If you're wearing a shirt or gown, just open it. Lean back comfortably and let gravity hold your baby against you; no need to lie on your back. A regular blanket over both of you is all you need. Study after study shows the importance of this skin-to-skin contact. Measurements, ointments, everything can wait. This is your time together. It comes once in both your lives. And it can shape both your lives. It's your right. And it's what your baby expects and needs. Skin-to-skin contact after birth helps to:

- Stabilize your baby's heart rate, breathing, and temperature
- Stabilize your own temperature
- Prevent baby blues later on
- Reduce your baby's stress (no, crying doesn't exercise a baby's lungs; it strains his heart and brain)
- Reduce your baby's pain from medical procedures
- Reduce your stress
- Increase interactions between you and your baby
- Increase the likelihood and length of breastfeeding

Nobody Told Me!

Despite childbirth classes and friends who've "been there," many little things about those early postpartum days aren't usually mentioned. So it might help you to know what's normal.

🔆 There aren't many diapers to change at first. The colostrum your baby gets from your breasts is small in quantity, which is perfect because his stomach is about the size of a large marble at birth. His first poop will be sticky and black—that's the meconium, the wastes that filled your baby's intestines before he was born. If you are planning to use cloth diapers, you might want to use disposables just long enough to get all the meconium, since it can stain cloth.

- ✧ You'll be having what seems like a heavy menstrual period that can last for a couple of weeks. This is called *lochia* and at times the flow can be really heavy. Standing up your first time can cause quite a gush. At first, you might want to use overnight pads and keep a pad or dark-colored towel on the bed.

- ✧ When you breastfeed your baby, your uterus will contract in response to the oxytocin released by the baby's suckling, and you may get a gush of blood each time. The cramps will soon fade—but they can be almost labor-strong sometimes.

- ✧ Unless you're recovering from surgery (and maybe even then), you'll probably be hungry after the birth. You've just had a real workout, and you deserve some real food. One mother told us, "A local restaurant had a dish called Once Around the Kitchen that had a little bit of everything on the menu. I had my husband order that for me right after each birth! It was the only time I ever ate that—but boy, was it good right then!"

- ✧ Your baby doesn't fit the books (not surprising, since babies can't read).

- ✧ You can't sleep. Part of it is the mental turmoil of having made the leap into motherhood. Then there's the shift in hormones—pregnancy levels of progesterone and estrogen drop quickly after birth. And being a new mother raises your radar so that you sleep more lightly and wake more easily, especially if your baby isn't with you. Keep your baby with you, and you'll probably sleep better.

- ✧ You might feel overwhelmed by visitors. If you're in a hospital, ask the staff to stop visitors at reception and suggest they visit when you get home. If you're at home, post your visiting hours (short ones!) on the door and just stay in your nightgown. If you behave as if you feel great (even if you do), people will treat you that way, and that's not in your best interests right now. You can use the refrigerator list in the Tear-Sheet Toolkit to direct visitors' energy in helpful ways.

- ✧ You start leaking from everywhere. We've already mentioned lochia. Some women also find they have temporary bladder issues—leaking a little urine if they cough or sneeze. As your milk comes in, you may find that you can't keep a shirt dry. Also temporary. You may sweat a whole lot at first, too, especially at night (keep extra PJs handy) while your body goes through hormonal changes and simultaneously tries to dump any IV fluids you might have been given. Once she starts getting a lot of milk, your baby will start filling a lot of diapers, so there are *her* fluids to deal with. And your eyes... well, they seem to tear up over just about anything! More than one former-CEO-turned-new-mother had to have someone else call for breastfeeding help because she couldn't keep from breaking down on the phone. While some tears and emotional days are normal, if you find you are feeling anxious and depressed for days at a time, be sure to talk to your doctor or midwife as soon as possible. This could be postpartum depression, and getting help quickly can help get you back to enjoying your baby.

- If you've been given a lot of IV fluids, you may look more pregnant after the birth than before, with swollen eyes, swollen fingers, swollen breasts, swollen everything. (An epidural can significantly reduce blood pressure, so the fluids were pumped in to help keep it in the normal range.) Eating protein or a lot of watermelon may help you unload the fluids. If you were on an IV for several days, expect to spend several weeks getting your basic body back, and be prepared for a possible delay in having your milk increase in volume.

- These first few nights can be tough! Take plenty of naps, even an evening nap, and prepare your bedtime nest. One mother unwrapped an energy bar before bed and set it on her bedside table, knowing that she wouldn't be able to manage the wrapper at three in the morning, when she was hungry. You might want to have water or juice beside your bed as well—new mothers can get very thirsty. Your nights will settle down, but not instantly.

- You may be stunned by how much you love your baby. Or you may be stunned that you don't. The first is what we're built for; the second often results from birth interventions. Two of this book's writers, Teresa and Diana, both fell in love with their babies instantly. The third, Diane, remembers looking at her son on the changing table and saying aloud to him, "I would defend you with my life, but I don't love you," and thinking what a curious thing that was for a mother to say. Love can come as a thunderbolt, or it can creep up on you over the first month or two. But it comes. It comes. Two years later, Diane watched her son run across a field and thought, "If anything were to happen to that child, I don't know how my heart could go on beating."

☀ *Being a mother is a twenty-four-hour-a-day job, and it can be hard.* Many mothers feel outraged and shell-shocked by the challenge of taking care of a new baby.

This is why a network is so important. You need people who will take care of you, so that you can mother your baby. Day by day you settle in, you learn new patterns, and life smooths out.

Nursing Habits: First Few Days

There are probably three questions on your mind right now: how long, which side, and how often.

How long? Your baby can nurse as long as he wants to. An unmedicated baby may nurse for an hour or more at a time in the first few days. A medicated, sleepy baby may need encouragement. Mothers have nursed twins, triplets, and even quadruplets, so your nipples are up to the task. If they're calling for relief, you might want to find that good La Leche League Leader or other breastfeeding helper and do some problem solving.

Which side? In these first few days, you may find that your nipple or your arm or your itchy nose makes you want to switch sides before your baby has stopped sucking. That's fine! Change sides—or don't change sides—for any reason you like. As long as it's comfortable, you can keep it up all day and only good will come of it. Do make use of both sides during the course of the day, but there's no need to obsess about giving equal time.

How often? So long as your baby is an active and eager nurser, you can feel free to nurse him as often as he wants to. Unmedicated babies who stay with their mothers tend to nurse more than the eight to twelve times a day you often hear about, interspersed with some serious napping. They're putting in their order for abundant milk.

If your baby is too zonked from birth medications or jaundice to wake on his own, you can wake him up every three hours or so, later in this chapter, counting from the beginning of one feeding to the beginning of the next (see "Should We Wake the Baby for Feedings,"). Start about six hours after birth and aim for *at least* eight feedings in twenty-four hours. He should be giving clear feeding signals within a week, once he can think straight, and then *you* can relax and follow *his* lead.

You don't need to feel trapped on the bed or couch with your baby. If you want to go to the bathroom or get a snack, just slip a finger in the corner of your baby's mouth to break the suction and do what you need to do. (One simple approach is to use a finger about the size of your nipple. Slide it into the corner of his mouth, between his gums, and turn your finger as you'd turn a screwdriver in a paint can lid. Then you can slide your nipple out without any risk of gums clamping on it.) Your baby may want to nurse again once you come back. Offer if he seems interested.

Bottom line: if your baby is latched on and positioned comfortably, you can nurse from the first breast until one of you wants to stop. Sometimes he'll take the other breast, and sometimes he won't, which is fine. If he falls asleep or stops nursing actively within a few minutes, you can encourage him to continue. If he's too fuzzy to manage on his own, hand expression can carry him along in these first few days.

> "I recently spent twelve days doing a project for the World Health Organization in Thailand. We saw a lot of abandoned plastic cots [bassinets] in the hospitals. I was told that despite rooming-in, there had been a problem with jaundice. They got rid of the cots, put the babies in the beds with their mothers, and the jaundice stopped. The mothers feed all day and the nurses walk around fine-tuning positioning and helping as required. Where were the hypoglycemia, engorgement, sore nipples, babies unable to latch, etc.? Not to be seen. I never heard a baby cry. That's frequent suckling, folks, not what we play around with."
> —Ros Escott, IBCLC, writing to her colleagues in 1995

Nights and Naps

If your baby was born in a hospital, there are three likely nighttime scenarios. One is a centralized nursery, although these are declining in number. Having your baby away from you is unnatural for both of you, day or night. You lose control over what happens to your baby and whether he is supplemented with sugar water or formula. If your baby isn't with you, his heart rate, breathing, and temperature are less stable, his feeding cues are likely to be missed, and your milk generally comes in more slowly and less fully. If you're bonding well with your baby, you'll hate being separated, and

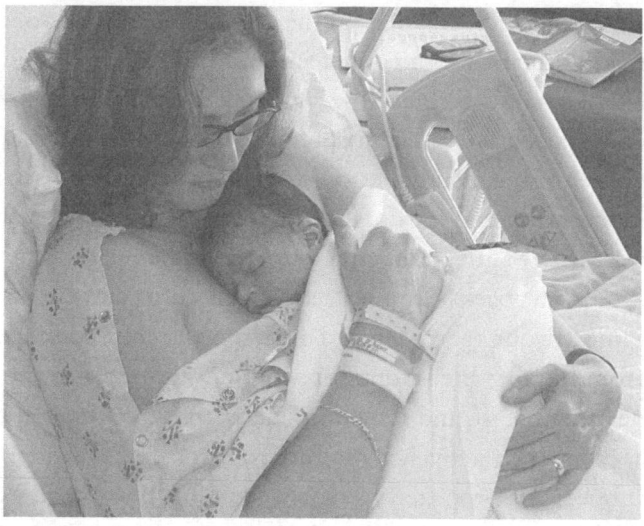

Keeping your baby skin-to-skin.

if you don't mind the separation, consider that that might be a reason for spending more time together!

Rooming-in is the more common arrangement today in hospitals, with the baby in a bassinet or Isolette in the same room as the mother. You can have your baby on your chest, in your arms, or at your side as much as you like during the day, but many hospitals don't want a mother to have her baby in her bed at night. Some hospitals are starting to use a "sidecar" bed for the baby, attached to the mother's hospital bed, instead of the "plastic box" approach. *Bedding-in* is increasingly common in some places. Mother and baby share the same bed both day and night, nursing as they choose, beginning to synchronize their sleep patterns, falling in love, and bringing in a faster, more abundant milk supply.

SHARING SLEEP SAFELY IN A HOSPITAL

If you're using painkillers, sleeping pills, or other consciousness-altering medications, your baby will be safer in someone else's arms or in a bedside bassinet when you feel drowsy or plan to sleep. Otherwise, sharing sleep safely in the hospital depends on the bed.

- Some hospitals now have double beds, enabling mother and baby and partner to sleep safely together simply by putting the baby in between the two adults at breast height, so that pillows aren't an issue.

- Rehabilitation centers often put a mattress on the floor for patients who don't want the confines of bed rails but who are at risk for falling. It's a thought!
- You can discuss arrangements with the friendliest nurse on that shift. You have the right to switch nurses if yours is a mismatch.

If you feel you just can't go against the grain, know that you'll be home in a couple of days, where you can use whatever arrangement you and your baby like best!

JUST A LITTLE FORMULA?
Concept courtesy of Marsha Walker, RN, IBCLC

Here's the problem. Your newborn's sterile intestines are open to whatever comes along. And they're truly "open," so that illness- or allergy-promoting substances can slip through into your baby's blood-stream. His intestines need two things right from the start: *your milk*, to help set up the right bacteria and provide a temporary seal against infections, and *time*, to mature and create his own solid seal against illness- and allergy-promoting "leaks."

Babies born by Cesarean, who don't pick up their normal bacteria during the birth, are at higher risk of picking up hospital bacteria and may be in even greater need of your presence and your milk. So giving your baby formula, for any reason, in these first days is not something to be taken lightly. It may mean that your baby's intestinal bacteria are never quite the protective ones that an *exclusively* breastfed baby has. A little formula after that can alter your baby's protective intestinal bacteria for a full month. A little formula anytime in the first few months, before the intestines are well sealed, can increase the risk of allergy and diabetes in susceptible children. The risk may be highest in the first few days and in babies born even a little early. If your milk isn't available, banked human colostrum or mature milk is the next best choice. More and more hospitals keep banked milk on hand because they realize the long-term importance of keeping a newborn exclusively on human milk. It pays to find out in advance what your birth place does. If they don't have banked milk, you could ask them to consider it...for the lifetime health of their smallest patients!

Minding Your Pees and Poos

What goes in must come out. In fact, for full-term babies what comes out is generally a good way to gauge what went in. At first, it's not much. In the first twenty-four hours, if you get nothing more than a slightly wet diaper and a black, tarry diaper, you and your baby are doing absolutely fine. By the next twenty-four hours, your baby will have had enough colostrum that she'll move most of that meconium out and will produce a little more urine. By the third day, expect to see real changes in the color of those poops. And by the end of the week, you'll probably be well into yellow poops and noticeably heavy diapers. You'll find a rough chart that you can tear out and follow in the Tear-Sheet Toolkit. Why doesn't the chart record pees? Because they're not as important. In fact, you may not see many wet diapers at all in the first few days, but you can figure that any bowel movements your baby has were accompanied by some urine.

There is one thing about the wet diapers to be aware of, though. About the third day, you may notice orange-red deposits in the diaper. This is commonly known as "brick dust" or *urate crystals* and is highly concentrated urine from not getting enough fluid. It's very normal for breastfed babies on the third day right before the milk comes in and will be gone as soon as the milk volume increases. It is often mistaken for bleeding after a baby boy's circumcision or a baby girl's normal vaginal bleeding from her mother's pregnancy hormones. If you continue to see these deposits after the fifth day, especially if your baby is having fewer than three poops a day, contact your baby's doctor and your breastfeeding helper.

Once your baby is old enough to have a track record—a solid pattern of growth—everyone stops looking at the details. But in the early days, you may be tempted to read and record all the signs you can track: left breast seventeen minutes, right breast six minutes, diaper at 2.24 a.m. Is all this record-keeping important? Not the details. You're keeping an eye on poopy diapers, and there's a section in the next chapter on how to know if your baby's doing well. Because every baby is different, doing a spreadsheet will just increase your concern, and can become so inhibiting that breastfeeding suffers. Our repeating song: if you have concerns, give your breastfeeding helper a call and talk it over!

Weight Watchers

Conventional wisdom these days says that babies shouldn't lose more than 7 percent of their body weight before they start gaining, absolutely shouldn't lose any more than 10 percent, and should be back at birth weight by two weeks. But there are some problems with these guidelines. The mother who's had a lot of IV fluids may deliver a baby who has also had a lot of IV fluids. He'll be born at an artificially high weight and seem to lose more than he really does. This is one of the reasons why babies born at home often register little or no weight loss. But babies are built to tolerate some initial fumbling while their new life gets under way. If your baby has lost considerable weight but is eager and organized when he eats, swallowing well, and starting to produce more diapers, then he's probably doing fine. Watch to make sure his good progress continues; it most likely will. If your baby has lost very little weight but is sleepy, not swallowing, and not pooping, then he probably needs some help digging himself out of a temporary hole. You may need to take charge of his meals by feeding him more often or express some extra milk if he's not nursing well. The extra milk expression will do two things: get more food into him so that he starts pooping, and wake your breasts up to remind them that there's a *baby* here! Check with an LLL Leader, other breastfeeding helper, or your doctor if you don't see a lot more pooping within a day or two. (A good helper will also be able to help you sort out when to visit the doctor. Remember that your baby's doctor is there whenever you need him—that's his job. Don't ever hesitate to call if you feel the need.)

Early-Days Issues

In today's birth world, it's not uncommon for problems—or what seem like problems—to crop up in the first days, and the problems come with a whole new and potentially confusing vocabulary. Hypothermia, hypo-glycemia, jaundice, engorgement, and excessive infant weight loss are all problems related to sleepiness and separation. And the best way to avoid sleepiness and separation is to bring your baby into the world unmedicated, and to keep him on or against your body most of the time in the early days. But if that isn't your reality, we have lots more information on coping with all these issues in Chapter 18.

Surviving on Your Own with Your First Baby

You're headed home from the hospital, or your helpers are headed home themselves, and suddenly, with no previous parenting experience, you're caring for a days-old baby! You may wonder how this can even be *legal* without some sort of advanced degree. Well, remember that this biologi-cal system called parenting was designed long ago to be accomplished by people who didn't know how to read. Your baby won't break if you hold him "wrong," or if you don't give him a bath for a month (really!), or if the water's a bit too cool, or if he coughs or sneezes or startles. Since he can't clear his throat yet, you may even hear some downright freaky sounds com-ing from him at times. But your baby is an excellent instructor, and your instincts and common sense are excellent students. You'll get all the truly important lessons. You'll even survive...The Second Night.

THE SECOND NIGHT (OR WHATEVER NIGHT YOUR BABY REALLY WAKES UP)
Contributed by Jan Barger, RN, IBCLC, FILCA

All of a sudden, your little one discovers that he's no longer back in the warmth and comfort of his womb, and it's SCARY out here! All sorts of people have been handling him, and he's not accustomed to the new noises, lights, sounds, and smells. He *has* found one thing, though, and that's his voice...and you notice that each time you take him off the breast where he comfortably drifted off to sleep, and put him down, he protests—loudly!

So you put him back on the breast and he nurses for a little bit, then goes to sleep. As you take him off and put him back to bed, he cries again and starts rooting around, looking for you. This can seem to go on for hours. A lot of moms are convinced it's because their milk isn't "in" yet, and the baby is starving. What's *really* happening is that your baby has realized that the most comforting and comfortable place for him to be is at your breast. It's the closest to "home" he can get. Breastfeeding helpers all over the world have seen babies do this even when the mother's milk came in early. Here are some ways to reduce his crying and increase your rest.

- When he drifts off to sleep at the breast, don't move him except to pillow his head more comfortably on your breast. Don't try to burp him—just snuggle with him until he falls into a deeper sleep with even breathing and no eyelid movement, so he's less likely to be disturbed by being moved. Better yet, just keep holding him!
- If he starts to root and act as though he wants to go back to the breast, that's fine—this is his way of settling and comforting.
- Babies feel comforted by touching with their hands, and his touch on your breast will increase your oxytocin levels and help boost your milk supply. So take the mittens off. He might scratch himself, but he's a fast healer.
- Sometimes babies just need some extra snuggling at the breast, because your breast is his home.

Concerns You May Have in the First Few Days

Here are some of the issues that mothers commonly call Leaders to ask about after the birth. No question is silly, any more than it's silly to ask for the French word for bread when you're trying to eat in France. You really are learning a new language. You'll be fluent soon, if you get your questions answered. If your questions aren't addressed here, you may find them in Chapter 18, "Tech Support." If they're not there either, look on the llli.org forums or call your local LLL Leader.

Should We Wake the Baby for Feedings?

Nature designed all mammal babies to sleep when they need to sleep and wake when they need to wake. We have all kinds of mothering instincts for all kinds of necessary situations, but waking a baby isn't one of them. All our instincts are geared toward soothing and encouraging sleep. If you had no medications, if your baby stays in physical contact with you, if he eats well when he eats, if he's gaining well, and yet he's sleeping longer than three hours at a stretch, that's probably just who he is. Keep an eye on his weight and enjoy reading that novel that the other new mothers don't have time for.

In some cases, though, the baby who sleeps more than three hours needs some intervention. That's because Nature never planned on birth medications or separating mother and baby. A baby away from his mother may shut down to conserve energy, and sleep longer than he normally would; a baby whose mother had birth medications may be unable to rouse himself normally for a while. If you had an epidural or other birth medications and your baby isn't waking at least every two or three hours, it's better to assume that it's the side effects of the medications keeping him asleep and get some food into him.

There are wake-able times and non-wake-able times. If you lift and then drop her arm and you feel some tension in it as it falls, if you see eye movement under those little lids, if her mouth is making little sucking movements, or if any part of her is making movements, waking will be easier. Here are some ideas to help wake her up:

- ☼ If there will be a bright light in her eyes, dim it. Is she facing a window? Pull the drape. It's much easier for her to keep her eyes open if she doesn't have to squint.
- ☼ Undress her. This may do the trick all by itself, but if it doesn't, put her skin-to-skin against your chest and see if that helps.
- ☼ Stroke her and call her name. Rub her feet. Maybe wipe her face with a damp cloth. Handle her gently.
- ☼ No luck? Lay her on the bed on her back, no wrappings, so that she can't feel you at all. That's unsettling enough to wake many babies. Gently roll her from side to side on the bed, from all the way on her left side

to all the way on her right side, back and forth. Almost all babies will open their eyes to see who's rocking their world.

- ☼ Or hold her along your forearms, head in your hands, feet at your elbows, and lift her so that she's more vertical, then lower your arms so that she's horizontal, up and down, up and down, talking to her gently as you do so.
- ☼ As a last resort, put a little colostrum or milk in her mouth—just a bit, waiting for her to swallow before adding more.
- ☼ The occasional baby will sleep through a whole meal or two this way. She might also latch and nurse in her sleep, especially if she's in a laid-back breastfeeding position. That's fine. Your real goal, after all, isn't to wake the baby up so much as it is to help her eat.

Should We Swaddle Him?

If your baby has been taken from you and comes back swaddled—wrapped up like a burrito—just unwrap him (he is, after all, *your* baby) and snuggle his bare or lightly clothed skin against yours, with your blankets over both of you. He'll quickly regain the heat he was losing, and you can keep him with you from that point on.

Swaddling is popular at the moment, but there's research that raises alarms. The swaddled newborn has poorer circulation. His temperature is lower, and so is his mother's. He gains weight more slowly, probably because he is less able to signal hunger and is maybe less aware that he *is* hungry. Mothers whose newborns are swaddled much of the time have more engorgement and lower initial supplies, and tend to handle their babies more roughly.

Some babies with special concerns are calmed by swaddling. There's no doubt that it has its uses. But not for ordinary babies. And certainly not in the first two hours, when the separation it creates can influence how gently you treat your baby for his first year of life! Keep in mind, too, that a swaddled baby is defenseless and can't move. Babies normally sleep safely with their mothers (see Chapter 12 for specifics), but sleeping with a swaddled baby is risky.

What Can I Do for Nipple Pain?

We can't say it too often: *breastfeeding is not supposed to hurt. Ever.* Your nipples are not supposed to crack or bleed. They're not supposed to come out of your baby's mouth creased or frayed or warped. They may be supersensitive at first, and you might feel some stinging here and there for a day or two. You may not want clothing rubbing them during this time. Some of these lesser sensations are the normal part of getting used to breastfeeding. But actual pain or damage? *NO.*

Getting rid of pain is often a simple matter of letting your baby lead the way more, or making small adjustments to his position or yours. If rearranging yourselves or taking another look at Chapter 4 doesn't help, we encourage you to find a helper—a *good* helper—as quickly as you can. Ask your friends for recommendations, call La Leche League, and think twice about anyone who uses phrases like "the right way," "you're doing it wrong," "but everything *looks* fine," "he's just being lazy," or anything else that feels like an absolute. The biology of breastfeeding is flexible, adaptable, and sturdy. And babies are no more lazy about feeding than they are about breathing. Getting good help earlier rather than later will most likely help you feel better faster, body and mind.

How Can I Tell if He's Really Eating?

Diapers tell you a lot, of course, and by three days or so you'll probably start to notice swallowing. Good swallowing of ample milk will usually sound like this: whisper the sound "keh…keh…keh" at about one "keh" per second. Some babies spend some time gulping (and there's no mistaking that); some may make the "keh" sound with every few sucks. But that whispered "keh" is usually a swallow.

During the first few days, you may not hear a steady, rhythmic swallowing sound; the amount of colostrum that a baby takes can vary a lot. Listen for the "keh" sound for practice—you'll hear it now and then—and you may notice that his lower jaw drops a little lower, maybe with a hesitation or pause when it drops. That drop-*pause*-close motion is also a swallow. Not every noise a nursing baby makes is a swallow, and some babies who nurse well are nearly silent. But watching and listening for swallows can be encouraging—colostrum and milk really are going from breast to baby. This really is working!

He won't swallow when he first latches. First he may make some quick, fluttery little sucks that mean he's organizing everything in his mouth and settling into a place where he can massage your breast and trigger a milk release. Call it *preparing* to nurse. Then he'll probably start some slower sucks, especially if he's getting nice mouthfuls of colostrum or milk.

They Say Everything's Fine, but I'm Petrified

Here are some basic concepts that can help get you through the scary beginning.

- Put the baby first. Maybe the house is a wreck, maybe the bills are due, maybe your mother-in-law wants to visit. Doesn't matter. *Put the baby first.* He needs to nurse, and he needs to be held, and those needs will be pretty intense and continuous for just a couple of weeks. The rest of your life can wait. Keep your baby supplies centralized, preferably where you're likely to be eating, sleeping, and nursing. Don't worry about organizing—put everything in piles. You'll have lots of time to streamline and organize as you go. Just go with the flow of this moment rather than trying to establish some perfect pattern from the start. Make several possible places to nurse, sleep, or eat. Kirsten had nursed Willem just fine in her flat, stiff hospital bed but somehow couldn't get it to work anywhere else. She put a pad of blankets on the living room floor and used that while they slowly learned other nursing positions. Whatever works, however silly it looks, go for it. There are no Breastfeeding Police who are going to come and check on you.
- Put yourself solidly next. You have healing to do, and that means rest, time with the baby, and something to eat and drink. You tend the baby, and let your partner, family, willing friend, or postpartum doula tend you.
- Your partner will inevitably be in third place for now. Check the next section for things your partner can do to help keep life going while everything is so new and unsettled. Reward him or her with a snuggly baby on the chest, provided the baby isn't looking for *your* chest at the moment.

Someone once said that bottle-feeding a baby is like riding a tricycle: you just get on and you do it. Breastfeeding is like riding a bicycle. You wobble at first, maybe you fall, and there's certainly a learning curve. But once you know how to ride a bicycle, would you *ever* go back to a tricycle?

What Can My Partner Do to Help Me Breastfeed?

Your own role is pretty clear: Feed the Baby. What about your partner's role? Share these ideas that can really make a difference:

- 💡 Feed the mother, and keep food on hand, especially no-fix, easy-to-eat, one-handed food, and foods high in fiber.
- 💡 Set up a sleeping arrangement that works for all of you. You may need to try a few different arrangements to find the best one, and it may involve separate sleeping spaces for a while. Be flexible!
- 💡 Monitor visitors. The mother may be too polite to chase them away. Read her signals, and shoo people out the door before they've overstayed. Or refer them to the job list on the refrigerator (see the Tear-Sheet Toolkit) to get a little work out of them before they go!
- 💡 Run errands. That may involve dropping off the mail, picking up groceries, or errands that you had no idea she usually ran.
- 💡 Call for breastfeeding help if she wants you to. Ordinarily, LLL Leaders and other breastfeeding helpers want the mother herself to call so we know she really wants our involvement. But when it's a few days post-birth and we hear her in the background giving you information to repeat to us, we know exactly what's going on. We've been there ourselves.

Trusting Yourself

Basic mothering is a combination of instinct and common sense. Your baby's cry prods you to respond to it because your baby needs you. You instinctively speak to him in a soft, high voice that babies instinctively find soothing. You put your baby against your shoulder to calm him because, well, it works. You learn ways of moving, holding, and nursing that no one tells you. It's motherhood by instinct, common sense, and trial and error. And it *works*.

Becoming a mother is kind of like learning to swim. At some point, you take a little deeper breath, let go of the edge, start to paddle...and realize you're doing it. Some of it is what you've learned, some of it is making the effort, and some of it is having faith in yourself.

These first few days, whatever they hold for you and your baby, are a time to enjoy each other. You two are both starting to let go of the edge of the pool. And you know what? Someday soon you'll realize that you love swimming...and you're *good* at it!

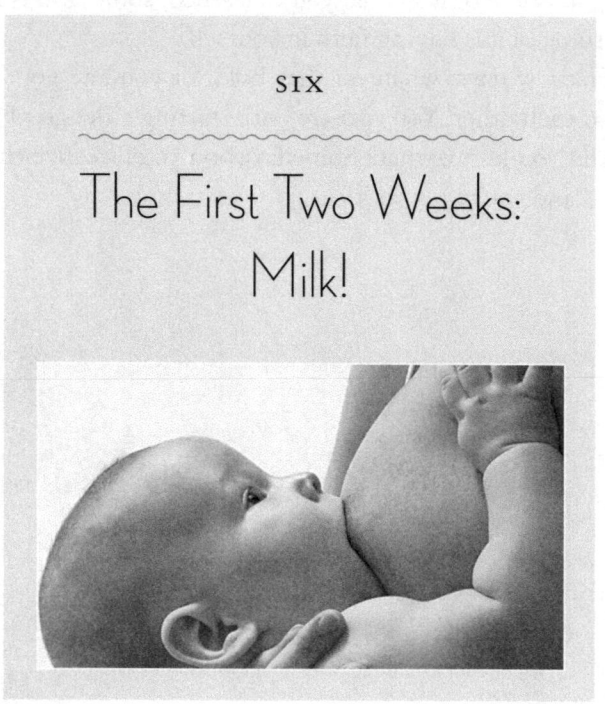

SIX

The First Two Weeks: Milk!

"*This baby girl of ours sighs and coos and squeaks and yells. And all that 'talking' obviously requires interpreting, so I present the following conversation between me and my ten-day-old infant, word for word, last night around three in the morning.*"

SOPHIA: *WAAAAAAH! STARVING BABY! HELP! HELP! DOESN'T ANY-ONE CARE? CALL UNICEF! HELP! HELP!*

ME *(scooping up one angry lump of baby): Hey there, sweetie. Hungry?*

SOPHIA: *OH, MOM, it was SO AWFUL! I woke up in that PLACE? You know the one? Where no one is holding the baby? And there isn't any milk? IT WAS THE WORST THING THAT EVER HAPPENED IN MY WHOLE LIFE!*

ME *(offers breast): Here you go.*

SOPHIA: *SO HUNGRY! (butts breast with her face)*
ME: *You have to open your mouth.*
SOPHIA: *WILL NO ONE THINK OF THE BABY?*
ME *(tickles her lip): It's okay, sweetie.*
SOPHIA: *SO HUNGR—oh. Snarf. Nom nom nom nom nom nom. MAN,*
    that's the stuff! Nom nom nom nom nom nom. SO GOOD. Nom nom
    nom nom. I almost DIED, you know. Nom nom nom nom.
ME: *Zzzzzzzzzz.*
SOPHIA *(head lolling back, mouth slack and dribbling milk):*
    Duuuuuude."   —Kira, remembering 2009

YOU'RE HOME! OR maybe you never left, but you're not in the home that existed before. You're in this new place, this restaurant that's open 24/7, where everything is about baby and breasts, where diaper contents are completely captivating, where time is measured in minutes at breast, minutes of sleep, minutes of calm. It's no wonder most of us cry at some point! Motherhood, we realize, isn't a job that ends at quitting time. There *is* no quitting time!

But there are those amazing moments, too, when you realize that you're still sustaining this little life with your breast, having sustained it within your belly; when he looks at you with wise and knowing eyes; when he sleeps peacefully and trustingly on your chest; when you can't believe what an extraordinary feat you've accomplished. You've made the one-way crossing into motherhood, a land with the most intense work and greatest pleasure you will ever have.

For now, though, the focus is on input, output, and rest. It's the same kind of process you went through when you learned to ride a bicycle. There was no hurrying it, but day by day, pedal by pedal, you got the hang of it and started to roll. The starting-to-roll feeling is something you and your baby will come to on your own. Here are some thoughts about the input, output, rest, and, well, the rest.

Nursing Habits: First Two Weeks

Here's what you can expect in a nursing session once your milk has increased, sometime after the first few days.

When your baby latches and begins sucking, you may still be feeling a moment of discomfort, but it should fade quickly, and it should be getting better every day. (If you haven't tried the laid-back breastfeeding described in Chapter 4, you might want to take another look!) She'll probably make fast, fluttering sucks at the beginning of a feed. She's getting everything arranged in her mouth so that she can hit the exact right spot to trigger your release of oxytocin and get your milk flowing. If she's having trouble getting enough breast in her mouth to release your milk, you'll find she does the little fluttery sucks, waits, does more little fluttery sucks, waits, has a swallow or two, and does more little fluttery sucks. (If nursings usually begin with a long series of fluttery sucks and pauses, check with your LLL Leader or other breastfeeding helper to troubleshoot.) Once your milk is flowing, those rapid sucks give way to longer, slower sucks with a whispered "keh" sound, a hitch or pause in the jaw motion, or an almost digging motion as her lower jaw circles forward into your breast. You'll probably notice a swallow with every one or two or maybe three sucks.

After a while, the steady sucking and swallowing stop completely. She rests, neither sucking nor letting go. Just like you, your baby likes to "put her fork down" now and then. It gives her a chance to collect herself, catch her breath, and wait for that next milk release! She may start in again without the rapid little fluttery sucks, or she may need to use them again to reorganize her mouth or release your milk. She knows what she's doing.

As her meal progresses, there are more sucks before each swallow. After some periods of slow, steady sucking and some pauses, her eyes usually close. She may relax so much that she starts to lose your nipple and gives a few sucks to draw it in again. But after a bit, sleep overcomes the pleasure of even these last, widely spaced swallows. Your nipple slides gently from her mouth, and she naps with her body against yours. Or she doesn't quite let go, but when you slide a finger gently into the corner of her mouth to release her grip, she doesn't rouse enough to complain. Or she finishes her meal in a state of calm alertness, enjoying the cuddle and the sights and sounds around her.

FINISH THE FIRST BREAST FIRST

There's no need to interrupt the feeding to switch breasts. You can let your baby nurse from the first breast until he comes off on his own by letting go or falling asleep. Sometimes he'll take your other breast if you offer, and sometimes he won't. That's just fine.

CCK

If she has fallen asleep nursing, it's partly because her level of *cholecystokinin* (CCK) has risen. In a newborn, a high level of this hormone makes a baby sleepy and tells her that she's full; a low level can wake her and tell her she's hungry. After maybe twenty minutes of sucking (*not necessarily eating*) your baby's CCK has risen enough to put her to sleep and give her a rest from all her hard work. About twenty minutes after she's stopped sucking, her CCK level has fallen again. Your baby may wake up (HELP! STARVING BABY!), convinced she's never eaten before in her life, giving her a chance to "top off her tank" with renewed energy. Another sucking bout, another CCK rise, and she's likely to zonk out completely.

CCK is a marvelous arrangement that keeps your baby from working too hard too long, but also acts as an alarm clock to give her a second or third (or fourth) chance if she needs a little more. And it allows a new and inefficient baby to come back for seconds and encourage your new milk supply—part of a system that helps ensure enough food for baby, enough production from Mama.

Sucking on a pacifier releases CCK, too. A baby can fall asleep with a pacifier, thinking she's been fed. But *really* she's been fooled out of a meal, and your breasts have lost a feeding's worth of milk removal. Result: slower weight gain and lower supply.

CCK is Nature's way of helping to make sleep happen and keeping your supply strong. Why mess with such a well-designed system? Save yourself a lot of effort, nurse the baby one last time, and odds are she'll start to snooze.

Here's another use. Your baby wants to nurse again and Aunt Franny is shaking her head? Just say, with great authority, "Well, you know, it's her CCK talking."

Cluster Feeding

Whether it's CCK, other hormones, or something about babies, you may find that nursings often cluster together, maybe especially at certain times of day. *Cluster feeding* means a clock is pretty useless in a normal breastfeeding relationship. The clock is valuable for keeping track of a sleepy baby to make sure she's eating often enough. But beyond that, young babies' needs are variable, unpredictable, and often clustered into a series of meals and a longer stretch. Evening especially is often a time of "nursing marathons," when nothing but another time at breast seems to work.

All this nursing right now makes sense. Your baby will never be less skilled at this than she is right now. She'll never have a smaller mouth, tongue, and stomach to work with than she has right now. Her intestines aren't very efficient yet. And yet she'll never grow faster than she'll be growing in the next few weeks. You can see why there's a whole lot of nursing going on. At the same time, your breasts are trying to figure out just who and how many they're going to be taking care of in the future. Having your baby put in a big order now will make everything much smoother later on.

So long as your baby is gaining well, cluster feedings are absolutely normal. If your baby routinely falls asleep at the breast, is waking up soon after and nursing again and again *and isn't gaining well,* see Chapter 18 and contact your local Leader or other breastfeeding helper to help you figure out possible reasons and solutions.

> What about the clever bracelet or iPhone app to remind you which side you nursed on last? Your breasts are probably a better guide—you'll sometimes see a nursing mother privately hefting first one breast and then the other before choosing a side.

Your Baby's Diaper Output

When milk goes in, diapers fill and the weight on the scale goes up. Once you know your baby better, diaper contents and scales won't seem nearly as important. But for now, it's important to keep an eye on diaper output for reassurance that he's getting enough milk. To help you keep track, there's a diaper log in the Tear-Sheet Toolkit.

The number of wet and poopy diapers should increase day by day through the first week to ten days. Basic rule of thumb: by the middle of the first week, it takes most babies *at least* three poops a day that are nearly the size of the "okay" circle you make with your thumb and forefinger in order to gain well—an "okay" sign for an okay diaper. More is fine. If you see fewer, check with your midwife or doctor. Don't be fooled if someone says, "Breastfed babies often stool only once every few days, so it's normal that your newborn is having so few stools." That may be true of an eight-week-old (see the next chapter). It's *almost never* true of a six-day-old.

In exclusively breastfed babies, most poopy diapers are mustard-colored (bright yellow or spicy brown) after the first few days. Some babies have diapers with stringy or watery mucus in them; some have what looks like small-curd cottage cheese. After the transition from meconium in the first few days, lots of green poops can result from too much milk (though if you let an ordinary yellowish poop sit for a while, it will turn greenish in color), a diet heavy in greens that are rich in iron, green food coloring, taking iron supplements (including prenatal vitamins containing iron), or bilirubin excretion during the first week or so. Scant green poops can be a sign of too little milk. And what some people call "green" others see as khaki, olive, or brown. The diapers of breastfed babies tend to smell like buttermilk, bread, even cheddar cheese or popcorn—yeasty or sharp, but not at all unpleasant. It makes sense. Your milk is designed to work hand in glove with your baby's intestinal bacteria. And Nature knows that the more attractive we find *everything* about our babies, the easier they are to take care of. All those scented baby lotions and powders? Most of them came on the market when formula-feeding and its accompanying, um, aromas became more common. An occasional exclusively breastfed baby does have poopy diapers that really don't smell good. It may signal a minor food sensitivity, and matters only if the baby thinks it does. Bottom line: color, consistency, and smell don't matter *at all* in a thriving, happy baby, but they can help in figuring out the problem if the baby isn't happy or thriving.

Notice we haven't talked about wet diapers. It's possible for a baby to fool you with diapers that seem sort of wet, without having many stools or much weight gain. But having ample stools means your baby is taking ample milk. If a baby has plenty of poopy diapers, you know automatically that he has plenty of wet diapers. A month or more from now, he may switch to less frequent (but larger) stools, but by then you'll have all sorts of ways of knowing that he's doing fine and the state of his diapers won't matter.

HOW TO KNOW YOUR BABY'S DOING WELL

- *Weight gain.* Look for a return to birth weight by two weeks. An average gain after that is roughly 1 ounce (30 g) a day, but your baby may gain somewhat more or less.
- *Diapers.* Look for *at least* three "okay" (thumb and forefinger circle size) diapers each day during the first month or so.
- *Your breasts.* Look for comfortable nipples, a milk release within a minute (usually *much* sooner), and noticeable softening by the end of most nursings.
- *Nursing behavior.* Look for open eyes when the feed starts, periods of slow (about one per second) sucks with periodic pauses, and finishing within a half hour at most feeds.
- *Disposition between nursings.* Look for the baby falling gently asleep toward the end of the nursing (or contentment for at least a while before he nurses again), limp hands, and an unworried expression most of the time.
- *What doesn't matter.* How many minutes on each breast, whether he falls asleep at the breast at the end of the feeding, or whether he nurses long enough to "get to the hindmilk."

The Weight Gain Smile Syndrome

You take your baby to the doctor when he's a week old, thinking that things are finally going pretty well after a rocky start…and the doctor says he's still losing weight and you need to supplement with formula. Don't panic!

Let's assume your baby was born in a hospital and that you leave the hospital on, say, the second day. Your baby has lost weight, and everyone says don't worry, that's normal. You go home, breastfeeding limps along for a few days, but then it starts to improve. Your baby seems happier, you hear more swallowing, he starts putting out the diapers…and now this?

Here's where the Smile Syndrome comes in. A weight chart for a baby who loses weight and then starts to gain would look something like a smile: down on the losing weight side, then up on the gaining weight side. If your baby was weighed near the higher part of the losing side before he left the hospital (Day Two), and then was weighed again near the lower side of the *gaining* side, after he had begun gaining weight but before he had gained very much, those two points, and the line connecting them, would look like this:

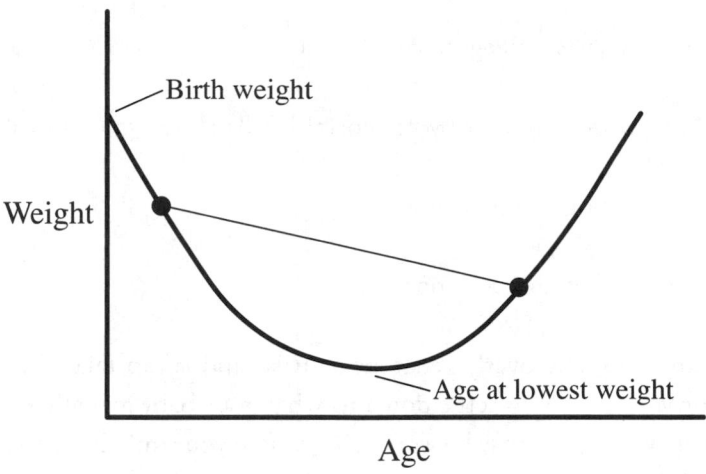

Smile Syndrome: Is your baby losing weight? Or gaining?

It looks as if your baby is losing weight, even though he has actually started to gain nicely. So you really can't tell what's going on from just a couple of points on a chart.

The section "How to Know Your Baby's Doing Well" will give you some positive signs to watch for. When your baby is weighed, also make sure that he's weighed on the same scale, naked or in very similar clothing, with his stomach about as full as it was last time.

Your Milk Output

These days, most women worry that they don't have enough milk. In fact, the opposite is usually true at first—most of us have more than enough.

Within the first few weeks post-birth, your breasts size up the situation and develop hormone receptors that work with your breastfeeding hormones to provide enough milk for the new baby or babies, based on how much milk is removed. This process *expects* milk to be taken out frequently and efficiently by the *baby,* but it responds to milk removal by *any* means—nursing, pumping, hand expressing. The more milk that is removed during this time, the higher your long-term milk supply will be. The process starts fresh with each baby.

There are only two things that matter about your nursing technique:

1. Are you and your baby comfortable? (He'll let you know if he isn't.)
2. Is he getting plenty of milk?

Beyond that, there are no rules!

Nature is usually overly generous at first, and it can take a month or more for your supply to settle down to what your baby actually needs. By around six weeks, you may be wondering where your milk has gone. It will still be there, but all the unnecessary early fluids will have packed up and gone away, and you'll be into comfortable, smooth, easy-running breastfeeding.

If you've been using both breasts at each nursing and you feel as if you could feed the world, see what happens if you just let the baby nurse on one breast as long as you and he like. Many, many babies are happy with just one breast at each nursing session, and it can help to diminish overabundant milk. For more information on the symptoms and solutions for oversupply, see Chapter 18.

Breast compressions can move more milk.

Breast Compressions: Simulating a Milk Release

One way to *increase* the amount of milk your baby gets during a feeding is by compressing (and holding) the breast while he's nursing (you can also do this while pumping). When one La Leche League Leader first learned about breast compressions, she asked the women at a meeting to try it and tell her whether it worked for them. To her surprise, about a third of the mothers replied, "Oh, we already do it." They'd simply figured it out on their own, for their own reasons.

During a sucking pause, with your fingers and thumb positioned well away from the areola, squeeze your breast gently (it shouldn't hurt) and hold the pressure. You can press your breast against your chest or cup it between thumb and fingers and squeeze, depending on your position and preference. Your baby should start swallowing again. When the renewed swallowing stops, release your hold to allow more milk to flow into the area you were compressing, then compress again. Shift your hand to compress different areas.

What's the point? It mimics a milk release by creating pressure within the breast. If your baby is frustrated that your milk isn't coming fast enough, this can help propel milk out of the breast. If your baby stops actively sucking, this can stimulate him to start sucking again. If you're increasing your milk supply, it can help ensure that your baby gets more of your available milk. If you have an oversupply, this can help bring down more fat for him (remember also to stay on one side for one or more nursings). If you're pumping, it may increase the amount of spurting and give you more milk. And if you're in a hurry to get somewhere, sometimes you can shorten a nursing. Worth a try, anyway!

Your Food Input

Life won't be like this forever, but it is for now. Which can make it hard for you to do *your* much-needed eating. And *that's* why the friends and relatives come to visit, whether they know it or not—to keep *you* fed! Here are some guidelines you can give them for food:

- *Healthy*—think whole grains, unprocessed meats, fresh or frozen fruits and vegetables, with smaller amounts of dairy
- *High-calorie*—think nut butters, olive and canola oils, whole-milk cheeses and yogurts, even that leftover birthday cake
- *One-handed*—think casseroles, sandwiches, finger foods, hummus-type dips, whole-grain crackers, pre-sliced nibblies, smoothies
- *Sturdy*—think freezable, reheatable, long refrigerator life

Downtime

There's the question of how to get naps and a good night's rest. And there's the question of where you sleep and where your baby sleeps. Your baby would answer them with one word: together.

Daytime Downtime

You've probably heard the suggestion to sleep when the baby sleeps, and you probably think, "With so much to do? The house is a mess, so's the kitchen, I need to fix supper, I haven't taken a shower, and the relatives come tomorrow!" Right now, rest is more important. Really. Maybe you can't always sleep. But you *can* rest.

Find several places in the house where you can comfortably practice "laid-back mothering," leaning back at a relaxed angle, fully supported by pillows as needed, your baby snoozing on your chest (with your shirt open when you can). If he wakes up to eat, he can take care of most of the job himself, without you getting carpal tunnel syndrome trying to support his body against gravity. Relax in that position as much as you can, whenever you can, whether he's eating or sleeping. Rest, with or without sleep, speeds healing and helps keep you from feeling overwhelmed.

Nighttime Downtime

It's amazing how many of us finally got some sleep when we just let our babies sleep on our own chest or beside us. Separating mothers and babies at night is a recent idea, not at all what Nature had in mind. Mothers and babies have slept together since the beginning of time. See Chapter 12 to learn about safe co-sleeping.

Even sharing sleep doesn't guarantee a good night's sleep at first. Your baby was probably used to partying at night before he was born (remember those kicks that woke you up at two in the morning?), and he may see no reason to stop now. Keeping the lights low and doing what you can to soothe him if he's lively or calm him if he's upset, with as little commotion as possible, may help. He may need a lot of nursing at night at the beginning, precisely because his clock is backward. But whatever time zone he believes he's living in, he'll gradually learn the difference between day and night. One nighttime job to work on during the day: learning to nurse lying down. It may be that you use laid-back breastfeeding all night. It may be that you prefer to nurse on your side, with the baby on his side next to you. Check out Chapter 4 for some hints on side-lying, and practice it during the day, not in the wee hours of the morning. And see Chapter 12 for much more about sleep.

> Accomplish one small thing a day. Maybe it's cleaning that counter, maybe it's writing one thank-you note. Don't make the task too difficult. For the rest, you're healing a uterus; adding millions of cells to your baby's brain (though it might sometimes feel as if they are being siphoned off from your own); developing his liver, heart, and lungs; boosting his immune system; and maintaining the integrity of his intestines…you're a busy lady! All while sprawled comfortably on the couch. Multi-tasking raised to an art form!

An Emotional Roller Coaster

After a normal birth and the easy start that normally follows, most new mothers are elated. If they have supportive people on all sides and confidence in what they're doing, a sense of calm elation and being in step with the baby can continue right through the early days and weeks. But even under these ideal circumstances, a new mother is including a new person in her life and learning to meet that person's unaccustomed needs, and that's challenging.

> *"We often think of the new mother as gentle, loving, and selfless, but the new mother is also tough. She delivers a baby and then proceeds to care for that baby around the clock. It took tough-minded resolve as well as love and tenderness for me to continue nursing [through our early problems], but the rewards have been unbelievably great. I gained a lot of confidence, not only as a mother but as a person."*
>
> —Cynthia

Baby Blues

Sometime in the first week or two after birth you may get hit with the *baby blues*—a day or a few days of "What have I gotten myself into? Where has my life gone? Everything is just wrong!" Now is when a partner or close friend can be extremely helpful—not necessarily by solving problems or having answers, but by being there, with a shoulder for you to cry on, an understanding ear, or gentle hands that you can trust your baby to for a bit. The baby blues may make you tearful, uncertain, forgetful, restless, or irritable. They may give you nightmares, or even give you negative feelings toward the baby. But they're gone—and good riddance!—within a few days or a week. Some of us have more troubling feelings; for information on postpartum depression and other emotional upheavals, see Chapter 18.

The Grandma Hour

As one new mother said, "What do you mean, hour?" It's that time late in the day when almost every new mother wishes someone else—like Grandma—could take over for a while. A lot of new babies are frazzled by now. They've spent the whole day taking in sharp and bright sounds and sights—new activities for them—and they're *up to here* with it all. The biggest comfort they know is nursing, and they know that comfort comes with milk. But even though your milk production is at its highest point of the day, your baby has worked his way to the bottom of the barrel. (Like having a bank account with a wicked high interest rate but a low balance!) Having less milk in your breasts also slows your milk flow. You can try breast compressions to help your baby get more milk faster and put a bit more oomph behind your milk release.

Many babies, though, don't even want the milk. Maybe they want to go back to the womb, or maybe they're trying to put themselves to sleep. Or maybe they feel that something different might break the end-of-the-day spell. This is a time when your baby may actually be settled more easily by a different person who offers a change of scenery and who doesn't smell of milk. Sometimes that change of scenery is all he needs to switch off and drift into a long sleep. Or maybe he just wants to keep nursing.

One idea for heading off the "grandma hour" is to try to take a nap together in the afternoon. Another is to try offering to nurse about an hour before he usually gets upset. Soothing him before he gets wired up may make for a more peaceful evening. At worst, it will give you both a little rest.

The Magic Baby Hold

Also called the *colic hold*, this has been a helpful calming technique for just about every well-fed but fussy baby we've met. Hold your baby's back against your chest, so the two of you are facing forward. Bring your left arm over your baby's left shoulder and hold his right thigh. He'll have one arm on either side of your arm, and you'll have a solid grip on his leg. You can hold him so that he faces the floor, hug him

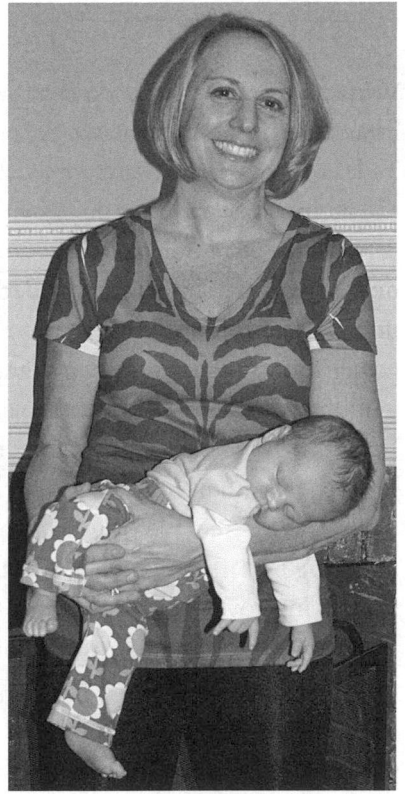

The "Magic Baby Hold" can be calming.

against you so that he faces out, or even rest your left hand, still holding his thigh, on your hip. Your shoulders are relaxed, and you have a hand free if you like. Using your left arm also puts your baby on his left side, which some babies find especially soothing.

Now add the *baby bounce*. You can start with swaying, but it may be that he needs at least a sway with a hitch in it. You won't be able to see your baby's face with this hold, but you'll feel his body's tension. If you see the back of his head start to wrinkle or his body start to tense, turn just a bit. Now he suddenly has completely new scenery in front of him. Most of the time, the baby bounce and the new scenery will help. Nothing really helps a baby who needs to nurse, though, except more nursing.

> *"When the baby is being really fussy at night, go out and look at the moon, and think about all the other mothers and babies out there under the same glowing moon."* —Margaret

Pre-Soothing

Why wait for the wail? Ron Barr, a professor of pediatrics who has studied infant crying around the world, recommends "Carry, Contact, Walk, and Talk" for soothing an unhappy baby, and has found that doing these *before* the crying starts will mean less crying overall. And don't hesitate to interrupt what you're doing to offer comfort—a quick response to your baby's unhappiness will mean he's settled again more readily. There's no need to doggedly pursue a diaper change on a shrieking baby. Think Baby First rather than tasks like diaper changes and baths. If your baby says it isn't working, *stop* to nurse and console, then try again. You'll both be happier. It won't be long before baths and diaper changes are playtime. In the meantime, there's no need to make them an added stress.

In the first couple of weeks, most of the fussy times are just the baby adjusting to Life on Earth. Offer to nurse yet again, and see if life doesn't start to improve as you and your baby settle in a bit more.

If you have a hard-to-settle baby for reasons you can't just figure out, life is tougher at first. It may help to put a smiley face on the calendar on those days when your baby was happier and look back over the calendar to see the positive trend. Like so many issues during the first few weeks, fussiness is almost always temporary. Enjoy your baby's moments of contentment, do your best to soothe his distresses, and know that he's no happier about his unhappiness than you are! There's information about colic, reflux, and other common causes of baby distress in Chapter 18. For more baby-soothing techniques, check the Tear-Sheet Toolkit at the back of the book.

Concerns You May Have in the First Two Weeks

These are some of the issues that are often raised at LLL meetings by mothers in the first two weeks after the birth. If your questions aren't addressed here, you'll probably find them in Chapter 18, "Tech Support." If they're not there, either, look on the llli.org forums or call your local LLL Leader.

How Often Do Babies Eat?

It's going to vary, not only from baby to baby but also from day to day and month to month as your baby grows. Instead of looking at frequency, try looking at how your baby behaves after a nursing. Does he stay awake for a bit after some nursings, looking at you calmly for a few minutes before wanting another snack? Does he drift off to sleep while nursing sometimes? Does his arm drop like a dead weight when you lift it as he sleeps? Those are all signs that he's setting his own pace just fine, just as any mammal baby would, even if it's much more frequent than you expected.

If you left the hospital still struggling with a medicated or very sleepy baby, assume that he'll need to eat at least every three hours, and more likely every two hours, through much of the day, and at least a couple of times through the night. Offer your breast, and if he keeps turning you down, see Chapter 18 and the Tear-Sheet Toolkit for suggestions on keeping a baby well fed during a wobbly start. As he becomes more alert over the next few days and begins to set his own pace, he'll let you know his needs. He may suddenly begin nursing much more often than you thought was normal. It probably *is* normal, especially if he's catching up.

How Long Should a Feeding Be?

That, too, is going to vary. (Don't you love these vague answers?) Your baby may want one, two, three, or even four sides, with a complete meal generally taking around twenty minutes and sometimes as long as forty (remember, most of your day at first is going to involve feeding and tending your baby, but that will change as he gains efficiency). An occasional baby can routinely zip through a whole feeding in five minutes in the early weeks and be satisfied for several hours. It's kind of tough on those babies, though. They get their milk so fast and end up so full that they don't have a chance to linger over dessert, snacking and napping in their mother's arms in typical newborn fashion. Check out the oversupply information in Chapter 18 if you feel your baby always gets too much too fast.

The baby who's getting plenty of milk usually has open eyes at the start, as if he has to pay attention (WOW!) to keep up. He may doze later in the feed and fall asleep at the end, maybe with some unswallowed drops of milk on his mouth, or with his body limp as a rag doll. One dad commented, "Well, that's it. He's gone galactic."

> *"Sometimes nursing relaxes Peter so much that it's like he's made out of rubber. I look down at him and always say the same thing: 'I've nursed his bones out.'"*
> —Jazz

In contrast, the baby who sleeps through most of his meals, which are usually long and slow, may be using numerous sucks to get every swallow of milk. It takes a lot of time and energy to eat that way, and these babies doze as much as they can. But take them off the breast and their eyes fly open. They watch you with a worried expression and do their best to get back on the breast, where they doze off again. Some of these babies sleep really well at night, not from contentment but to conserve energy, and they usually aren't gaining enough. If this describes your baby, see "Weight Gain Worries" in Chapter 18.

TRUST THE FISTS

When a baby is hungry, he tends to clench his fists tightly and bring them toward his face. If he falls asleep hungry, his fists usually stay clenched. But when he gets milk he relaxes, starting with his face. Then his shoulders relax, and finally those fists unclench. Eventually they're as limp as the rest of him. Think of his hands as his built-in fuel gauge!

Should I Offer Both Breasts?

Mammal mothers don't worry about minutes, milk transfer, or changing sides. They nurse as long as they feel comfortable in that position, and they change positions when *they* want to, or when the baby stops being happy with what's happening. Think of a breast as a "serving." Some babies want two servings right in a row; some fall asleep after the first one and save the second breast for later. Some, who are trying to build up your milk supply, take three or four or more breasts (yes, all of them yours) before dozing off. Since you'll be nursing your baby again whenever he tells you he needs it, it doesn't really matter how many breasts or servings he takes in a row, as long as he's satisfied when he's finished. You can trust that your breasts will let you know if you're not feeding enough from one side. If you go too long without emptying one breast, it's going to start feeling uncomfortable, signaling that it's time to have the baby nurse from that side.

How Long Does He Have to Nurse to Get to the Hindmilk?

You may have heard that *foremilk* is the thin, low-fat milk that comes at the beginning of the feeding, and *hindmilk* is the creamy, high-fat milk that finishes the feeding. Well…

Your breasts make only one kind of milk. The reason it can *seem* different is that cream rises. If you nurse really often, it all stays swirled together. Wait a little longer between feedings, and some of the fat in your milk can creep back up the ducts, leaving a lower-fat milk behind. At the next nursing, the fat gets squeezed down again, gradually mixing back in. It's all nutritious, and the fat variations give your baby some variety and maybe even some control over how many calories he gets and when. It isn't an issue, except for the babies who find themselves with too much collected "soup" to work through to get to "dessert."

Even that's not a problem most of the time; *all* your milk is good milk. If your baby does plenty of swallowing but seems unhappy or has green or frothy diapers, see "Oversupply" in Chapter 18. Otherwise, know that the system is built to have variations, and yes, *all* your milk is good milk.

Won't My Baby Grow Better if I Wait Until He's Really Hungry?

He probably won't grow nearly as well!

We adults aren't trying to grow. Yet we still eat several large meals a day with snacks and beverages interspersed. Give us a two-hour plane ride without something to nibble and we get cranky. Even as non-growers, we like to eat often.

Babies simply need to eat more often than we do. But how often? Well, they eat one food, and it's a food that digests really, really quickly; sixty to ninety minutes and it's gone. If they eat a meal, then wait until it's well digested to eat another, but Mama doesn't make the offer, they're in serious trouble. If they really pig out and overload their stomachs, they risk indigestion, gas, cramps. But if they stay somewhere in the middle, with frequent snacks, never fully empty, never excruciatingly full, their stomachs are happier, they feel safer... and they can grow the way they're built to.

Our milk supplies are designed for the same system. If we wait until our breasts feel really full, they've already started to slow down production. Our milk production stays highest when we nurse before we *need* to.

But Won't She Eat Better if She's Really Hungry?

Probably not. A baby starts with subtle nursing cues—eyelids fluttering open, hands coming toward her face, mouth movements. Then she adds more obvious ones—rooting toward your chest, whimpering. If you offer to nurse by then, she'll probably take your breast gently and easily. As her hunger builds, her body and mouth tense. She gets distracted and starts to cry. By the time she's crying, she can be too stressed to eat and harder to calm. The nursing will actually take longer and may be uncomfortable. As the American Academy of Pediatrics states, "Crying is a *late* indicator of hunger."

Responding to requests (and offering, echoing LLL, without requests whenever you like) rather than waiting for demands means you're not waiting for your breasts to signal you, which is also a good way to go.

Do I Have Enough Milk?

Breastfeeding is a mother-baby dance that mothers often take too much responsibility for. Yes, there are women who simply can't produce enough milk for their babies, but if you feel your baby isn't getting enough, it's much more likely that something else is going on. Here are some of the most likely issues:

- ☿ Nothing's wrong at all. You just didn't expect that your baby would need to eat this often.
- ☿ It's all in your perspective. Now that you know about CCK and cluster feeding, take another look at how your day is going. For every woman

who says, "I think something's wrong. If I'm not holding him or nursing him, he's crying," there's another who says, "I figured it out! All I have to do is hold him and nurse him and he's happy as a clam." These early weeks are a time for getting your milk supply and your baby's growth well established. Life will get simpler. For now, expect newborn inefficiency, follow your baby's lead, and take another look to see if he's actually more content than you thought.

- Someone is scaring you. Having someone at your elbow saying, "Are you sure he's getting enough? I don't think he's getting enough. He shouldn't be eating again. Are you *sure* he's getting enough?" is enough to make any new mother worry. Try instead to surround yourself with women who've enjoyed breastfeeding and who know good nursing when they see it. (La Leche League meetings are a great place to find exactly this kind of support.) It doesn't make sense to learn from people who weren't successful themselves!

- Your baby isn't taking your breast as well as he might. You might be holding the baby too far away, too high, too low—all things that can keep him from getting milk easily. Sore nipples are a major tip-off that things can be improved; they often signal less-than-adequate milk removal. Lots of sucking without much swallowing is another tip-off. For starters, you could try the laid-back positioning described in Chapter 4; most babies do a much better job of proper positioning on their own than we can invent for them. If you don't find a big improvement in comfort and begin to see a change in the way your baby nurses when you follow his lead instead of having him follow yours, check with a breastfeeding helper.

- Maybe your baby *can't* suck effectively because he has a minor issue himself. One cause is tongue-tie, which is usually dealt with quickly and easily. See Chapter 18 for more information.

- You're following a book, parenting program, or schedule that doesn't fit you and your baby. Babies come with differing stomachs, sizes, activity levels, sleep needs, and levels of efficiency, and if your breasts didn't happen to come with a lot of storage space (an issue not visible from the outside), it's going to take more than nursing every two to three hours to keep your milk flow strong. Try going totally with your baby and you'll probably see a happier baby and more poopy diapers within a day or two, though it can take longer to turn a milk supply around if it's dipped too low. Cookie-cutter instructions are for cookies, not people. You've probably seen that in a lot of other areas in your life; it's true for babies, too.

- ☌ You have a fussy or colicky baby. Some babies have periods of crying that are hard to figure out or soothe. If your baby seems to have signed up for the "frequent crier program," you may worry that your milk is the source of his fussiness. It may not have anything to do with feeding at all—it might be just his temperament or a temporary stage. Many a fussy newborn blossoms into a sunny six-month-old. Pay attention to the other signs such as poopy diapers and weight gain to reassure yourself. And see the "Colic" section in Chapter 18.

Whatever your situation, before you panic and open up a can of formula, check out Chapter 18, "Tech Support," and talk with an experienced breastfeeding helper as soon as you can. You and your baby deserve quick and skilled help.

Are There Special Milk-Making Foods or Drinks?

Yes and no. Many cultures have their own foods or recipes that have been used for centuries to support milk production, and many mothers swear by them. Certain herbs and foods also have been used throughout the world to increase milk production (see Chapter 18). But there's nothing in particular that you need to eat to make enough nutritious milk.

Likewise, you don't need to drink anything in particular—it doesn't take milk to make milk. Dairy cows make gallons and gallons of milk without ever drinking it! You don't need more fluids than you want in order to make milk, and your supply won't decrease if you're mildly dehydrated. If your urine is medium to pale yellow, then you're doing fine. Oxytocin release *can* make you suddenly thirsty (carrying a water bottle helps).

Calories are pretty simple, too. Eating more won't make more milk, and not eating enough won't make less milk. You don't need a perfect diet to keep your milk nutritious. Your milk is made from your blood. If you haven't been worrying about the quality of your blood lately, there's no need at all to worry about the quality of your milk! The healthy food guidelines are mainly to keep *you* healthy enough to take care of your baby and yourself. If you're a vegetarian or vegan, make sure you understand how to keep up your vitamin B_{12} levels. It's important to eat well so that *you* feel good. So eat when you're hungry, don't do more than glance at your scale for the first month or so, and you'll probably find that at least some of those extra pounds drop away in the first few weeks without any effort, even though you're eating like a horse at times.

If your baby is fussy, don't automatically blame it on your diet—much more likely culprits are discussed later in this chapter. Some cultures whose diet includes spicy foods have a special, milder diet for nursing mothers for the first month or so. But after about the first month most babies are not bothered by *any* foods in their mother's diet. Your favorite foods will flavor your milk somewhat, and your baby will learn the family menu through breastfeeding.

If your baby comes from an allergic family (yours or his dad's), you might want to avoid or go light on common allergens in your own diet at first, easing into them slowly to see how your baby does. If there is a food problem, the most likely culprits are cow milk and dairy products. Even babies who are made fussy by, say, dairy may be fine as long as their mothers don't eat large quantities at one time.

Go easy on caffeine for the first month or so while your baby's body is still maturing enough to handle it. Watch him for jitteriness once you add it, and go light enough that you can nap easily when you get the chance.

Is It Normal for Breastfed Babies to Have This Much Gas?

All mammals have intestinal gas every day, just because they're alive. We adults are (usually) just more discreet about it. The baby who's gassy and who isn't bothered by it is fine. But sometimes gas makes a baby truly uncomfortable. Nursing, using the Magic Baby Hold described above, and carrying the baby upright against your chest or shoulder can all help move those gas bubbles around painful intestinal corners. If your baby is frequently gassy and uncomfortable, he might be getting too much milk—see "Oversupply" in Chapter 18 for more information.

How Do I Burp My Baby?

Each baby is built differently from the next, so the most effective burping position is something you just have to learn. Or not! Cultures that carry their babies don't understand the notion of burping a baby. The baby who is carried upright most of the time will naturally burp when he needs to. Burping a baby is probably something we developed when we started laying them down after a big meal, which tends to trap air in their stomachs. (How do *you* feel when you lie down after a big meal?) Some babies seem to squirm a bit shortly into the feeding, especially if the milk comes out fast and they are noisily gulping. They may need a quick burp early on in the feed, so that air doesn't get trapped below all that milk.

If your baby needs to burp, try holding him against your shoulder (which you might want to cover with a cloth to catch any spit-up) and rub or pat his back gently. No need to pound. You can also sit him up in your lap, bending him slightly forward while you gently pat his back.

What Can I Do About Spitting Up?

Many babies don't seem to be the least bit bothered by spitting up, and the amount of milk they lose usually looks like a lot more than it really is. It can happen as a result of larger meals at longer intervals, so try offering more often. Your baby will take less each time and may keep it down better. Carrying your baby upright, especially after nursings, can also help. Those cultures that carry their babies and offer small snacks more than hourly do seem to have some answers for us. If spitting up makes your baby uncomfortable, see "Fussy Baby Ideas" in Chapter 20 for more information.

I Need Help Getting My Sling to Work

Slings are designed to carry babies from birth through toddlerhood, so it's no surprise that they can be awkward at first. Your newborn will probably do best in a snug sling, so that he's stabilized in a fairly upright position with his head at about the level of your breasts, not down by your waist. Babies usually hate being dropped into a "black hole," which squeezes their head, keeps them from being able to see out, and can interfere with breathing. So arrange your baby with his face above the level of the sling. Start moving as soon as he's settled, patting him through the fabric and talking to him. Being in a sling is a new experience for *your* baby, but babies around the world have used slings for eons and most come to adore them. A few other starting thoughts:

- 💡 Non-adjustable slings can be shifted to find a good angle. They may need a thin blanket in the bottom for a newborn. Be careful that the baby is not curled up with his chin against his chest, which can restrict his breathing.
- 💡 Ring slings can be worn with your newborn upright and facing you, with legs crisscrossed inside the sling or dangling outside of it. To make the sling snug, pull the loose fabric through the rings or just use a rubber band to gather the extra fabric quickly and simply. If you wear him "hammock style," he'll probably want his head higher than his feet.
- 💡 Wrap slings can also hold the baby upright against you.

For more help with your sling, check for instructions or videos online, ask for suggestions at an LLL meeting, and keep experimenting. If you feel it simply doesn't work, try again in a week or two. Like so much else in this chapter, the answer sometimes is "maybe not yet, but soon."

SOME GOOD BOOKS FOR THE FIRST TWO WEEKS

A Ride on Mother's Back, by Emery Bernhard
Attached at the Heart, by Barbara Nicholson and Lysa Parker
Babywearing, by Maria Blois
Mothering the New Mother: Women's Feelings and Needs After Childbirth, by Sally Placksin
Permission to Mother: Going Beyond the Standard-of-Care to Nurture Our Children, by Denise Punger
What Mothers Do: Especially When It Looks Like Nothing, by Naomi Stadlen

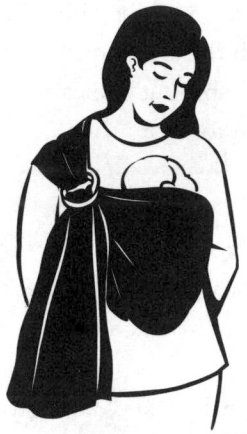
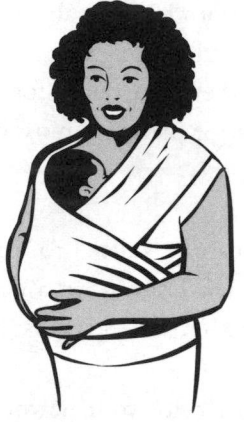
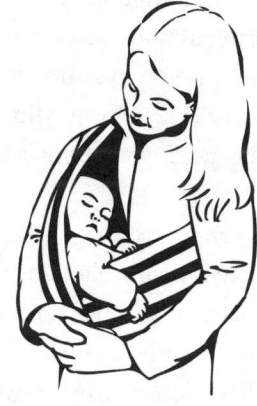

Ring sling—feet in or out.

Wrap style—one newborn position.

Non-adjustable sling— baby can see out.

Should I Be Using a Pacifier?

Pacifiers, also called dummies, have their place, but not necessarily in *your* baby's mouth. They were designed to substitute for your breast, and they sometimes do it too well. Remember how twenty minutes of sucking raises a baby's CCK so that he thinks he's full? Sucking on a pacifier can trick the CCK system and the baby's weight gain will suffer. In the early weeks especially, if a baby wants to suck, he wants to eat, pure and simple. A pacifier is like sugarless gum for someone who's trying to double his weight in a matter of months. It can reduce intake at a time when a baby is meant to grow quickly.

Pacifiers are linked to early weaning, though the reason for the connection isn't clear. They may be associated with sucking problems, too, especially if they're started in the first few days, though again the reason isn't clear. What *is* clear is that if you're tempted to use a pacifier, it makes more sense to reach for the phone and call a helper to see what's going on.

Mothers who rely on pacifiers tend to develop fewer baby-calming skills of their own. Children who use pacifiers in day care are more prone to thrush and ear infections. Latex pacifiers have been linked to latex allergies. Prolonged use can affect mouth development, raising a child's palate and crowding his teeth, as well as narrowing his nasal passages and leading to an increased risk of sleep apnea and later speech problems. "Orthodontic" and "exercise" pacifiers really aren't. While they're sometimes recommended for nighttime use in a breastfed baby, we have to wonder why a breast isn't recommended instead. Nursing, after all, meets those sucking needs fully, with emotional needs, good jaw development, and a full tummy thrown in!

How Soon Can I Get My Baby on a Schedule?

At first, feeding the baby looms larger than anything else in your shaky new world. It takes time and effort to organize and carry out feedings, and you can't do anything else at the same time. You might think that if you could schedule the feedings, life would get back to normal faster.

Ah, but feeding a baby will soon be a really *minor* event—one of the easiest, quickest, most casual, and most flexible parts of your day! You'll be able to fit it in among other things. If you schedule the feedings, you end up trying to fit more complicated events around baby's meals. And despite all that extra work, your baby will almost certainly not grow as well! Many babies simply can't wait the length of time the books propose, or they can't do it and gain weight *and* keep your supply in good shape. Setting up a schedule risks an underfed baby and early weaning—and a more complicated life.

Here's unscheduled nursing two months from now: Going to the grocery store? Top the baby off with a quick nursing before you go and you can shop longer without stopping. (Babies rarely refuse these little extras when you offer. In fact, the little extras are what really make them grow.) Paying the bills? Talking on the phone? Watching TV? Writing the definitive work on Tolstoy? You can do any of these and more while you nurse the baby. One of this book's writers, Diana, wrote most of her first book with a nursing baby in her lap. Nursing, once you and your baby have had some practice, is just not that big a deal.

Nursing babies were around long, long before clocks were, when life was truly hard. Nursing had to fit into a day of finding food (often unpredictable), tending animals (ditto), and avoiding sudden dangers (ditto again). *Raising a baby had to be all about flexibility, and it was, and it worked just fine.*

Is It Possible to Spoil a Baby?

No. Babies aren't manipulative, perceptive, sneaky, or subversive. They just...are.

As you grew up, would you have felt secure if gravity had been unreliable? If when you let go of a book it had been just as likely to fall up as down? Providing for our babies is like that. Meeting their needs gives them a totally reliable base from which to begin to explore and make sense of the world. At this young age, their wants are the same as their needs. We can meet either one without worrying in the slightest about spoiling.

When that same baby is two years old, sometimes his wants and needs will be different. He may not know the difference, and it will be up to us to help him sort it out—to help him learn patience, tolerance, kindness. But for now? All he needs to learn is love.

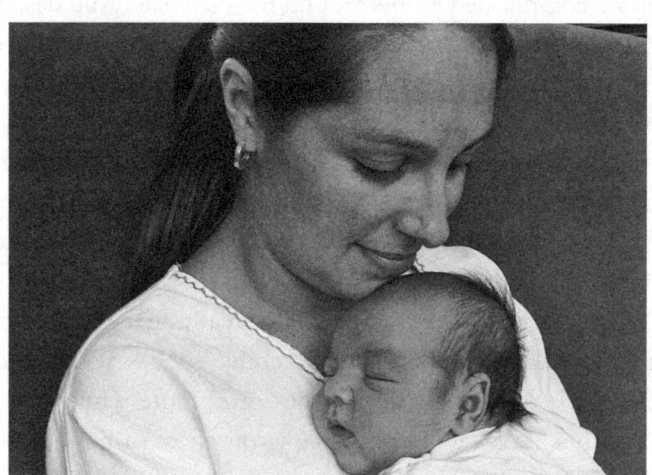

SEVEN

Two to Six Weeks: Butterfly Smiles

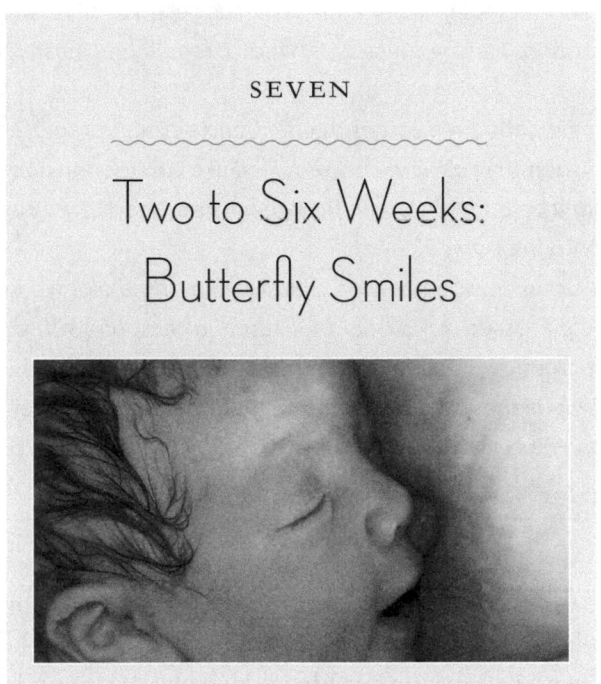

"*As a nurse in the hospital nursery in 1952, I had practiced all the then-current breastfeeding routines. Predictably, when I had my own baby, I ended up with excruciatingly painful, damaged nipples. By ten days, I quit, vowing to do better the next time. Same painful, damaged nipples on day five with baby number two. With baby number three, I decided that I would stay in the hospital for a full five days, so I could get it right this time. Wrong! My ego was utterly crushed. Nearly all my ancestors had been able to breastfeed, and here I was, the 'Golden Girl,' the first one to go beyond high school, and I couldn't succeed at it!*

"*By 1959, when baby number four joined our family, a La Leche League Group had formed in our town. As a professional obstetrical nurse, I was too proud to think much about this group of 'laywomen' before I delivered. Fortunately, a nursing school classmate was on their phone counseling committee. I called her up nine days in a row till she got me over the hump. She understood my feelings and discomforts, encouraging me daily with gentle new suggestions to replace all my misinformation. Her gentleness is what I remember most fifty years later.*

"At one month, I remember my husband sitting at the other end of the couch, admiring us as we nursed. I felt like a madonna painting with the spotlight on both of us; with the other three it had always shifted off me and onto the baby alone.

"That summer, when he was about five months old, we lay on the bed, barely dressed, on a beautiful sunny afternoon, with the breeze blowing across us as we nursed. I can clearly remember my inner dialogue. 'With all the pleasures of the flesh this world celebrates, why is it that no one has ever talked about this bodily pleasure before?'"

—Jean, remembering 1959

YOU'RE PROBABLY NOT feeling on top of things yet. Most likely the fog you've been in since the birth has lifted a little, and you've begun to discover some new rhythms in your life with a baby. But your days probably aren't fully smooth and comfortable yet. New mothers in our culture often say it takes them six weeks or more to feel "settled."

Why "in our culture"? Because most of the world's breastfeeding cultures give a mother a much-needed "babymoon"—a honeymoon-type month or so of help with housework and meals so that she can connect with her baby, recover, get breastfeeding going, and adjust to motherhood. And in most of those cultures, because she's watched breastfeeding mothers since childhood, nursing comes easily.

Most of us aren't lucky enough to have a "babymoon," and even if we do, there are still lots of little things to learn. Who is this new person? What do her sounds mean? Is this normal? It takes time to get to know the little individual who has joined your family, but as you do, you become more confident in your mothering.

Nursing Habits: Two to Six Weeks

Babies at this age are still a bit awkward about latching, mainly because their nerve impulses are still pretty primitive. But you've probably noticed that both of you are faster at it now—that even if you lead, your baby follows with rarely a missed beat, making the process smoother and simpler.

A baby this age is generally all business when he's eating, but you'll also see quick and gentle "butterfly smiles" flit across his face when he's feeling good after a nursing or at times in between. These early eyes-closed smiles signal emotional comfort, not gas. By six weeks, you may even begin to see social smiles, with eyes open and looking right at you, a very big reward for your many weeks of nurturing.

If your nipples are still bothering you after two weeks, check with an LLL Leader or other skilled breastfeeding helper. Pain is a signal that something needs to be different, no matter how good "the latch" looks! If you haven't tried that laid-back breastfeeding position, give it a whirl. You may find that it makes breastfeeding much more comfortable and relaxing.

I Still Don't Know When to Nurse Him

When you're at a party, the hostess doesn't usually ask if you're hungry before she passes the snack tray. She offers frequently, and *you* decide whether to eat or pass it on. You're the one with the breast "snack tray"; why not be a good hostess and offer whenever your baby seems unsettled? No need to force the issue if you guessed wrong. But your baby can't nurse if the offer isn't made.

Whim Nursing

It can be your baby's whim, or it can be your whim. You can offer to nurse for no other reason than that it feels as if it's been a while. Or you miss him. Or you want to finish reading that article. Or you just...feel like it! Those are all *perfectly good reasons,* even if your baby isn't asking. It can be his whim, too. Maybe he's just had a scary dream (how would you know?). Or maybe he has a bubble of gas and nursing will help his intestines move the bubble somewhere more comfortable. Again, how would you know? But it doesn't really matter what his reason is. If it makes your baby happy, that's good enough.

But Why Does My Baby Need to Nurse Twice as Often as My Friend's?

You can search for the reason, or you can just accept the difference. Some babies can't get milk as efficiently as others, or tire before they're really full. They do absolutely fine, so long as they can eat frequently. Some mothers simply can't store a lot of milk. Nursing frequently not only fills their babies better but also keeps their milk supplies in better shape. Sometimes it's just a personality difference. As long as your baby is gaining well and you're okay with the extra nursing, all's well. If you're not okay with it, your baby isn't gaining well, or you suspect there's a bigger problem, don't hesitate to talk to a Leader or your baby's doctor.

Also keep in mind that maybe your friend's baby isn't nursing *enough*. Maybe your baby is the one nursing appropriately!

Shouldn't I Watch the Clock?

In the past, mothers were often told to feed on a schedule—every three or four hours. When research showed that this led to breastfeeding problems, and we came to understand better how breastfeeding works, the recommendation changed to "feed the baby when he gives you hunger cues." Trouble is, the idea of the schedule still lingers in many minds: "Feed the baby on cue, about every two [or three, or four] hours."

Some mothers say they're feeding "on cue"...so long as they feel it's been "long enough." They may bounce the baby, change a diaper, try a pacifier—anything other than nursing. The baby may be fussing, even crying, but the mother keeps checking the clock and thinking, "It's only been an hour; how can he possibly want to nurse again?" But if nursing isn't what your baby wants, he'll tell you. Go ahead and offer. He may respond with relief, as if to say, "Well, *finally*! Weren't you *listening*?" If he's been crying for a while, he may be too upset to nurse, so give him some cuddling and soothing, then offer again.

Putting your baby to breast when he cries will not spoil him. Your baby's physiology is geared to constant holding and frequent feeding. Your milk is geared to the same. Deliberately holding a baby off interferes with his physiology and yours. It has not been shown to provide benefits of any kind, and slows weight gain in the long run.

Interestingly, the same mothers who wait until it's "time to nurse again"—closet clock watchers—are often uneasy about their baby's weight gain. Remember, *a baby can't gain weight well if he doesn't take in plenty of milk,* and all those little "whim" nursings are what allow him to take in plenty of milk. Maybe your baby is gaining all the doctor says he needs to gain. But maybe he wants to gain more! Some babies are built to grow faster than those lines on the chart, and holding them to an approved rate of gain just doesn't meet with *their* approval.

It's also normal for a baby to cluster-feed at times, meaning he takes several short feedings during an hour or two, often tanking up in preparation for a longer sleep.

So we encourage you to throw the whole idea of schedules out, and offer to nurse whenever your baby is unsettled, even if you nursed just ten minutes ago. As nursing becomes harmonious, you may find that whim nursing quickly begins to include conversational nursing.

Conversational Nursing

Nursing is your baby's first human relationship. It's how she first communicates with you, and how you communicate with her. Those deep gazes that the two of you share at times are communication, too, but you've probably found that they're short-lived at this age. Nursing represents your longest conversations, and you can hold them whenever you and your baby like.

You've probably already found that sometimes you kiss your baby for no reason. Did you look at the clock before you did? What would you think if you were told to kiss your baby only once or twice a day? Actually, in the early 1900s, some books did advise mothers to handle their babies as little as possible and refrain from showing them affection. There were some very unhappy mothers and babies as a result. Whim nursing, conversational nursing—what you're providing with these just-because nursings—puts those healthy rolls on your baby's arms, makes both you and your baby feel secure and happy, gets your lifelong relationship off to a close and connected beginning, gives your milk supply a solid base, and makes your job soooo much easier!

Isn't He Just Using Me as a Pacifier?

Not at all! Nursing feeds him, pacifies him, puts him to sleep, comforts, reassures, and relaxes him. If you offer your breast only as food and not as a "pacifier," you'll cut out all the calories he gets along with those other reasons, you're more likely to end up with supply problems, and you'll lose the pleasure of—literally—going with the flow. The phrase "he's just using you as a pacifier" works against confident, smooth-running breastfeeding. Nursing is how a baby grows; why hold back?

Other Concerns You May Have Between Two and Six Weeks

These are some of the other issues that are often raised at LLL meetings by mothers with babies between two and six weeks old. If your questions aren't addressed here, you'll probably find them in Chapter 18, "Tech Support." If they're not there, either, look on the llli.org forums. Then it's time to put the books and the Internet aside and call your local LLL Leader. Printed words can take you only so far. You deserve real people, too.

Help! My Breasts Are Soft!

Remember how in the early days your breasts felt full and firm if the baby went very long between feedings? The difference in fullness before and after feeding was really noticeable. By six weeks, though, many women find that their breasts don't feel full anymore. Their breasts feel fairly soft most of the time, and feel full only if the baby goes longer than usual between nursings. If you used to leak a lot, you may not be leaking as much anymore, either. Supply and demand have balanced. Excess fluids, excess milk, and unneeded circulation have packed up and gone away, and breastfeeding's now running smoothly.

Your breasts are also getting more efficient at releasing milk only when your baby is actually at your breast. In the early days, you probably felt your milk releasing (and maybe leaking) at random times or whenever you were especially full. But as the weeks go by, milk begins to flow only at your baby's request (although sometimes a baby's cry or even thinking about your baby when you're apart can still lead to a milk release, and of course pumping can release milk, too). It's nice not to worry about leaking anymore, and as long as your baby continues to gain well, you can relax about your milk supply, too. Maybe you're thinking, "My baby is gaining well, but my breasts have *always* been soft!" That can be because you have a lot of storage capacity, or because your baby nurses often enough to keep them from overfilling. So don't worry if your breasts are softer now, or if they never were very full. The same guideline applies: a happy, thriving baby who's growing well and filling diapers is nursing just fine.

> "I remember getting breast pads because they were on the list of essential equipment and regularly putting them into my (too big) bra, where they scrunched up and became uncomfortable. After about three weeks I asked a friend what these breast pads were for. She just looked at me. 'To catch the leaks, of course.' 'But I don't leak,' I told her. 'Then don't use them!' she said."   —Jill

A THRIVING BABY

Most mothers today worry about their milk supplies in the early weeks. Most of them don't have to. Here are some signs of a thriving baby at this age. Your baby:

- Begins gaining weight after your milk comes in.
- Passes birth weight by at least ten to fourteen days.
- Is gaining weight appropriately. The average rate is roughly 1 ounce (about 30 g) per day during the early months, but remember that's only an average and your baby may gain more or less than that. Your doctor or midwife will monitor the baby's weight gain during regular visits.

- Has at least three yellow poops (about the size of the circle your thumb and forefinger make—an "okay" sign for an "okay" diaper) and five colorless, odorless, and heavy wet diapers each day.
- Doesn't have trouble latching on, and doesn't have trouble staying attached.
- Generally has his eyes open and looks interested for the first part of the nursing.
- Has slow, steady sucks for part of every nursing, beginning soon after the feeding starts.
- Is content for at least a few minutes after nursing.
- Can almost always be consoled by nursing again.
- Sometimes has calm, alert times between feedings.
- Is visibly filling out, with plumper thighs, fuller cheeks, and deepening creases on her wrists. Her skin looks smooth, not loose or baggy.
- Is growing in length and head circumference.

If any of these signs aren't happening for your baby, check with an LLL Leader or your baby's doctor.

How Much Milk Is He Getting?

The amount of milk a baby requires varies hugely from baby to baby. By about four weeks of age, most exclusively breastfed babies take about 25 to 27 ounces (750–800 ml) of milk a day. By the end of the first week, mothers are already producing about three-quarters of that amount! By two weeks, they're nearing their long-running peak.

But do precise figures matter? Not at all. How much milk do you put on your cereal? Do you measure it? Or do you just use "enough"? Your baby does the same. The amount he takes varies from nursing to nursing, day to day. Your supply bounces up a little or down a little, to accommodate his desires. Is it hot? He might want a bit more to quench his thirst. Is he really hungry? He'll take both sides and maybe go back to the first again to get more fat. And so on. So knowing that your baby took 2½ ounces (75 ml) still doesn't tell you how full he's likely to be, or how many calories he got, or when he'll want to eat again. He knows his own appetite just as surely as you know yours, and you can trust him to let you know how he's doing. So long as he's gaining well, you can forget the numbers, watch your baby, and let him tell you what he needs and when he needs it.

He Suddenly Started Nursing a Lot! He's Really Hungry! Am I Losing My Supply?

As long as your baby's diaper output stays high, there's no need to panic. In fact, this is most likely a sign that your baby is going through a *growth spurt,* which is a great sign that he's getting lots of milk and growing just the way he should.

Babies don't grow steadily. They grow in fits and starts that include growth spurts or, as some call them, "frequency days," when they suddenly seem endlessly hungry. Emptying a breast more thoroughly and more often increases its output, so this sudden feeding frenzy boosts your supply—but only during the growth spurt itself, not permanently. After two or three days, he'll suddenly go back to his normal feeding pattern and might even nap more than usual to rest from all that growing. And there you sit with two breasts full of milk and no takers! (Don't worry, your milk production will adjust again within a day or so.)

When do growth spurs occur? You may hear that you should expect them around ten days, three weeks, six weeks, three months, six months, and so on, but they can happen just about anytime. But here's a secret: if you're nursing your baby whenever either of you likes, you may never notice them at all. And here's another secret: they're a wonderful thing to blame fussy behavior on. Your little sweetie isn't being very sociable for Aunt Franny? Just give her a knowing smile and say, "I think he's having a growth spurt." Most likely all will be forgiven.

I'm Still Worried About My Milk Supply

We use the term *milk supply* throughout this book because it's what most people say and we couldn't come up with another term, but there really isn't any such thing. To say that a mother has a *milk supply* is to imply that it's pretty rigidly set. It isn't. Take milk out and more milk will be made; take less out and less is made. There's an upper limit, of course, and there are some women who are never able to provide all the milk their babies need. There's a discussion of milk production issues in Chapter 18, "Tech Support," but if you're concerned about your milk supply, understand that it isn't something that Just Has to Be. The sooner you deal with it, the easier it will be to turn around. Your body uses the early weeks to establish its expected milk production capacity, so if you're truly worried, read Chapter 18 and get help *now*.

I Feel Like I Have Too Much Milk!

Welcome to a very large club! Probably a third (!) of us felt the same way. Your body has lots of "backup systems" for living—two lungs, two eyes, two kidneys…and two breasts. If you had to, you could probably feed your baby with just one breast. And just in case there are problems (or twins), our breasts make extra milk at the start. By the end of these first six weeks, most of us have settled down uneventfully to what our babies need. But some of us have breasts that just don't want to quit—that may need a little persuasion to cut back. Chapter 18 will give you ideas on how to do this. We just want to add one reminder here: those of us with oversupplies grow so accustomed to overly full, dripping breasts and choking babies that we think we're losing our supply when it stops happening. Check the earlier section on thriving babies. Yours almost certainly is.

My Baby's Unhappy But Doesn't Want to Nurse Right Now

Try some other things. Some babies despise a wet diaper, while some don't care at all. Some babies need a change of position, a change of view, or a change of motion. Try taking your baby out into the fresh air, singing a song to him, or dancing with him. In between all your attempts, offer to nurse again. Nursing solves a multitude of baby problems besides hunger. At some point, most likely nursing will be your baby's answer, even if it wasn't his original question.

My Baby's Less and Less Willing to Nurse At All

Does your baby get flooded every time your milk releases? Any signs of illness or extreme stuffiness? Are there any white patches in his mouth? Has he been getting bottles? These are a few reasons for a baby becoming less and less comfortable with nursing as time passes. You'll find more information on breast refusal in Chapter 18, but this can also be a good time to touch base with your LLL Leader.

SOME GOOD BOOKS ABOUT FUSSY BABIES

The Fussy Baby Book, by William Sears and Martha Sears
Colic Solved, by Bryan Vartabedian

What Are Some Causes of Crying Besides Hunger?

Babies come in all styles. Your baby's personality now isn't necessarily what it will be later, especially if you meet his needs, whatever they seem to be. The single most common cause of crying is simply a baby missing his mother, which is why babies who aren't held cry significantly more than babies who are (especially around six weeks). Other common (and some more unusual) causes of frequent crying are discussed in detail in Chapter 18. William and Martha Sears's book *The Fussy Baby* has still more ideas, including an "I Love U" massage that may help. If *none* of those seems to be the problem and you have a truly unhappy baby, check with your baby's doctor.

You probably won't need it much longer, but for now it may still help to post "Fussy Baby Ideas," a tear sheet from the back of the book, on your refrigerator, so that when your baby is fussy, nursing hasn't helped yet, and you're looking for other solutions, you have somewhere to turn. There are usually at least partial solutions to chronic fussiness, including time. Sometimes the last solution to be tried is the one that gets the credit, when really the baby simply outgrew a difficult beginning!

SPARKLERS AND ORCHIDS

Just like us, babies come in all kinds of personalities. "Sparklers" are babies who are doing, fussing, and demanding *all the time*. They often have minor physical discomforts that they need distraction from—a food sensitivity or cranky intestines—or maybe it's just their personality. Tantrums come easily because they're already slightly on edge. They are high-energy and high-maintenance, always seeking brain stimulation in order to shine their brightest.

"Orchids" are also high-need. They may find many environments overly stimulating, confusing, or scary and they need their mother's soothing presence more than some other babies. These are the babies who can't leave their mother's lap easily, who don't rush over to the other children at nursery school, who maybe can't *handle* nursery school at an age when other kids can. They wilt if they're yelled at or overstressed, and they blossom with tender care. Just like an orchid.

The time you put into a high-energy or high-need baby is never wasted. You're helping him lay down nerve pathways that may land him that PhD when he's older. Do your best to keep him happy so that you're both happier, and know that a little growth and maturation go a long way toward lessening the needs. Respect your "sparkler" or "orchid" for who he is: a baby who needs you (at first) to help him cope with his reality, and who will ultimately shine or blossom as a result.

People Say I Shouldn't Pick Him Up Every Time He Cries

You might ask them what their concern is. Spoiling? Whether your baby is crying for a physical or emotional need, he isn't trying to "get his way" or control you; he's just asking for help because he can't help himself. He's like a visitor on a strange planet—he doesn't speak the language, the gravity is too strong for him to be able to move around on his own, and he's disoriented from the trip. He needs you to respond quickly and reliably when he tells you he needs help. This builds trust in you, confidence in the world, and lifetime resiliency, and it wires his brain to cope with stress positively. Ultimately, this makes him able to be secure and independent sooner than if he had to manage all on his own.

We've learned a whole lot about infant biology, neurology, and physiology since the days of "don't spoil the baby." Lauren Porter, a child development specialist in New Zealand, points out that babies spend their early years laying down many, many nerve pathways. Some pathways result in anxiety and stress, and some result in confidence and coping. Research indicates that the way a mother responds to her baby greatly influences whether her child will respond automatically with calm or stress to the world around him as he matures. Refusing to answer his cries for help lays down "no one cares" pathways, decreasing his trust; making him feel neglected, hopeless, and despairing; decreasing his feelings of self-worth; and wiring his brain to react to future stresses more intensely. The children raised on the old "exercise their lungs, let them cry it out, teach them independence from the start" methods can become adults experiencing high rates of anxiety, low self-esteem, and stress-related illness.

But you already *know* that ignoring your crying baby doesn't feel right. Mothers are hardwired to respond because it's Nature's design to keep babies protected, cared for, and thriving.

No, you can't spoil your baby by responding to his needs. It's not possible at this age. What you *can* do by responding quickly and reliably is to help develop the neural pathways in his brain that with make him a secure, resilient person for the rest of his life.

> *Mothers ask the people they trust for information (mothers, mothers-in-law, pediatricians) and often get real misinformation. They worry that they are doing something horribly wrong in following their instincts. This makes them feel that their instincts are wrong, and society confirms their doubts.*
>
> *Encouraging mothers to trust themselves—validating that my body hurts when my baby cries for a biologically imperative reason—is one of the things La Leche League does that is the most vital, in my opinion!*
>
> *—Cassandra*

I'm Just Not Enjoying Any of This

Some babies and some breastfeeding situations take more work than others, but this is also the time when postpartum depression can make its first unwanted appearance. If feelings of anxiety, unhappiness, or depression continue for more than a few days, talk to your doctor. There's information on symptoms and treatments during breastfeeding in Chapter 18, "Tech Support."

When Can I Take My Baby Out?

Back in the heyday of formula, the official word was usually to keep new babies at home for weeks or months. It wasn't a bad idea; a formula-fed baby's immune system is so limited that he's much more susceptible to illness. Your breastfed baby is sturdy right from the start. As soon as you want to be out and about, your healthy baby can certainly join you. When Teresa's first daughter, Lisa, arrived, Teresa couldn't wait to go out and buy some girly clothes for her, so she tucked her in a sling and went to the store. Another woman stopped to admire the baby. "How old is she?" she asked. Teresa replied, "About fifteen hours."

It's not going out that makes a baby sick; it's being held by sick people. Encourage others to wash their hands before holding the baby, and follow your instincts on whether or not you want to pass him around.

Is It Really Okay to Nurse in Public?

Absolutely! We know of no province, state, or country that prohibits it, and there are many that specifically protect this natural right of mothers and babies.

Your partner may worry that strangers will see your breasts. Most likely they won't get more than a brief glimpse of skin, though they may notice that you're nursing. The more often breastfeeding is noticed, the more completely it will be accepted, even by our own families!

Many of us nurse for the first time in public because we suddenly don't have a choice—hungry baby, public setting. Some things you can try to make it simpler:

- Practice at home or with friends—in front of a mirror if you want to see what others see.
- Wear clothes that you can nurse in comfortably. They don't have to be

special nursing clothes; two-piece outfits with tops that you can pull up from the bottom work just as well. Your baby's body will hide almost all the bare skin.

- 💡 A cardigan sweater covers anything your baby's body doesn't.
- 💡 You can also wear a tank top underneath your top, with circles cut out for nursing. Your outer shirt covers the circles, and the rest of the tank top covers anything that your outer shirt doesn't. This is especially helpful with twins.
- 💡 Dark-colored prints help to hide any wet spots.
- 💡 When nursing on one side, press your forearm against the other side to prevent leaking. If that isn't enough, pull the side baby isn't nursing on up just a bit so that when you settle your clothes, the wet spot isn't a bull's-eye around your nipple.
- 💡 The most awkward moment is when your baby actually latches on. Turn your body away briefly. Or turn your head away for that moment, and it's unlikely anyone will notice at all because they'll be following your eyes, which are looking in another direction.
- 💡 Meet others' eyes with a friendly, open expression, or casually avoid eye contact. Most people will automatically match your behavior.
- 💡 A blanket or specially designed shawl or cover-up is *much* more attention-attracting than just nursing.

Limiting nursing to very private situations can limit nursing, which limits your baby's food. Another reason to nurse in public: we learn best by watching other mothers nurse, so by modeling successful breastfeeding, you may be teaching someone you never even notice how to breastfeed confidently.

> "When my daughter Bridget was a newborn and we were very new at breastfeeding, I nearly had to undress in order to get her latched on. One day I was visiting my parents and she was clearly hungry but my dad was in the room. I said, 'Dad, I have to nurse the baby now, but I nearly have to take my blouse off to do it.' He said okay and left the room. I got her latched and my dad blundered back in. He took one look at me and said, 'Honey, that's the most beautiful sight in the world—a mother nursing her baby.'

> It made me cry then and it makes me teary now. I never asked him to
> leave the room again."   —Sherrie

What About Bottles?

If your baby isn't gaining well at any age, a bottle can be used very successfully—or very unsuccessfully—for supplementation. See Chapter 18, "Tech Support," for ways to use a bottle that support breastfeeding.

If you want to use a bottle because you're going back to work, consider waiting until both you and your baby love breastfeeding and feel like old pros at it. There's no magic window of opportunity, and this reduces the risk that bottles will take over. There's a lot more information in Chapters 14 and 15.

If you want to have some emergency milk in the freezer, you can express it and store it without having to get your baby used to a bottle. Giving a daily or weekly bottle "just in case" to an otherwise fully breastfed baby is usually much more of a problem than a solution. Store some milk if you want to; in an emergency, your baby will eat.

Having someone else give a bottle in order to participate in feeding misses a key point about breastfeeding. It's a way to fill a stomach, yes, but it's a relationship that *only* a mother and baby have. Partners are the ones who teach babies that there are relationships beyond breastfeeding—that love doesn't always come with something to eat.

If you do use a bottle from time to time for casual reasons, it's well worth the extra effort to use your own milk in it. The intestinal changes and illness and allergy risks that accompany even occasional formula mean that it's something to be used only if no human milk is available.

People Are Saying I Need to Get Away from My Baby

Mothers hear this a lot, but by this point in the burgeoning breastfeeding relationship they don't usually feel like going. Did you feel you needed time away from your partner when you were falling in love? No, you probably couldn't be with each other enough. This is the falling-in-love stage with your baby, and togetherness is really important as you get to know each other.

The best thing about babies at this age is that they are very portable. You can get out with your partner to dinner, the movies, bowling, or just about any activity you like and your baby can come along contentedly. Babies often sleep through movies, and if they don't, you can nurse in the dark without anyone noticing. You don't have to leave your baby to get out of the house. Bring him with you and you'll both have a better time.

> *"I clearly remember my first restaurant meal after Jill was born—it was one of the best-tasting meals I ever had. It was wonderful. We went at four in the afternoon and took Jill with us. She slept through the entire meal, and we were able to sit and enjoy ourselves. All we wanted to do was talk about the baby anyway.... and she was right there with us."*
>
> —Janette

What About Sex?

Will you ever make love again? Sure. Many mothers already have at this point. And if sex is at the very bottom of your wish list, that's common, too. There's a very, very wide range of normal experiences. And remember: the way things are now is NOT the way they'll always be from now on. See Chapters 8 and 12 for more about reestablishing touch and intimacy with your partner.

Being Home So Much Can Be Lonely

If you're feeling alone right now, this is a prime time to get to an LLL meeting. Motherhood isn't supposed to be something you do by yourself. Throughout time, mothers have gathered together to share information, reassurance, and friendship. When mothers get together, there's an added bonus that doesn't get talked about much. Research indicates that women don't have a fight-or-flight response to stress; ours is called "tend and befriend." When we're under stress, we release oxytocin, and it makes us want to take care of our children and seek the company of others. Oxytocin, stress, tending our children, seeking friends? La Leche League is a natural!

At LLL meetings, you'll meet women who may have very different backgrounds but who are dealing with your same new-mother learning curve.

You can watch the more experienced mothers to see how they nurse, carry, and hold their babies, you can pick up little streamlining hints; you'll find that other babies are making the same sounds and faces and diapers as your own. New motherhood is different from any other club. We all flounder at least a little, and we all have at least a little something to give. You'll find you actually feel better about your own concerns if you have a chance to help someone else with hers. As one mother said after her first meeting, "I was going from here to the pediatrician's to get some of these questions answered. Now I think I'll just go home and enjoy my baby!"

If you don't have an LLL Group in your area, look for a childbirth class reunion or a made-for-mothers meeting of any kind. Or consider asking some friendly-looking mothers if they'd like to form a playgroup with you. They're most likely looking for company just as much as you are. If they're already in a group, they'll probably be happy to have you join. Really!

Any of these gatherings can be the glue that holds a mother together. The friendships often last for decades. After all, once you've compared bras and diaper contents with another woman, you've bonded for life!

Your baby will probably enjoy going to a mothers' group, too. Babies are born expecting a lively community around their mothers, with voices, breezes, leaves, dogs, laughter, busyness. Even a small baby can get bored at home. But a mothers' group? Now we're talking! You may find yourself saying about your fuss-free or peacefully sleeping baby at playgroup, "But he's not like this at home!" That's because you've found the community both of you need.

> *"My advice to new mothers? That after six or eight weeks everything is a lot better."*
> —Kasey

Follow Your Heart

This whole book is pretty much an expansion on this phrase. Every ordinary mammal mother comes fully equipped to raise her ordinary baby. Special circumstances may call for some specialized knowledge, but even there, the bedrock of that specialized knowledge is instinct. We're unsettled by the sound of a baby crying, so we pick that baby up and stabilize him on our chest, near our breasts. How smart we are! And yet that reaction was pure instinct.

All your life, you've had to learn new rules that go with each new role or skill. School, job, even running a microwave or using a phone—they all have rule books. Now you're starting the most complicated job of your life, and you may think they left out the rule book! No, they didn't. It's right in front of you, slightly cross-eyed and terribly cute. And it's right *inside* you, because *you think* he's terribly cute. Your instincts make you think that, and because you do, you'll take care of him. And because he knows how to complain if he's in need, and because you have an urge to respond when he complains, the two of you can work out the details as you go. Bottom line: follow your heart.

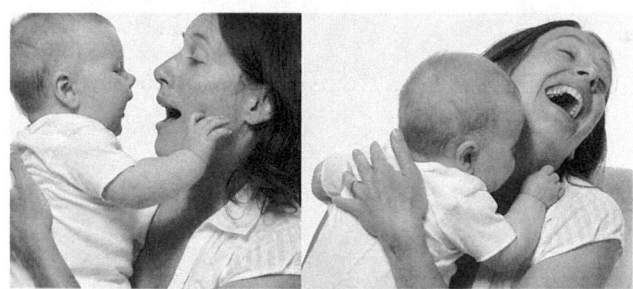

EIGHT

Six Weeks to Four Months: Hitting Your Stride

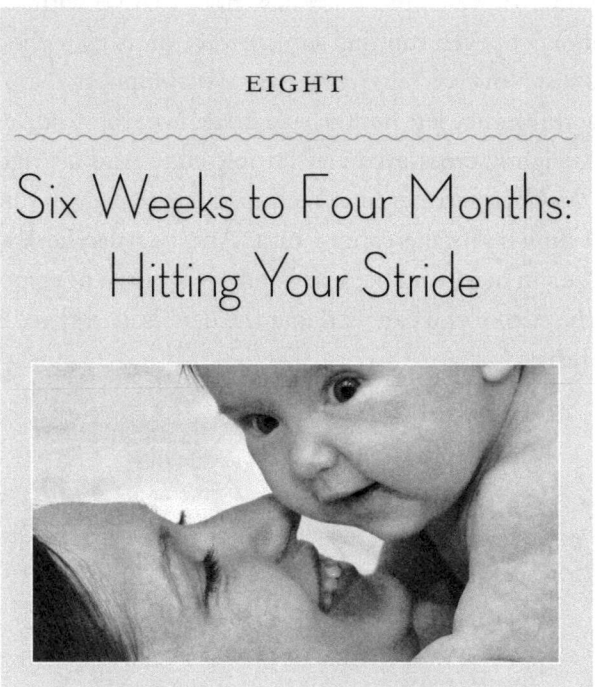

"When my first baby was about six weeks old, friends insisted that my husband and I should get out for a date. 'You need it for your marriage!' My husband also put pressure on me to do this, so I agreed. We left the baby with friends and went to dinner. I was miserable and could not enjoy the restaurant meal or being out on a date with my husband, because every second I was thinking about the baby, worried that he was crying for me. I really tried to enjoy myself but I couldn't. I could not WAIT to get back. I rushed in when we got there. I remember the feeling of relief to gather him back into my arms. THEN I could look at my husband and think about having a conversation with him, meeting some of his needs, with the baby in my arms. Things were NOT RIGHT when the baby was not with me. I never let that happen again. Dinner out without the baby did nothing good for my marriage.

"With babies number two and three, there was no way you could pry me away from them for many months. We had dates when we had each new baby, and we hired a sitter. But the sitter was for the OLDER children! We would go to the fanciest restaurants in town and the baby came along.

"We don't have to completely sacrifice the needs of one person in the family to meet someone else's needs. Everybody bends a little and everybody gets their basic needs met. The person who is the most dependent gets more of his or her needs met because he or she is less developed or less able to cope.

"I'm far from a perfect mom, but breastfeeding my children and keeping them close those early years is something I did right, and it really worked."   —Jane, remembering 1975

REMEMBER HOW STRANGE and challenging breastfeeding seemed when your baby was a newborn? There was so much to learn. By now, you're such an expert that you can help other mothers! You've likely become more confident about your milk production and have proudly watched your baby gain weight and flourish on your milk.

Your baby has wakened to the world, too. Social smiles begin to come more and more frequently. When he really gets going, his whole *body* smiles; by four months he may even be into giggles. And talking! Would you have guessed that your baby would be talking this soon? It's not words, but it's definitely speech—controlled sounds that he tries to produce evenly, with careful lips and furrowed brow. And while your baby works on *your* basic sounds, you've learned to recognize *his* cues—to nurse, change sides, burp—and often you're not even aware of what you're doing, you just respond, two people increasingly in sync.

You're still tired, of course, and there are many days when you *can't* figure out what the baby wants or why he's crying. Crying tends to peak around six to eight weeks, so you may find your baby seems inexplicably fussy at times, especially in the evenings. You might still find it easiest just to get comfy on the couch with some snacks and a favorite book, TV show, or DVD and plan to nurse on and off for the next few hours when you hit one of these fussy times. A long walk in the fresh air with your baby in a sling or carrier often helps, too. By now, you may have experienced growth spurts—fussier, needier times when your baby may nurse more than usual to build up your supply for a few days. Many mothers feel they occur somewhere around ten days, two weeks, three weeks, six weeks, and three months, but you can see from that frequency that the term is useful for explaining *any* fussy day to your aunt Franny.

Nursing Habits: Six Weeks to Four Months

The nursing behavior that's dearest to many mothers' hearts begins somewhere in here. Your baby, nursing busily, catches your eye, smiles, and starts to leak milk around the smile. She has to hurry up and suck again, but those moments tell you how much she adores you and loves nursing. She may begin patting or thumping your breast while she nurses, and may even stroke your face with her hand. Talk about heart melting!

> *"One of my favorite breastfeeding memories was when my son was around two months old. He was nursing and pulled off to give me a milky smile and my milk kept flowing; there was a little waterfall down my breast onto my stomach. My son turned his head and started licking the underside of my breast as the milk continued to flow."*   —Macy

The Four-Month Fussies

Your baby's growing awareness has its temporary downside. At an LLL meeting a while back, a mother arrived with a four-month-old, saying he had begun "nursing funny." Another mother in the room said, "My baby's four months old, too, and *she's* started nursing funny." And another mother spoke up with the same age baby and same concern. We dubbed it the "Four-Month Fussies" but didn't have a perfect solution for them beyond nursing in a quiet room, minimizing distractions, time, and nursing in whatever position the baby seemed to need. The group concluded that by around four months, babies had gained enough intellectual ability to tune in to the room around them but didn't yet have enough gray matter to tune in *and* nurse well.

Two of the mothers came back a few months later. "Are your babies still nursing funny?" we asked. They didn't know what we were talking about! It had passed so quickly that they had forgotten about it.

With some sensitive babies, this stage can be a bit more frustrating and challenging. Very distractible babies may let go or stop nursing every time they hear a new sound or catch some movement out of the corner of their eye. One mother remembered having to nurse alone with a fan on, to block out other sounds, for several weeks. But these babies, too, will settle down to nurse easily again when they get a little older.

Changes in Sleeping Patterns

Some babies may start sleeping through the night at some point in the first four months, especially if they sleep alone. But when they start going through the Four-Month Fussies, they may need nighttime nursings for a substantial part of their food. Sleeping through the night may result in a reduced milk supply and slowed weight gain. And sleeping for shorter periods and waking more frequently will keep your baby from spending too much time in deep sleep states, reducing his risk of SIDS.

But don't worry that you'll lose those easy nights forever if you follow your baby's lead. *Most* babies sleep more at night, then less, then more, with a gradual shift in the direction of longer and more reliable unbroken sleep. Take the good nights when you get them, and if they stop, remember that they'll come again!

Softening to Motherhood

Most of us are used to being in charge, if not of a department or workstation, then at least of how we structure the loose ends of our day. And we're probably used to working with fairly logical people. A baby changes that. Your baby is who she is; there's no changing her basic personality. And she is also, as one father described it, "a bundle of primal urges." She needs you when she needs you, for reasons you can't always fathom, in amounts you probably weren't prepared for. Some of us spend the early weeks trying to keep to our old ways—to make the baby's day fit ours. And some babies go along with that. But many simply can't, and they let you know that this plan just isn't working. At some point you may find yourself giving in and letting go . . . and suddenly everything is easier. It's like learning to swim, when you realize that struggling to keep your feet under you isn't helping you move forward. For Meredith, it was the moment when she thought, "Where is it written that I have to have eight hours of unbroken sleep?" and her blood-shot eyes cleared up. For Fatima, it was the moment when she thought, "What law says I can't just nurse him again?" and her baby quieted. For Lisa, it was hearing advice that she *knew* didn't fit her life, and realizing that no one knew her life or her baby better than she did.

Despite all the books and advice, ours is not a baby-knowledgeable culture. Maybe that's *why* we have so many books and so much advice. Your baby comes very well equipped to find her way in the world, and you come very well equipped to be her guide, once you start listening to your baby and let your feet leave the bottom of the pool.

Concerns You May Have Between Six Weeks and Four Months

These issues come up frequently at LLL meetings among mothers with babies between six weeks and four months old. If your questions aren't addressed here, you may find them in Chapter 18, "Tech Support," or the llli.org forums. And always feel free to call your local LLL Leader for information and support!

My Baby Hasn't Pooped in a Week! Is She Constipated?

For the first few weeks, every really messy diaper is a cause for celebration and a sign that your baby is getting enough milk. Around six weeks or so, though, some babies stop having the several bowel movements each day that are expected up until this point. Some start pooping once a day; some wait several days; some have a week or so of poop-free days. The change can be as abrupt as flipping a switch and can really throw a mother who'd stopped thinking about her baby's diaper output.

What's going on with the ones who poop only every week or so but continue to gain weight and seem active and healthy? We don't really know! Some experts feel infrequent stooling can be a sign of digestive problems or allergies to something in the mother's diet. Other experts think this is a normal variation since when they do finally poop, it is still very soft, not the hard stools you'd see in a constipated baby. What we do know is that this is *not* a reason to add formula, corn syrup, prune juice, or other foods to the baby's diet.

Of course, if it's been several days or longer since your baby last pooped, the results can be really messy—a blowout instead of skid marks. After a week, expect a mudslide. Sometimes these deliveries are made over the course of a day. The mothers of very predictable babies may not even bother with a diaper bag for much of the week, but they plan to stay home on Poop Day.

Some of these babies start to feel uncomfortable and cranky as they work up to having a big bowel movement. Nursing may help; being at the breast stimulates the baby's digestive system to move things along. But sometimes the uncomfortable baby refuses the breast, maybe because it just makes her tummy hurt even worse. You can try holding her in an upright or squatting position to see if that helps, or try bicycling her legs or massaging her belly gently. You might also want to try sitting the baby in a warm, shallow bath. (Be prepared—you'll need to wash out the tub if this works!)

Will Exercising Affect My Milk?

Exercising is basic to mammals—because their lives depend on it. Mice, desperate to stay alive, have always run from cats...and then nursed their babies. Cats, desperate to eat, have always run after mice...and then nursed their babies. It would be a fragile system indeed if babies suffered every time their mothers ran to catch their dinner, or ran to avoid *being* dinner, or ran on a treadmill! Not surprisingly, most studies have found no significant difference in the volume, taste, or composition of milk after exercise; babies were just as willing to drink it as at other times.

But would it really *matter* if your baby wasn't thrilled with the taste of your post-exercise milk? It may well be that your baby also isn't thrilled with the taste of, say, cinnamon or butterscotch in your milk. No problem. If a baby takes less than usual at one nursing, he'll just take more than usual at the next. Since babies never take all the available milk in a breast, there's always a reserve for the baby who wants more.

There are, of course, plenty of benefits to exercising and staying fit while you are breastfeeding. Working out can improve your mood, give you more energy, and help you sleep better at night. So go ahead and develop an exercise plan that fits into your day with your baby. You might:

- Breastfeed your baby before you work out so that your breasts are less full.
- Wear a supportive bra to help you feel comfortable. Some women wear two, for more support.
- Wear breast pads if leaking is still an issue.
- Take a quick shower or towel-dry before you nurse if your baby doesn't like nursing when you're sweaty.

What if you're training to the point that you might, in your childless days, have stopped having periods? That means you're exercising to the point that your body wouldn't even try to raise a baby, and your milk production may be affected. One of the reasons we gain weight during pregnancy is to sustain an infant during possible famine. You might want to wait until next year to aim for the Olympics, but you can certainly train for a slower-than-usual marathon.

Modest exercise is fine, too. A long or even short walk with your baby in a sling or carrier can be a good way to start. Finding a walking partner helps make walks a regular event. Fitness centers often have programs for pregnant woman and new mothers to which you can bring your baby. Some even work the baby into the routine. You're already doing weight-bearing exercise just toting your baby around...and the weight increases daily!

What About Dieting?

Many women lose around 1.75 pounds (0.8 kg) per month during the first six months of breastfeeding. Most of the rest of us find that we're at least holding our own. A bonus is that during breastfeeding, we tend to lose weight from our hips and thighs—something we're less able to do at other times.

If you're dieting, aim for losing no more than about 1 pound (0.5 kg) a week. Losing weight rapidly during breastfeeding can release the environmental pollutants stored in your fat into your milk. It's not a problem at a slow and steady rate, but a rapid weight loss can unload a lot in a hurry.

Are There Environmental Pollutants in My Milk?

Oh, we're glad you brought that up! Stories about the high levels of environmental pollutants in human milk hit the news every now and then. They're true, but don't let them worry you. There are *thousands* of studies to show that formula-fed babies end up with lower IQs, poorer health, and higher rates of cancer, diabetes, and heart disease than babies who breastfeed. Formula also contains environmental contaminants from cow milk and other ingredients, processing, and packaging. The reality is that contaminants are everywhere, in just about all the foods we eat. *By far* the safest, healthiest food for your baby is your milk.

Do Breastfed Babies Need Immunizations? Won't Breastfeeding Alone Protect My Child?

The breastfed child has an immune system that's nearly as good as her mother's, and way better than that of a formula-fed or even partially breastfed child. But the antibodies that you've acquired against diseases that can be immunized against—either from having had the diseases yourself or from vaccinations—aren't transmitted through your milk in large enough doses to protect your baby. Diphtheria, chicken pox, measles, mumps, and so on were around long before formula was, and fully breastfed children have always been susceptible to them. On the other hand, research indicates that the formula-fed baby, whose weaker immune system can't mount as long and strong a defense, won't be as well protected by a vaccine as your breastfed baby will be. A good guide for navigating the complex immunization issues is Dr. Robert Sears's *The Vaccine Book*.

**SOME GOOD BOOKS FOR MOTHERS OF
SIX-WEEK-OLD TO FOUR-MONTH-OLD BABIES**

Eat Well, Lose Weight While Breastfeeding, by Eileen Behan
The Attachment Parenting Book, by William Sears and Martha
    Sears
*The Baby Book: Everything You Need to Know About Your Baby
    from Birth to Age Two,* by William Sears, Martha Sears, Robert
    Sears, and James Sears
Attachment Parenting, by Katie Allison Granju
Attached at the Heart, by Barbara Nicholson and Lysa Parker

Should I Be Giving My Baby Vitamin D?

Recent research has shown that most of us, including our exclusively breast-fed babies, need additional vitamin D. Some public health groups say this supplementation should start at birth, while others say it should start by two months. What's right?

Here's the scoop: we are designed to manufacture our own vitamin D in our skin by exposure to sunlight, not to get it from food, and throughout most of human history that worked fine. But getting enough sun on our skins has gotten tougher. The thinning ozone layer makes sun exposure so potent that people tend to use sunscreen generously when they're outdoors. Modern lifestyles mean most of us spend most of our time indoors. Some women who are covered for religious reasons may protect even their faces from the sun. Adequate vitamin D isn't made from sunlight above certain latitudes in the winter. And people with dark skin need even more time outside to acquire enough vitamin D.

Vitamin D helps us absorb and use calcium properly and keep our immune system strong, which may be why so many folks in colder climates are susceptible to colds and flu during winter, when the sun is low. And we're learning that too little vitamin D may put us at higher risk of such problems as diabetes and cancer before we see such obvious problems as rickets.

It isn't possible to get too much vitamin D from sunlight. It *is* possible to get too much through supplements and enriched foods, but it turns out we've been too cautious with supplements in the past. The first and best way to get more vitamin D into your baby is to expose her to more sunshine, but in ways that minimize the chance of sunburn. Here are some ideas: If you carry your baby in a car seat, there's no need to throw a blanket over the whole thing unless it's a really cold winter day. Run errands with your baby—all that dashing in and out of stores, babe in arms, contributes to her vitamin D supply for the week. Use sunscreen very sparingly until your baby is six months old and then only if his exposure will be prolonged. If your baby is dark-skinned, his need for sunscreen is even less.

Talk to your doctor about increasing the level of vitamin D in your milk by taking a vitamin D supplement yourself. Recent research suggests 4,000 IU per day may be the amount needed to get enough into your milk. Discuss your particular situation with the doctor to decide if your baby needs vitamin D supplementation, look for a brand of drops that is *only* vitamin D. You can put the drops on your nipple and let the baby nurse them off.

Does My Baby Need Other Vitamins and Minerals?

Other than his access to sunlight for vitamin D, a breastfed baby's life hasn't changed that much over the millennia, and neither has his food supply. Your milk contains what your baby needs.

You might be told that your baby needs extra iron, but that's because *formula-fed* babies need extra iron. There isn't a lot of iron in your milk, but there isn't supposed to be. It's much more completely absorbed by your baby than the kind in formula, baby cereal, or iron supplements. If your breastfed baby gets too much iron, it will end up feeding the wrong bacteria in his intestines. Your amazing milk contains a protein called *lactoferrin* that binds to extra iron that your baby doesn't use, keeping it from feeding harmful intestinal bacteria. Iron supplements can overwhelm the lactoferrin so that the bacteria thrive, often resulting in diarrhea and even microscopic bleeding.

Formula is a different story. The kind of iron in formula isn't readily absorbed by the baby, so more has to be put in to compensate, and formula-fed babies' intestines routinely have too much iron. The result can be microscopic intestinal bleeding that ends up reducing their overall iron. It's tough to get iron, or *any* vitamins or minerals, well balanced in formula!

So, after generations of formula-feeding, you can see why doctors with little experience in breastfeeding may recommend unnecessary vitamin or mineral supplements for their breastfed patients.

There are a few exceptions:

- 💡 If your baby's cord was cut before it stopped pulsing, he missed out on up to a third of his intended blood supply. That's a lot of iron to lose. He should be fine for the first half year, and will probably be fine from then on as well, but when he starts solids look for iron-rich foods such as meats, dark green leafy vegetables, and beets (much better than the type of iron in baby cereal).
- 💡 If your baby is started on solids prematurely—before he would start eating them on his own—his iron stores may drop. Some fruits and vegetables can bind with the iron in your milk before the baby has a chance to absorb it.
- 💡 If your baby was born prematurely, he may not have been born with the same nutrient stores as a full-term baby, and the same guidelines may not apply.

If iron supplements are suggested, you can't increase the levels in your milk by taking iron supplements yourself or eating more iron-rich foods, but you can ask for a blood test for your baby to confirm the need. Your baby's finger or heel shouldn't be squeezed, which can skew the results. Keep in mind, though, that tests show only one part of a larger picture of overall health, and should always be viewed that way.

What About Traveling with My Baby?

Traveling really makes you appreciate the ease of breastfeeding! And if your baby is accustomed to sleeping with you, she'll feel at home wherever you go.

Once you get to your destination, you may want to avoid passing her around at first. Even a very young baby can be frightened by a group of loud, excited strangers all clamoring to take her away from you. Wait until she settles in a bit, and you may find that she adores all the hubbub (though probably mainly from the safety of your arms). Lay whatever ground rules you're comfortable with. You may be going to visit your mother, but this is *your* baby and you're the boss!

Car Travel

Travel by car with a breastfed baby doesn't take much advance preparation—no formula or bottles to pack, and any poopy diapers aren't too stinky if you can't throw them out right away. But when your baby wants to nurse? That's a tough one. There's just no completely safe way to feed a baby in a moving car, breast or bottle; if your baby is hungry, you'll need to pull over. But don't assume that you'll have to take the baby out of the seat! Some mothers find the stop is shorter and the baby happier if they lean over to nurse the baby right where he is. All that taking out and putting back can rouse a baby who's fallen blissfully asleep in your arms. If you're *really* creative and flexible, you may be able to nurse from both breasts without taking the baby out or moving to the other side of the car seat. Or you may both appreciate the in-arms time a stop allows. Staying in the backseat if you're not driving lets you interact, sing endless verses of silly songs, and pass over soft toys. Some mothers of chronically unhappy travelers keep a pacifier in the car.

Plane Travel

One advantage to traveling with a breastfeeding baby is the ease of "nursing up and nursing down" to avoid those plugged ears that make so many children cry when the plane is taking off or landing. Many mothers have nursed their babies during these parts of the flight, and other passengers aren't even aware of what's going on—they're just very happy that the baby is quiet! If you brought the car seat along, nursing during takeoff and landing isn't possible; this is another place where a pacifier might have a use.

Will you be traveling with another adult? Bring a newspaper, and you can create your own private cubicle by sitting near the window with your traveling companion on the aisle. All he or she has to do is open the newspaper wide to read, and your seats are completely private.

"I was at the first session of a breastfeeding peer counselor training program. Everyone was introducing themselves and saying something about their breastfeeding experience. One mother said that she had

felt uncertain about nursing her baby in public until she saw me in the waiting room of her doctor's office when she was pregnant. I was nursing my two-year-old and she decided that if I could do that, then she could certainly nurse her newborn. I remembered hoping at the time that no one would notice what I was doing. But someone did notice, and it made her life easier. Maybe we shouldn't be quite so invisible."

—Lesley

I Still Have Too Much Milk!

By about six weeks, you probably have a good sense of whether your supply has fallen into line with your baby or whether you're dealing with true oversupply. There's a whole discussion of oversupply in Chapter 18; if you haven't tried it yet, a first step is using just one breast at each nursing. You and your baby will both be happier once you get this sorted out.

If everything's going fine except for leaking…well, it's not a huge deal. Nuisance that it is, leaking does reduce your risk of plugged ducts from extra milk. You may need to wear breast pads and keep an extra pad on the bed for a little while longer. If you're still wearing breast shells (see Chapter 18), that could be what's encouraging the extra flow—time to put them away.

Is It a Problem That My Baby Is So Easygoing?

Having a happy, easygoing baby can make the first weeks and months of motherhood a lot easier. Your baby feels perfectly in sync with you and he's happy to be your baby. Just don't forget him! Sometimes quiet babies start out gaining well when you're paying close attention to every signal. But later, when you're back to getting errands and chores done, you don't always notice their very subtle feeding cues, and they're too polite to complain when a meal is missed or delayed. This is especially true in day care settings, where the fussy, demanding babies get most of the attention.

So definitely enjoy your happy baby, but even though he doesn't insist on constant holding, it will probably help to keep him close to you as much as possible, and offer to nurse whenever it strikes your fancy or his. He can always say no when you offer, and you may be surprised at how happily he says yes.

I'm Still Dealing with a Fussy Baby

You don't even want to HEAR about those calm contented babies, because yours sure isn't one. He's thriving, but still fussy and demanding. It may be worth taking another look at the possibility of oversupply, food sensitivities, and other possibilities such as sensory integration and reflux (see Chapter 18) with an LLL Leader or other breastfeeding helper. Or it just may be his personality. Maybe you've got a sparkler—an intense, sensitive baby who needs input, input, input! His only settings are high and off. That's the downside. The upside is how truly bright and curious he is likely to become. You'll work hard as a mother to this baby. Look for other mothers of sparklers, to share notes with. Keep your sense of humor and try not to compare your busy days with those of your placid-baby friends. And keep your little sparkler close to you—your presence and touch will often go a long way toward calming him.

WHEN YOU REALLY LOSE IT

All mothers have days when they try everything and the baby is still crying and they're exhausted and absolutely at their limit. So what's your backup plan? Is there someone you can call to come over and take the baby for a walk or who will just talk to you and reassure you over the phone? Can you call an LLL Leader for some comforting words? Can you do something for yourself—have a warm bath (with baby), enjoy a special snack or treat, or put some music on and dance with the baby? One mother kept a stash of chocolate for use only when her baby was pushing her over the edge. She almost started to look forward to those fussy times!

If you're feeling desperate, put your crying baby down in a safe place and step outside for a moment. Breathe deeply and take a few minutes to calm down. Imagine how amazing he'll be at twelve years old when he helps you cook, carries in your groceries, and gives you special handmade Mother's Day cards. When you're ready, go back inside, pick him up, and smell the top of his head—that amazing smell that only he has. And bring your breastfeeding network into play! You have friends out there who are happy to help. Even if you haven't met them yet.

I'm Going Through the Motions, but I Don't Love This Baby Yet

Maybe you feel that this baby is on loan, or just isn't yours. For some of us, love takes a while to grow. Remember the woman in Chapter 3 who said, "I feel as though I adopted Edwin and he is not biologically mine"? A few years later, she was amazed that she had written that, and could barely remember the feeling. But other women have a long-term sense of emotional distance, sometimes part of the price we pay for medicalized births and early separations. One thing we don't get much chance to do today is talk through the birth—what happened, how we felt about it—and process it.

You might take reassurance from this comment from a lactation consultant: Her client sobbed that she hadn't even wanted to *see* her baby for the first twenty-four hours because of a traumatic birth. "You know," said the lactation consultant, "after a birth like that, if you'd been a bear, you'd have *eaten* her!" We do manage far better than the average mammal mother after a disruptive start!

If you sense that love is growing, give yourself more time. If that disconnected feeling keeps coming between you and your baby, though, it can help a lot to find someone who understands—a counselor or friend, or maybe a support group related to birth, breastfeeding, or early parenting. Keep looking until you're satisfied with the person you find and the results you feel. You deserve to enjoy and feel fulfilled by motherhood.

Should My Baby Be on a Schedule by Now?

The mothers of long ago had jobs to do and food to prepare, and no safe place to keep the baby except at their side. Baby Uhr just had to nap on Mama's back...and he did. They didn't have clocks, so schedules didn't happen. Mothers today have busy lives, too, and thankfully babies are born with the expectation that they'll fit naps and feedings around whatever else needs to happen.

Sometime in these first few months, you may realize that your day has fallen into a fairly reliable rhythm, but it won't be something you can set your watch by. There are still days when your baby eats all day, and days when he naps all day. Add to that the fussy days, busy days, errand days, lazy days, and it may seem that every day is an exception to the rule. But more and more, your baby is able to fall in with your changing plans, entertaining himself with new sights and sounds or relaxing in a sling or car seat as he takes a nap. Most babies are flexible above all else.

An actual schedule would only make things more complicated, and spacing out nursings to suit a clock jeopardizes your milk supply. So expect that while you can nudge your baby toward predictability, there will still be a certain amount of unpredictability. The good news is that unpredictability is a close relative of adaptability; the baby who won't nap at the expected time today is the same baby who'll obligingly sleep through a frantic last-minute errand tomorrow. As one mother said, "We have a routine, but we don't have a schedule. A schedule would mean he naps at three. A routine means we usually have a bath after supper."

What About Sleep Training?

When your baby is older, you may be able to encourage him to sleep longer stretches at night. Right now, though, most babies still get a hefty portion of their calories at night. Unless a baby has chosen it on his own, sleeping through the night can slow his rate of growth and risks early weaning. But we know how important sleep is right now, which is why Chapter 12 is all about how you and your baby can get more of it.

But I'm Starting Work Soon!

It's a difficult situation: a mother who has to get up to an alarm clock and a baby who can't tell time. Absolutely not fair, and not something most working mothers of the world have to contend with in the first year! For starters, you could try taking the baby to bed with you an hour earlier than you would normally turn in. That extra hour of being horizontal in a dark room, even if you don't sleep through all of it, can mean you're much better rested the next day. For many more ideas and a thorough discussion of going back to work, see Chapters 12 and 14.

What About Solids?

For this period of your baby's life, you don't have to give it a thought. Aunt Franny may be eager for your baby to taste ice cream, but hold her off. Your baby isn't ready on the inside until she's ready on the outside, and it's the rare four-month-old who's able to sit up, pick up food, put it in her mouth, chew it, swallow it, and reach for more. The World Health Organization, the American Academy of Pediatrics, and the Canadian Paediatric Society all agree—under normal circumstances, babies don't need solids before about six months. Early solids can cause digestive problems, reduce a baby's iron stores, and increase the risk of obesity and allergies. Might as well save yourself another few months' work and wait until she starts grabbing the food off your plate. See Chapter 13 to enter the brave new world of solids in all its detail.

Teething

Most babies begin teething sometime after four months, but some babies do get teeth early, and some are even born with them. For the most part, teeth are irrelevant to breastfeeding. You may have to wiggle your baby into a more comfortable nursing position at times when the teeth first come through. And some babies try to bite down while nursing, particularly during those sore times when the teeth are trying to surface. Check out Chapter 9, which discusses the period from four to nine months, when teeth are most likely to appear. And there's a discussion about cavities and night nursing in Chapter 12.

For now, even if your baby isn't ready for teeth, she may be *getting* ready for teeth. And with this, you gain one more all-purpose mothering excuse: teething. Everyone understands that teething makes babies uncomfortable. Say the magic words "Well, you know, he's teething," and even Aunt Franny will back off.

Actual teething may involve fist gnawing, a lot of drooling, vague unhappiness, and occasionally pain during nursing. Before you reach for something to numb your baby's gums, remember that any numbness is going to make nursing feel mighty funny to her, and possibly even to you. Instead of medication, you could try an ice cube wrapped in a wet washcloth and secured with a strong rubber band, a frozen washcloth or teething toy, or any teething toy with lots of projections or holes. These teethers allow your still-awkward little one to be able to hold on to them anywhere and get something satisfying into her mouth.

What About Sex?

Some of you are thinking, "What about it? We've been back at it for weeks," and others are thinking, "Sex? Why would I even *think* about sex?" The timetable for reestablishing *any* form of intimacy with your partner varies hugely, depending on the simplicity of the birth, how breastfeeding is going, your baby's personality and needs, and at least as many other issues as there are couples.

You may find that your new body and role are a real aphrodisiac for both of you. Or you may find that romance of *any* kind goes out the window completely for a while! If you fall into the second group, you can reassure your partner and yourself that this part of life hasn't ended and that, like a good bottle of wine, it's going to be all the better for having been on the shelf for a bit. In the meantime, a pat or squeeze from either one of you to the other is a way of saying, "I know you're still there."

You may find that anything more than that is beyond your abilities at first. But eventually a simple dinner for two (and a half) can feel luxuriously sexy, even if it's just a candle and a can of soup. So can (eventually) a sexy bra, a nightgown that shows only the best of your (ahem) new curves, and anything that pleasures the needier of the two of you. Sex without intercourse can be a fine place to start. From there, stretch your mutual entertainment envelope as far as you want—after all, everything else has stretched!

This is a chance to rediscover sex. What you enjoy and to what extent may have changed. Your breasts may be more tender, especially in the first few months, but they may also feel and look sexier. And of course they now contain milk. If you want to keep milk *out* of your lovemaking, nurse the baby on both sides ahead of time. But milk can be a plaything for the two of you as well. Where there's orgasm there may be milk. In fact, that very same hormone (and the milk it can trigger these days) just might be released by having a great meal, seeing old friends, hugging a pet, or even (one of us blushes to say) successfully arguing a bill with the electrician. When good times happen, sometimes milk happens. You and your partner can squirt it, massage with it, joke about it. Since you've got it, you might as well flaunt it. It's a sweet and special time in your life.

Some of us find we need extra vaginal lubrication because the low estrogen associated with breastfeeding can cause vaginal dryness. Try an over-the-counter lubricant rather than an estrogen-containing one, to avoid any possible effect on milk supply. Unaccustomed fluid up top and unaccustomed dryness below—not the body you had a year ago! Enjoy exploring the new pleasures of your new body, don't rush, and keep your sense of humor intact.

And where is your new little sweetie in the meantime? Some babies nap soundly and are most easily moved to where you want them when they're in a car seat or infant seat. You can even start your romantic moment with a drive that puts the baby to sleep! or if your bed is big enough, you can just leave him on one side while you two enjoy each other. Remember, *the baby doesn't care what's going on*. It may be that you're uncomfortable with an audience, but an infant's only concern is that his needs for food and comfort are met, and during these early months he may stay asleep best if you're not far away. Babies do seem to have a sort of radar, however, and may wake up when you least expect—or want—them to. Your hand on his back may be all he needs to settle him back to sleep.

What if you're not interested in sex? Some of us find we feel "touched out." After spending all day being intimate with the baby, giving him our body, time, and mind, we don't have anything left over. The time that you're devoting to your baby is time well spent—an investment in your family's future well-being and, yes, happiness. You partner's understanding, patience, and help can make a huge difference as you lay the foundation for your new future.

Your love life is just one more area where things have changed for now. The words to remember are *for now*. Life with Baby *will* gradually become less intense, and the sex life you previously enjoyed *will* gradually resume. Creativity, flexibility, and a strong sense of humor go a long way toward rekindling the physical side of your relationship while there's a baby in the house.

My first episiotomy hurt unbelievably for MONTHS—it was over a year before I was comfortable with intercourse. I even saw a doc about it who couldn't see anything wrong. Took ages before I could actually enjoy it and wasn't gritting my teeth and thinking about England and the Queen. And no, I really, truly don't think it was a psychological issue!   —Janette

---

We first made love at three days. I guess that's not typical, but I felt really ready.   —Myra

---

I remember the doctor telling me at my six-week checkup with Emily that I could "start relations" again. I didn't mention we'd already started them. That first time was very memorable for me, as I had a milk release in the middle—the only time this ever happened. Fortunately, we found this hilarious. I don't remember when we resumed such activities with the other three, but I think it was months rather than weeks.   —Sarah

---

I was totally ready to roll by four weeks. My husband, on the other hand, had zero interest for many months postpartum.   —Cassandra

Can I Get Pregnant?

If you want to avoid another pregnancy, the Lactational Amenorrhea Method, or LAM for short, is 98 to 99 percent effective (about the same as the pill) in preventing pregnancy when *all* three of the following are true:

- Your baby is under six months old AND
- Your periods haven't resumed (before day fifty-six postpartum, bleeding, spotting, or vaginal discharge with some blood is not a period) AND
- Your baby is breastfeeding exclusively, without regularly receiving any other food or drink, including water

There's strong biological logic behind LAM. The baby who's getting all his food, day and night, from his mother, isn't ready to share her. His mother's body isn't ready to take on a second intense job.

If we fool Nature by formula-feeding the baby so that the mother's hormones don't know there *is* a baby; or if we train him to sleep through the night so that he routinely goes more than six hours without nursing, like an older baby; or if we give him a pacifier and reduce his time at breast, like a baby who's weaning, our bodies may assume it's safe to add another baby, and pregnancy becomes possible. Even having a job during those first six months that separates you from your baby for four or more hours a day reduces the effectiveness of LAM because pumping is not as effective as a baby at suppressing ovulation.

If you want to use another kind of birth control, it's a good idea to steer clear of all hormonal methods—the pill, contraceptive implants, hormone-impregnated IUDs—for at least the first six months because of their potential effect on milk supply. Many women using these methods continue to breastfeed with no decrease in supply, but some find they don't recover from the supply drop that can result. The possibility of a decreased supply is much lower after about six months.

Breastfeeding can continue to provide good pregnancy protection beyond six months, provided your periods have not returned and your baby still nurses frequently day and night, but the effectiveness isn't as certain and declines further over time. Three good resources are Toni Weschler's *Taking Charge of Your Fertility,* Sheila Kippley's *The Seven Standards of Ecological Breastfeeding by Sheila Kippley,* and the Academy of Breastfeeding Medicine's Protocol 13, at bfmed.org/Resources/Protocols.aspx.

I Haven't Been Away from My Baby Since He Was Born

We're back to the beginning of this chapter! Many mothers are torn between a sense of guilt that they *should* "get away from the baby"—for their own well-being, for the sake of their marriage, because Grandma's visiting and can watch the baby—and a sense that they just don't *want* to be away from their baby. Over the past weeks or months of hard work and little sleep, this wee one has become so woven into your life that you miss her when you're not with her. That's *normal*. It's the spell a baby weaves so that you won't leave her behind, which is wildly unsafe from the baby's perspective. If you don't want to leave her, don't feel you need to! Those solid mothering instincts have worked on behalf of mothers and babies for millennia. There's nothing to say you have to resist them now! Soon enough, your child will be headed off to slumber parties. But a little baby isn't built, stomach or soul, to be away from her source of all things good—*you*.

Everyone is different, and you may find you want or need to be away from your baby for a period of time. If that's your situation, plan ahead to leave your milk so the caregiver can provide your baby with her safe and familiar food. Feel free to check in as often as you want and, if possible, plan so you can come home early if the baby needs you.

> *"I finally realized that if I would just abandon myself to my baby and relieve myself of expectations (usually other people's) of how she 'should' behave, then everything would be so much easier and so much more enjoyable and I just wouldn't care what other people thought. This took a few months, but it changed my life!"* —Barbara

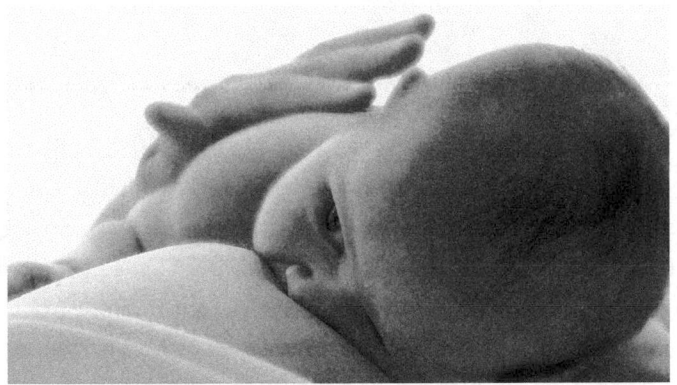

NINE

Four to Nine Months: In the Zone

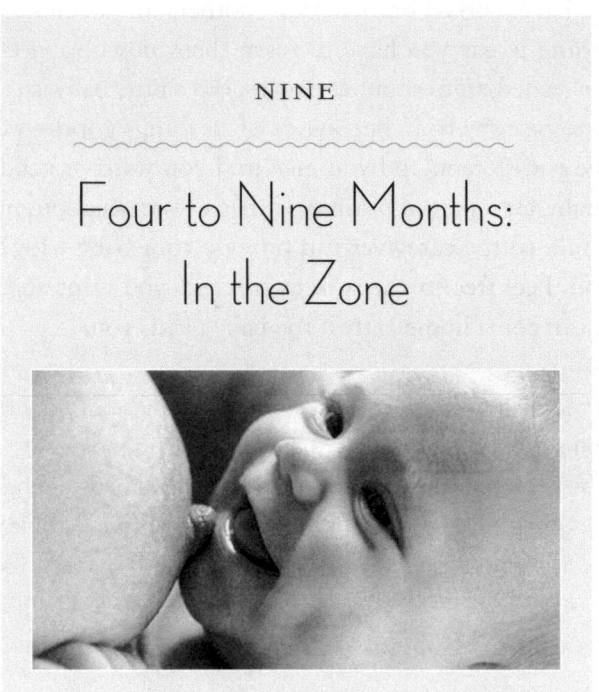

"My first was a very happy, easy baby. When my second was born, it was clear he was a different child completely. He needed constant nursing and constant contact. I nicknamed him my barnacle baby. As long as he was held, especially by me, he was happy and contented. He literally lived in the sling while I kept track of his two-year-old sister. If I put him down to use the bathroom, he would scream. He hated the swing and the bouncy seat. I learned to take the fastest showers on earth. I figured this is what it meant to have a high-need child.

"Then one day, when he was four and a half months old, he started to crawl. He was able to move on his own and he moved away from me. I was astounded. He was happy and became a very quick crawler. I could put him down and he'd zoom across the floor, usually in the direc-

tion of his sister. It was amazing to see this little guy get around. He still
nursed more than his sister had. A good thing, because that's the only
time I got to hold him!"   —Sherrie, remembering 1997

YOU MIGHT ALREADY have people asking you, "So, when are you going to wean?" Yet you probably feel you're really in the zone with breastfeeding at last. You've solved any early problems, stopped worrying about weight gain or milk production or latch, and...and your baby looks at you with those eyes when he nurses! How could you stop now? And why would you?

Life with Baby continues to change. If you've been using a sling or carrier, you may find that your baby wants to face forward at this point, his back against you, legs crossed tailor-style. (If the sling didn't work for you at first, you might want to shake the dust off it and try again.) He can see the house as you work inside or the scenery as you shop. He can chew on the front edge, lean to the side to nap, and get plenty of attention! Watch him taking in the clerks and crowds, following faces and conversations. By contrast, a baby in a stroller does a study of kneecaps and counter walls. (Not all babies like all that attention and stimulation, and yours may be one who prefers a sling position facing you that shelters him from the noise and bustle of the world.)

Nursing Habits: Four to Nine Months

Your very proficient nursling may be able to knock back a whole meal in five minutes, so some nursings now are over almost as soon as they begin, leaving you wondering whether your child ate anything at all. But nursing is increasingly a social time, too, as her flirting and fiddling demonstrate. The milk-leaking smiles continue, and the happy satisfaction you feel with each other makes nursing almost like a conversation. While your baby used to focus completely on nursing, her little hands splayed or curled against your breast or body, now she might begin to touch your mouth or face with one hand or play with your hair while nursing. She may massage or pat or knead your breast; both babies and kittens figure out that this can trigger another milk release. As her aim improves, she may be captivated by your nostrils or a mole on your chest. She may provide dental exams and explore your face with less-than-gentle fingers.

Okay, so nursing isn't always perfectly peaceful anymore and a few of her nursing fiddles can be downright irritating. She may twiddle or pinch the other nipple, twist a hand into your bra strap, pinch your skin. Any of these ways of touching can quickly become part of a baby's nursing routine, especially when she's tired or going to sleep, so it's worth putting a stop to the bothersome ones, holding your baby's hand or guiding it into a more agreeable activity. You're actually practicing early discipline—gently encouraging an alternative activity, substituting an acceptable object or activity for an unacceptable one, distracting your child to head off a problem. A decade from now, you'll be saying, "I know you're disappointed that Sadie can't come over today. Why don't we make some cookies that you two can share tomorrow?" The same technique, and you're practicing now!

> Alison's toddler had developed the habit of fiddling with the other nipple, which probably brings on a milk release but which most mothers dislike because it's such an intense feeling. Her solution was to string some of his chunky wooden beads together to make a "nursing necklace." She would slip it over her head before they nursed—in public she'd wear a scarf or fancy necklace instead—and he would fiddle away happily with the beads.
>
> Melanie had a mole under her left breast that her daughter loved to pick at idly while she nursed. Melanie started wearing a small adhesive bandage over it. Problem solved.
>
> Tiffany's son loved to wind his arm through her nursing bra. She would grab his hand and kiss it when he started; once her milk released, he was more likely to forget the bra.

The early days of a baby who has to eat *immediately* are over. Your baby has a small scrap of patience now, an ability to be distracted briefly, that can mean a reduction in any tears or tensions. She's learned to trust that even if there is a brief delay, the breast will be there for her. Your own tensions about nursing have probably relaxed, too. This is a fun time to be nursing for both you and your baby!

> "I remember that one day when Omer was four months old he suddenly smiled and stopped nursing, the nipple fell out of his month with a drop of milk on it, and he held me tight as if to say, 'Thank you, Mom,' and then he latched again."
>
> —Vered

> "Nursing is almost like cheating because it makes mothering (bedtime, naptime, boo-boos) so easy. Breastfeeding is fun and endlessly amusing."
>
> —Zafira

Two Steps Forward, One Step Back

These are exciting months for your baby. Think about it: teeth to experiment with, the phenomenal pleasure of being able to get from A to B with some speed and competence, sitting steadily enough to pass a toy from one hand to the other, legs that are more and more able to support him, starting to cruise around tables and furniture. For a baby it must feel like a lot to master, a lot to savor…and a lot to think about, day and night. It's no wonder they go through patches of increased neediness. *It's all very well to be able to crawl, but please, Mama, I need reassurance. Can we nurse?*

Slowed Weight Gain

At around four months old, breastfed babies begin slowing down their weight gain from a previous average of 1 ounce (30 g) a day to an average of about 0.6 ounce (18 g) a day. Between seven and nine months, this slows even further, to an average of about 0.4 ounce (12 g) a day. Only the World Health Organization (WHO) weight gain charts reflect these normal changes in the weight gain rate of breastfed babies, so if your doctor raises a red flag about weight gain, check to make sure she's using the right chart for your breastfed baby.

Concerns You May Have Between Four and Nine Months

These issues come up frequently at LLL meetings among mothers with babies between four and nine months old. If your questions aren't addressed here, you may find them in Chapter 18, "Tech Support," or the llli.org forums. And always feel free to call your local La Leche League Leader for information and support!

How Often Can I Expect My Baby to Nurse?

It's both normal and healthy for a baby from four to nine months to nurse frequently throughout the day and probably at least once at night. His body is growing really fast, and so is his mind. Nursing is conversation, entertainment, and a place to learn, explore, and play, and those reasons are just as worthy as hunger and thirst. How often he nurses varies depending on how quickly and easily he's able to fill his tummy, what his personality and sucking needs are, and what else is going on in his life. Some babies naturally begin to cut back the number of nursings between four and nine months; encouraging this, though, can lead to early weaning.

> *Elizabeth could put her hunger on hold if I wasn't around. She wouldn't act hungry for Scott, but the minute she saw me walk in the door she would cry and desperately want to nurse. We thought she could go three to four hours between each meal, but she really shouldn't have, and as soon as we realized it, she didn't anymore.*   —Laura

Is My Supply Dropping? Is My Baby Weaning?

If feedings were restricted or limited (for whatever reason) in the early weeks, milk supply may begin to drop at four months or so. By now, you've probably seen many of your friends with babies the same age who are starting to supplement with formula. Fortunately, there are many ways to increase your milk supply—see Chapter 18 for strategies.

Sometimes your supply is fine until eight or nine months—a common time for mothers to call La Leche League saying, "Help! I think he's weaning, and I was trying to nurse for a year!" The underlying reasons are often negotiated nursings ("you'll have to persuade me that you really need to nurse") and contract nursings ("the clock says it isn't time yet")—both recipes for a faltering milk supply or premature weaning.

If you want to nurse your baby according to a schedule (if it's two o'clock, then we nurse), it's like nursing by contract. If your baby has to convince you, maybe by working up to full-blown crying, that she really does want to nurse, she's having to negotiate her nursings. It's like she's saying, *If I cry, will you let me?* Neither one is very much fun for either of you... and both are hazardous to breastfeeding.

Imagine that you have to have lunch at your workplace cafeteria every day. But when you step up to the counter, you're always quizzed as to why you want to eat and why you want, say, a hamburger instead of a veggie burger. You put up with it because the food is really good and it's the only place you can eat lunch. But then one day they expand the cafeteria and put in a second counter. At the other counter, you ask for food and you get all you want, with a smile, no questions asked. Which counter will you go to?

It's the same for a baby who's always been asked why he wants to nurse. "You can't be hungry yet; it's only been an hour and a half," or "You're probably just tired. Let me rock you to sleep," or "Not now. Here's a pacifier." Then one day he starts getting a bottle to hold on to, or a spoonful of solids that he's encouraged to eat, even praised for eating. Now he feels as if he and his mother are on the same side. Nursings—and the milk supply that goes with them—start to fade away until it's just easier to give the bottle or offer the crackers than it is to fight about nursing.

If you feel you're losing your nursing relationship to negotiations and contracts, it's not too late. Make nursing fun and spontaneous again: nurse in the bathtub, take naps together, offer to nurse for no reason at all, make it silly, play with his toes and hands. It can take some time and patience to convince your baby that the rules are gone, but many mothers have turned a faltering nursing relationship into something they enjoy for many months or years to come. Make yours the lunch counter with the welcoming smile.

Should My Baby Take Naps?

Some babies nap frequently and easily; some resist sleep; some barely nap during the day but wake up only once at night. Basically, whatever your baby is doing is normal for him. Babies who are carried for much of the day usually sleep when they need to without fuss, dozing while their mothers move about. "Putting him down for a nap" works beautifully for some babies and not at all for others. In fact, many babies at this age sleep well only when they're carried or held or are sleeping on or next to an adult. Rest assured that all these babies will sleep like logs as older children and will be nearly unrousable as teens, no matter what patterns you try to establish now. So do whatever is the least stressful for you and your baby, and don't expect a schedule at this age. In fact, the least stressful approach right now may be *sharing* that nap when you can!

"Some people are closet nursers of older children. However, it is nap-time that I have yet to 'come out' with. I tell people that Lauren naps fine. What I don't tell them is that I hold her during her naps. That's right, I'm a closet holder. I can't help it. My heart melts when she falls asleep in my arms nursing, her breathing becoming slow and heavy, her face relaxed and beautiful. How could I possibly miss a minute of that? It's intoxicating and I can't give it up. Not yet.

"I have missed parties, movies, dinners, and hours on the treadmill because I can't lay Lauren down and get away while she naps. I've made up countless excuses to avoid confessing, but it has all been worth it. When Lauren is an adult and on her own, I will have the memories of the hours I spent smelling her hair and feeling her breathe while she slept peacefully on my chest. I will always remember watching her drowsily wake up with hot rosy cheeks only to look at me lazily and snuggle back into my neck or into my breast to nurse again into dreamland.

"Lauren will soon outgrow my arms, especially with a new baby on the way. This has made me hold on to and treasure our naptime even more. I have well-meaning friends who tell me, 'Try not to pick Lauren up so much. If you keep picking her up all the time, she'll have a hard time adjusting to the new baby.' I just nod. If only they knew." —Heidi

When Do We Start Solids?

Starting solids isn't quite like starting college, but it's still a big step. Your baby has probably been mouthing things for as long as he's been able to pick them up, but it's pretty obviously not been an attempt to chew and swallow them. As your baby learns to sit (around the middle of the first year), give him a place at the family table or some other regular access to solid food. At the right moment, he'll reach for food (probably off your own plate), chew it, swallow it, and reach for more. *That's* when solids start. (The World Health Organization and many other big organizations, having studied the research, agree. They could just have asked the babies!) This is not something you have to do *for* him, it doesn't require any special baby foods at all, and starting before six months (unless your baby does it herself) has minuses without pluses. It's also fine if your baby doesn't want solids for a good while yet.

Some babies, eager to imitate other family members, will be reaching for your cup or water bottle about the time they start on solid foods. Others push the cup away or use it as a toy, and prefer to breastfeed when they're thirsty. If your baby starts by sipping from your own glass at the table, with your help, he'll begin to understand how fluid behaves when it's not in a breast.

You'll find lots more information about solids and ideas for first foods in Chapter 13.

How Long Will My Baby Be Teething?

The fist chewing, gum rubbing, drooling, and sometimes fussiness that you might be seeing now may continue off and on for months, but it probably means there's a new tooth somewhere in the works. Nights may be especially restless at times, because pain probably seems worse at night when there is nothing to distract him from it. And teething really does cause a lot of misery for some babies. That's the downside. The upside is that it's such a wonderful excuse! "Well, he's teething" is an excuse that can last for many months and explain away many fussy times.

Beware of teething medications that contain numbing agents, because they can also numb your baby's tongue, possibly making nursing difficult for him.

What About Teething Rashes?

When some babies start actively teething, their saliva seems to increase and even become more acidic. This can cause a rash on their face, on their bottom, or on your areola. Rinsing breast, bottom, and face a few times a day can help.

My Baby Has His First Tooth!

First teeth may come before or after the six-month mark—some babies are born with teeth, some don't get them until after their first birthday. That first tooth has an entry in almost every baby book. It's quite a milestone, and milestones often change things. They are, of course, part of a baby preparing for solid food, but they aren't the *signal* to start solids. That signal, as we mentioned, is simply the baby grabbing food and eating it successfully.

The biggest change that a tooth makes from the moment it appears is in what you give him to teethe on. A single little sharp new tooth can be remarkably efficient at nipping off something that the rest of the baby's mouth isn't equipped to grind up, like a piece of raw carrot. So you'll probably want to stick with the frozen wet washcloth or soft toy teethers from now on.

Now, let's talk about what you *thought* we were going to talk about.

Will She Bite Me?

Many babies never ever bite, while some bite once or twice and a few go through a true biting phase. When a baby clamps, teeth or no teeth, she always gets her tongue out of the way first, or she'd bite herself. She can't suck and bite at the same time, so as long as she's actively nursing, you're safe. But when she does bite down, especially once she has those lower incisors, it really gets your attention. There are *upper* incisors, too, and they leave teeth marks on your skin! But those tooth marks rarely cause any discomfort at all because the upper jaw doesn't move and can't clamp.

Sometimes you'll find your baby gradually clamping more over time, maybe even biting, for a surprising reason: if you're holding her in a way that doesn't accommodate her growing body, she may have to tuck her chin in order to stay attached now. Way back in Chapter 4, we talked about how a baby can't nurse well if her chin is tucked. Her clamping can be an attempt to nurse in an awkward position. Try shifting her position so that her head tilts back a bit more. That may be all you need to do.

Or not. Other reasons for biting can include teething, earaches, a stuffy nose, allergies, and The Great Unknown. One mother eventually discovered a bit of facial tissue stuck to the roof of her baby's mouth. For some reason, it made him want to bite.

Remember that babies don't have a clue that their clamping or biting hurts you, so be gentle and consider these tactics:

- ☼ Take him off as soon as he bites, and set him down gently, breaking all physical contact. Then pick him up again and offer to nurse. This sends the message that the nursing has ended because of the biting; you will start a new nursing now.
- ☼ If he tends to bite at the start, try a little nipple fiddling of your own or a breast compression to hasten that first milk release to start him swallowing.
- ☼ Remember that he can't bite if his tongue's in the way. If you feel his tongue shift, either take him off or just say his name. Sometimes the momentary distraction makes him forget he had biting in mind, and the moment passes.
- ☼ Pull him in closer, which makes it harder for him to breathe and makes him let go.
- ☼ If he tends to bite at the end, just stop a little sooner for a while, or switch sides. Or keep a finger positioned right by the corner of his mouth, ready to slip in between his gums.
- ☼ Avoid pacifiers and bottles, which don't react if they're bitten. Otherwise it's a lot for a little brain to keep straight: one sucking source can be chewed all he wants, but another sucking source can't.

Biting is almost never a cause for weaning and rarely involves skin damage. If it does, you can wash with gentle soap and use a bit of household antibiotic ointment. Call a La Leche League Leader or other breastfeeding helper if biting becomes a problem.

"My daughter bit when she was teething, sometime between five and seven months old, usually at the end of the nursing session when her tummy was full but her gums ached and my nipple just happened to be handy. I learned to sense when the end of the session was approaching and had my pinkie finger poised to stop the chomp. If I was really organized, I'd have a cool teether or chewy toy available for her to gnaw on.

"My son bit when he was just under a year. He would get a big reaction from me, then he'd giggle like it was the funniest thing on earth. I was not amused. I put him on the floor facing away from me. He still wanted to nurse and he still wanted attention, but I didn't give it to him. I had a little talk with him about not biting the 'na-nas.' It took one or two more sessions of 'isolating' him briefly and he never bit me again."

—Sherrie

Will Night Nursing Cause Cavities?

There's really no need to worry. You'll find a full discussion of this in Chapter 12, but the gist of it is that research shows that human milk itself rarely contributes to decay and actually has tooth-strengthening properties.

My Baby Suddenly Stopped Nursing. Is It a Nursing Strike?

True weaning happens gradually. An abrupt, unexpected end to nursing is almost certainly a "nursing strike." Something in your baby's world has caused his favorite activity to become scary or distressing; that's not the same as his wanting to give it up for good. You'll find lots more information on possible causes and solutions in Chapter 18. Almost all nursing strikes end happily, but they usually don't end instantly, and it may be a lot easier if you stay in touch with a La Leche League Leader or other knowledgeable cheerleader who can suggest approaches and help you sort out your own feelings in the meantime.

"Sam got a stuffy nose when he was nine months old. I think he began to connect nursing with not being able to breathe, because he just

stopped nursing. Even after his nose cleared he'd turn away when I offered. I expressed milk for him, which he drank from a cup, and he really stepped up his solids.

"My relatives said it was the perfect time to wean, but I didn't think that was what he was trying to say. I tried everything I could think of, which wasn't much. The books said to nurse him in his sleep, but that wasn't something he usually did, and it didn't work now. I was holding him during a nap on the fifth day when his head tipped back and his mouth fell open. I squirted milk into it, thinking, not very charitably, that he'd either swallow or drown. He swallowed. Then he opened his eyes, turned toward me . . . and nursed just fine.

"That wasn't the end of the strike. We had to nurse that way—Sam falling asleep, me squirting milk into his mouth, Sam waking up and nursing—for another day or so. And then we went on as if nothing had happened. He nursed for two more years." —Jenny

How Do I Nurse in Public Now?

It's both easier and more challenging now. You're practically a breast-feeding expert and have probably figured out nursing in all kinds of situations—from sitting cross-legged on the floor at a friend's house to nursing while eating in a nice restaurant. Furthermore, your baby has a bit more patience and stomach capacity and now can get through outings that would have required at least one snack a few months ago.

On the other hand, he may be more wiggly and take pleasure in lifting your shirt higher than you wanted. If you've been using a cover-up, now you may risk having your baby just fling it off. It may be time to put it away. Holding his hand while he nurses can help settle him, and of course he's finished sooner these days; you can probably top him off and barely miss a beat.

You're helping out *future* nursing mothers by nursing in public. Every mother seen nursing makes it easier for the next one to do the same. And a private thumbs-up to other nursing mothers lets them know they have your support, too.

Any Traveling Tips?

This may be the easiest age for taking trips with your baby for a while. He's not yet walking, which means his tolerance for sitting in a car or plane is still fairly high. He has enough interest in his surroundings that you can distract him for at least a bit when sitting begins to get tiresome. You don't need to bring solid food along, beyond what you might be eating yourself. His diaper contents are still pleasant. And he's still a fairly small parcel to nurse in a limited space when sitting and distractions aren't enough. Take that trip now, before he starts walking!

> *"I held off on solids because we were planning a trip to a distant country when Brian would be seven months old. I didn't want to have to fuss with other foods, and I wasn't sure about the water supply. Brian would have been happy to start sooner, I think; while we were there he kept an eye on our forks. In fact, I finally let him have a stale roll, which delighted him. But I'm so glad we waited. He was an easygoing traveler. Just starting to crawl, but not so into it that he wouldn't stay happily in my lap."*
>
> —Lynne

Am I Still Protected Against Pregnancy?

The Lactational Amenorrhea Method gives 98 to 99 percent pregnancy protection for the first six months, provided you're nursing freely day and night without feeding other foods or liquids or using a pacifier regularly, and your periods haven't returned. Protection remains extremely good during the next six months if your periods don't return and if you don't often go more than four hours between nursings during the day or six hours at night. Many women do choose to add another method at six months.

Your return to fertility doesn't exactly coincide with your return to periods. Very occasionally a woman becomes pregnant before her first period, apparently releasing a fertile egg the very first time. And many women who have begun to have periods again have a few month of cycles that are too hormonally weak to support a pregnancy. But in general, once your periods return you can consider yourself fully fertile. If you are using a natural family planning method, you can begin charting your symptoms and temperature and see for yourself when ovulation returns. If your favorite method of birth control is hormonal, it's much less likely to affect your milk supply after the first six months.

My Baby Is (Choose One) Too Clingy/Too Irritable/Too Placid/Other

Most likely, what you're seeing isn't a problem but a personality. By now, your baby is beginning to announce clearly who she is. Our personalities are rounded out by our environment, but there's always a kernel that isn't. Each child is unique. You may be able to help your baby adapt a bit, but often the simplest approach is to accept your child for who she is, trust her as she lets you know what she needs, and follow your own instincts. We're guessing that Thomas Edison's mother couldn't get him to take naps; certainly the inventor of the lightbulb, phonograph, and movie camera was known for not needing much sleep as an adult!

How Can I Make Him More Independent?

Does a shy baby now mean an insecure adult if you don't start pushing him toward independence? Not at all! Independence comes from feeling secure, and your role right now is to continue to provide that secure base, just as you have been. Some babies simply need a secure base longer. Wise parents have often said, "Meet the need, and the need goes away. Ignore the need, and the need remains." Spoiling is still not a possibility at this age. Now's the time when you *get* to hold your baby a lot. He may not be looking for it as often when he's older.

What Do I Do with Him?

Babies are built to *fit into* our busy days, not to be the center of them. Do your work. Clean house, run errands, fix your lunch, go places, and include your baby. A trip to the grocery store gives far more stimulation for him than the most elaborate toy. It's sometimes called "benign neglect"— a mother focusing on her own tasks, meeting her baby's needs almost absentmindedly, but meeting them all the same. You can talk about how cold the frozen peas are, or carry him in the laundry basket, and never break stride. Your baby will probably love it.

My Baby Is (Choose One) Too Thin/Too Fat

Just like personality, some of this is built in. Most breastfed babies taper off their growth at around four months, so don't expect to see the rapid growth you probably saw at first.

Growth charts don't say how big a particular baby *should* be; they simply show how big most babies *are*. Someone will always be the biggest on a chart and someone will always be the smallest. It's not possible to have it any other way.

The most important factor is knowing if your baby is growing appropriately *for a breastfed baby*. The World Health Organization recently published growth charts based on exclusively breastfed babies around the world (whereas lots of other growth charts are based on a mixture of formula-fed and breastfed babies in just one region). You can download the WHO charts at who.int/childgrowth/standards/chart_catalogue/en/index.html. They show that breastfed babies actually grow a little faster, on average, in the first three to four months and a little slower in the period from four to twelve months, compared to formula-fed babies. You can share these charts with your health care provider if she isn't using them already (especially if your baby's weight gain is normal on the WHO charts but not the older charts).

If your baby is on the chubby side, don't worry. No evidence links roly-poly breastfed babies to later obesity. Some breastfed babies shoot almost straight up on the chart for a while, then coast with little or no weight gain for many months, and finally begin to grow slowly again as toddlers. The baby whose legs looked too massive to stand with slims down magically and begins scooting around, indistinguishable from his equally active friends. In fact, research has shown that breastfeeding ultimately protects against adult obesity. *Access* to a good milk supply and healthy solids when he's ready for them are all your breastfeeding baby needs in the way of dietary monitoring. He takes care of the rest according to a blueprint that you may (or may not) see in some of his adult relatives, and he doesn't need to have his intake controlled.

In the same way, some babies are destined to be petite. If your baby is active and on the lean side, he's probably doing just fine. No need to rush into solids or supplements to make him fatter.

If your baby truly seems to have a health problem that's affecting growth, his doctor can help you sort it out. If you feel you're not producing as much milk as your baby would like, an LLL Leader or breastfeeding helper can help you find ways to boost it. A starting point is to look at how often you've been nursing. If the growth problem is recent, perhaps you've just been forgetting to nurse as often as your baby might like.

How Do I Handle Criticism?

We can think of three causes for the criticism that nursing mothers often receive from family and others. One is a culture's sense of investment in children. Maybe it's built into us because we're a social species, but from the time strangers try to put a hand on your pregnant belly, others will sometimes behave as if your child is theirs. In a sense, he is. A society is built from all its members, and children are a society's future. On some unconscious level mothers seem to want to conform to society's child-raising ideals (the reason you may see a goth-attired mother holding a baby who's wearing a pink frilly bonnet), and society wants to make sure we do (the reason her friends gave her that bonnet). Another reason for criticism may be that not doing it the way our mothers or mothers-in-law did it feels to them like a slap in the face—a rejection of their own cherished ideas. And a third reason may be that some people are honestly fearful that what we're doing is harmful, often because they lack information about breastfeeding.

Knowing that the criticisms are based on faulty or incomplete information doesn't make them any easier to live with. So what can you do to defuse it? Mothers have found each of the following approaches helpful, depending on the situation:

- Ask to hear *their* stories, in detail and without criticism from you. Sometimes a relative or friend will lose interest in *your* story after having a chance to tell his or hers.
- Offer information. Invite your mother or mother-in-law to a La Leche League meeting, or share a news article or book chapter with her.

- ☀ Find some way to agree.
- ☀ When someone asks about weaning, the response "We're working on it" is true from the moment you start solids until whenever weaning is completed, maybe years later.
- ☀ Turn it around. Choose one: "Are you concerned? Why do you ask? Are you familiar with breastfed babies? Don't you think he seems happy and healthy?"
- ☀ Pick your battles. Sometimes you may just want to use a different room; other times it might make more sense to talk it through.
- ☀ Preempt the criticism: "I know the way Josh and I are raising Emily is different from the way you raised Josh. It means everything to me that you're so understanding."
- ☀ Agree to differ: "I know this doesn't fit with your own child-raising ideas. You can be sure we're doing our best, and this is what's working for us."
- ☀ It's your call: "We find that this works best for us."

Any activity is easier and more relaxed when the people around you can support what you're doing. If you can't get that support from family and friends, it can make a huge difference to get it from somewhere. It may help you to find friends whose philosophies are in step with yours, and find ways to spend time with them. Whether it's a La Leche League meeting, a playgroup, or a favorite understanding relative, having people who can "refill your reservoirs" can make this fun age even more fun.

> *"Babies have a knack for knowing when their mother needs to relax. When I was really stressed, Emma would nurse longer, which helped me unwind because I knew that there was nothing else as important as taking the time to nurse and hold her."* —Anne

TEN

Nine to Eighteen Months: On the Move

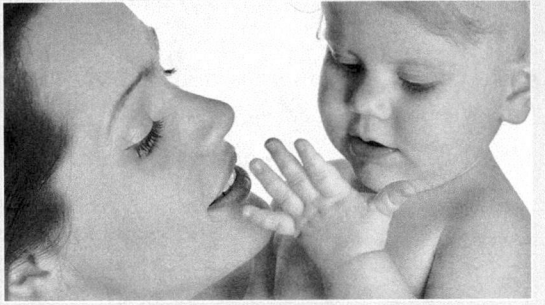

"*A few weeks ago, my baby gave me a flower. Never mind that he needed Daddy's help to pick it, or that it was missing a few petals, or that he wasn't entirely sure he wanted to let it go. It was—and is—the most gorgeous flower ever given or received. Silver and gold wouldn't buy it from me.*

"*Later, I pressed it into his baby book. I watched myself, a woman at her kitchen table flattening a wilted daffodil onto a page, and I was amazed. When in the past nine months of midnight nursings and teething and drooly kisses did I become a mother? For so long I saw my hands as the hands of a working woman on her own, hands making a living. Now I saw hands that have changed hundreds of diapers, washed and folded a thousand tiny socks and shirts, held a tiny, searching mouth to my breast late at night, held my baby dancing in the kitchen, and eased him down into sleep.*

"Seeing those hands, I understood something that has been at the edge of my consciousness since I first took my son in my arms and inhaled his newborn smell. These aren't just my hands anymore; they belong to a lineage of mothers a planet wide and millennia old. I was a woman on an April evening in a kitchen in my corner of the world, catching time between the pages of a baby book, and at the same time, I was my mother, her mother, a mother somewhere on another continent carefully tucking a flower into the pocket of her skirt, a flower you couldn't buy from her with silver or gold. We don't know each other, but all over the world and all through time, we're gathering up wilted flowers and misspelled love notes, and every single one of us knows the fierce, singular ache that's love and pride and sadness all mixed into one.

"I thought I'd become a mother the day my baby was born. It isn't so. Mothers join the ranks slowly, gradually, one caress, one diaper, one feeding at a time. And then one day we look down, and there they are: the hands of a mother, gently and with enormous strength doing the most important work on earth."   —Laura, remembering 2008

NOT LONG AGO your baby could get around only with your help. Now he can probably crawl, and by the end of this stage most babies will be walking—even running. His new mobility opens up a world of exploration. At the same time, his fine motor skills are improving. He can sit alone and play with toys. He can pick up tiny bits of food with his thumb and forefinger and pop them into his mouth. His first word might be "duh" or "buh" or "hah"—probably something that only his family understands, referring to some fascination such as dogs or birds or hot coffee. Don't be disappointed if that first word *isn't* "mama." You are a part of him, his everything; take it as a compliment!

Nursing Habits: Nine to Eighteen Months

Your nursling has opinions on breastfeeding now, not just when but sometimes where and which side, maybe sitting up abruptly and announcing,

"Side!" to indicate that this side is finished, thank you, and it's time to switch. He may joke with you about nursing. The jokes are pretty simple at first: peek-a-boo with your shirt, or exclaiming *"Hot!"* as he starts to latch but pulls away, using the only word in his vocabulary and laughing at his own silliness. It doesn't take a very big vocabulary to play!

"Gymnastic nursing" can take on an Olympic quality, with your child standing, twisting, and bending, all without letting go of your breast. Naps and bedtime become more sophisticated, maybe with books before, after, or during the nursing that is still, for most, the cornerstone of going to sleep.

By nine months, most babies are eating some solid foods, although some may not yet have started, and the quantity will gradually increase as they pass the one-year mark. Your baby will soon be sharing most of the foods you eat, even though the amounts might still be tiny. As the months go by, other foods become an increasingly important part of his total nutrition. That doesn't mean your baby isn't still getting many or most of his essential nutrients and immune factors from your milk. If your child were to stop nursing right now, the increase in his thirst and appetite might surprise you; you may be providing much more food and drink through nursing than you would guess.

As he takes more solids and your supply begins to decline, the concentration of antibodies in your milk actually increases. The proportions of some nutrients in your milk also change as your baby grows, to meet his changing needs.

The gradual shift in balance between your milk and family foods helps your child transition to the healthy diet you want him to keep eating as he grows. Or maybe he still isn't doing much more than finger-painting with solid foods. That's fine, too. For more on the shift from milk to solids, see Chapter 13.

> *"Once she could crawl, Madeline was too busy to cuddle. Even her nursings were short. She does sleep in my lap still, but I miss those long nursings. Now that she's a year old, she's starting to like to look at books. Maybe reading will be the new cuddle time."* —Danielle

Beyond Water

You probably introduced water several months ago, along with your baby's first solids, but what about other beverages?

There's certainly no need to introduce milk from other species like cow or goat as long as your child is breastfeeding well; many families never drink cow or goat milk at all. They aren't necessary for humans. If you do decide to give your child cow or goat milk, it's a good idea to wait until your baby is a year old, to reduce the risk of allergies. The same goes for soy milk, since some babies seem also to be sensitive to soy. Rice milk should be safer, but some babies are even allergic to that. Just like introducing solids, it's best to introduce these milks slowly to watch for allergic reactions. And there's some evidence that families with a predisposition for diabetes do best by waiting until a year to introduce cow milk. Fruit juices can be a treat at this age, but whole fruits are generally a better choice, since they provide more fiber and nutrients. If you do give juice, consider limiting it to between a quarter and a half cup each day, and possibly diluting it with water. Sipping juice off and on through the day can increase the risk of cavities. There's also no need to buy special baby juices or toddler drinks.

Toddlers tend to have small appetites, so filling them up with juice or water can mean they have less interest in eating more nutritious foods.

Slowed Milk Release

One of the nursing comments you may hear from your baby is, "Turn it on, Mama!" Most of us find our milk release happens less quickly as the calendar pages turn, probably because the volume has slowed down. So some of your toddler discussions may include the slowness with which the faucet turns on, when it was so ready to spill forth in the checkout line at three weeks. Think of it as one of your child's early lessons in patience.

Slowed Weight Gain

Between nine and twelve months, breastfed babies begin slowing down their weight gain even more, to an average of about 0.3 ounce (9 g) a day. As mentioned in the last chapter, only the World Health Organization (WHO) weight gain charts reflect these normal changes in the weight gain rate of breastfed babies, so if your doctor raises a red flag about weight gain, check to make sure she's using the right chart for your breastfed baby.

Concerns You May Have Between Nine and Eighteen Months

Here are some of the topics that often come up at LLL meetings from mothers with babies between nine and eighteen months old. If your questions aren't addressed here, you'll probably find them in Chapter 18 or the llli.org forums. And always feel free to call your local LLL Leader!

My Period Has Started Again

Sometime between nine and eighteen months is a common time for fertility to return, and ovulation can happen in the weeks before you see your first period. Your periods may be different from before: longer or shorter, or (if you're lucky) trailing into view over a day or two rather than appearing out of the blue at public functions in full force. While some mothers find that they have more discomfort than before, or that their breasts and nipples are more sensitive at ovulation, others find that former menstrual problems have eased.

Some mothers feel that their milk supply drops a bit during their periods, or that their older baby objects to a change in taste or expresses frustration because the milk lets down more slowly. Happily, these changes are short-lived each month, and solids are there to make up the difference. A daily dose of 500 to 1,000 mg of a calcium and magnesium supplement from the middle of your cycle through the first three days of your period may help minimize any drop in supply.

> *"I told a friend who doesn't have kids that I still hadn't had my period because of breastfeeding, and she said that made her a lot more interested in breastfeeding!"*
> —Beth

He's Not Nursing Very Often—Is He Weaning?

By now, some nursings are probably just a few minutes long, and solid foods may be greeted with enthusiasm at every meal. It's easy to forget how important breastfeeding continues to be, nutritionally and emotionally, and it may seem like the ideal time to wean. The American Academy of Pediatrics encourages nursing for *at least* a year, not weaning *at* a year; the Canadian Paediatric Society, the United Kingdom's Department of Health, and the World Health Organization all encourage nursing for *two or more* years. A child who's nearly one year old still doesn't have a very effective digestive or immune system. While he *can* manage without human milk, he isn't really designed to.

As your baby learns to crawl and walk, you may find he starts waking more at night, especially whenever he acquires a new skill. His days are so busy and exciting that he may need to tank up at night. This is not the time to night-wean; he's using these nursings for fuel, just as he did when he was tiny. If he doesn't nurse at night and doesn't make time to nurse during the day, he may not get the milk his body needs. So how can you keep breastfeeding going with one of these busy babies?

Remember that "don't offer, don't refuse" is actually weaning advice. Your baby may not think to ask for nursings. So if he's fussy or cranky, or you just feel he hasn't had a snuggle or a snack in a while, make the offer! You'll probably get in several more quick nursings a day this way, and that can make a significant difference in your relationship as well as your milk supply. Make room for a few more leisurely nursings, too, at a time and place where you can minimize distractions. Early morning, naptime, and bedtime are often good choices, and a sleepy baby is more likely to relax and nurse longer.

He's Still Fiddling with My Nipple

As nipple fiddling during nursing becomes more sophisticated, so do the solutions. If your baby has started to twist a lock of your hair between his fingers, you might see if he'd accept a doll with long hair or a blanket with a silky binding to keep his hands busy as he nurses. Having a small, squeezable toy to hold might distract the child who likes to knead your other nipple. You'll probably have to experiment to find an acceptable substitute. After a while, a child may bring his "fiddly" object to you when he wants to nurse!

My Baby Is Scared of Strangers

Smart baby! A baby's fear of strangers seems to develop just about the time he becomes mobile. It makes sense. A babe in arms is automatically safe, because his mother knows what's safe. But once he can crawl, he has to start making decisions for himself. The wise baby knows he isn't very wise yet, and errs on the side of caution. "I don't know this person or place. Where's my mother?"

It's not just strangers. Babies often have mixed feelings about being mobile. You might be sitting on the floor while your baby crawls around, staying fairly close to you. Then she spots the cat in the hallway and crawls off after him. A few minutes later, she comes back and climbs onto your lap to nurse. After just a few sucks she rolls away and heads out again—this time to investigate the bookcase. If you leave the room while your baby is off on one of her little adventures, she may be really upset. It's okay for her to crawl away from you, but not at all okay for you to leave the room!

Child development experts describe the mother as both the secure base from which a child dares to venture new things and the welcoming shore to which she returns from having adventured. Nursing serves both roles automatically. These "touching base" nursings are cute, they're flattering, they're an integral part of typical milk maintenance, and as far as your baby is concerned, they're part of playing it safe.

"I taught a yoga class for new moms when my son was ten months old. We all sat on the floor, and Tyler played nearby. While I was talking, he

> *crawled over to my lap. I gathered him in, still talking, and offered to nurse him, but he arched away. So I offered him a different toy, still talking, and he accepted it and crawled off. I realized later that I was 'mothering on the fly'—having a complete conversation with my son without having to stop my adult conversation!"*   —Michelle

What About Naps?

After the little-baby stage, some children just don't "do naps" again until the preschool years, and even then may consider them nothing but quiet time. But as children move from baby to toddler, most of them do consolidate their naps more and more. The baby who slept for ten minutes here and there may become a toddler who lives hard and plays hard for several hours at a time, then sleeps for a reliable and useable chunk of time.... provided he can nurse to sleep.

Does nursing to sleep create a bad habit? Not at all. It's very normal at this age. A small baby wants only nursing to sleep. An older baby may want nursing and a book. Older still, and the book is enough. Like all developmental stages, falling asleep on our own happens automatically in its proper time, no "training" needed. Before that time, most nursing mothers find that their child can fall asleep for someone else without nursing if Mom is out, but really *needs* to nurse if his mother is in the house. No need to rush a child out of naptime and bedtime nursings. They are one of the last luxuries of babyhood. For more about naps and nighttime, see Chapter 12.

Life Is Busy

Remember those early days, when you could barely get a snack eaten because taking care of your baby took up all your time? Your efficiency has undoubtedly skyrocketed since then, but life with a baby is always life in the fast lane. Some days you may want your little baby back, but other days you may wish your baby were six years old and not so needy! Here are some thoughts from mothers who've been there:

☀ The cute stories are starting to pile up. But your resolve to make baby book entries, like New Year's resolutions, lasts only so long. A low-tech alternative: anytime something cute is said or done, scribble it on a scrap of paper *and date it* (that's the important part). Have a place (it can just be a cardboard box) where you store the scraps. Since they're dated, orderliness doesn't matter; you can do something clever with them later. If you use a high-tech storage space—blog, Twitter, Facebook, cell phone, laptop, or BlackBerry—you may want to print the stories out so you don't lose them to fast-changing technology.

- Pick one thing a week to accomplish from your own list of goals. Maybe it's reading (or writing!) a chapter in a novel, cleaning out a dresser drawer, or attending a martial arts class. Do at least that one thing for yourself—you're important, too, and sometimes building an entire child from your milk and a few scraps of toast just doesn't feel like enough.
- Clean the bathroom while the children are in the tub (once they are old enough and you don't have to have a hand on the baby at all times). A steamy bathroom is easy to clean, you get something done, and you can still watch the kids.
- Dinnertime is tough—tired kids, tired parents. So make dinner in the morning and either use a slow cooker or put it in the fridge to reheat in the evening. Or cook in bulk once or twice a week.

What About Wants and Needs? Are They Still the Same Thing?

As your child starts to separate physically from you, the simple days of wants and needs being the same thing get a little murky. She really wants to nurse to sleep. Is that a need? Yes—in fact, nursing to sleep probably covers several needs: for milk, for relaxation, for closeness to you. She really wants your cell phone. Is *that* a need? Probably not! That was an easy one; the tests get harder and harder.

Happily, the gentle discipline you've been learning and using at the breast stands you in good stead. Substituting a safe object for an unsafe one, distraction, and removing the baby from the scene will cover almost all situations at first.

My Baby's a Biter—of Other People

It may be teething, stress, or experimentation, or maybe he just likes the salty taste of human flesh! Even an allergy can make some children want to chew. Whatever his reason, it can be a horrible embarrassment to discover that your child has taken to chomping on playmates. You can be sure that at this age it isn't prompted by meanness, anger at you, or bully tendencies. (One sensitive young man remembers smacking a playmate on the head with a stick purely because he wanted to see if the stick would bounce!)

Your best strategy may be to remove your child from potentially crunchy situations before crunch time. If you watch closely, you may be able to catch your toddler in time to prevent the biting. You can ask other mothers to help you—they may appreciate having permission to scoop your child up and deliver him to you when circumstances call for it. It really is a stage, it really will end…and it really is embarrassing until it does. But it *doesn't* say anything at all about your child's future personality or your parenting. Quick action, distraction, and patience are your best tools.

SOME GOOD BOOKS FOR TODDLER TIMES

Adventures in Gentle Discipline, by Hilary Flower
Healthiest Kid in the Neighborhood, by Martha Sears and William Sears
Mothering Your Nursing Toddler, by Norma Jane Bumgarner

We Get Even More Criticism Now

If you haven't heard it before, you're probably hearing it now: "If your baby can ask for it, he's too old to be nursing." "A baby with teeth is too old to nurse." "Mothers who nurse past a year are doing it for themselves." "You're making your baby too dependent on you." "There's no value to human milk after [choose one] three months, six months, a year…"

A simple "Thanks, but this is right for us" may be your best response. Your nursing relationship is your own and your child's, no one else's. The world's best health organizations are on your side, even if Aunt Franny isn't! For more thoughts on handling criticism, see Chapters 9 and 16.

I Suddenly Have Sore Nipples!

You've been nursing your baby happily for close to a year or more and *now* you have sore nipples? You can be sure that sudden sore nipples at this point, after many months of comfortable nursing, aren't just "one of those things."

One possibility is thrush, a yeast infection that's discussed in Chapter 18, "Tech Support." Could you be pregnant again? Breastfeeding is less and less effective in preventing conception at this stage. So even if you haven't had a period yet, pregnancy is a possibility. (Does this mean you need to wean? Almost never. See Chapter 16 for more information on nursing during pregnancy.)

Is a chipped tooth causing nipple pain? Baby teeth chip easily, but the razor sharpness that can result is also easily dealt with. A few seconds with an emery board will usually smooth any sharp edges. Your toddler may appreciate the result as much as you do!

Maybe your toddler's "gymnastic nursing" isn't always a gold-medal performance. Has she been pulling at your breast without breaking the suction, so it pops or smacks loudly when she releases it? Yowch! The same solutions suggested for biting in Chapter 9 may help end the game of Pop Goes the Nipple, starting by letting that be the end of that particular nursing.

If you have any food sensitivities and your toddler decides he'd like a little nursing for dessert after eating something you react to—peanut butter, citrus fruits, and dairy products are common irritants—you may end up with an uncomfortable rash. If you think this is the cause, ask your toddler to have a little drink of water before nursing, and use a damp cloth to wipe his face before breastfeeding and your breasts afterward.

Do you have a white spot or blister on the tip of your nipple? It could be a bleb or milk blister, both of which are discussed in Chapter 18.

If none of these reasons seems to be behind your sudden nipple soreness, your local LLL Leader can help you sift through other possibilities. Sore nipples at this stage tend to heal quickly once the culprit is found. You may have to ask your baby to go easy for a while, though. You can let her know when it hurts you and tell her she needs to be gentle. Or try saying, "SOFT mouth, honey," or "W-I-D-E mouth, W-I-D-E mouth, sweetie." A younger baby wouldn't have a clue what you were talking about. It's surprising how much your older baby or toddler understands!

What's Ahead?

By now you may have nursed longer than many of your friends. In fact, you may feel as if you're reaching the limits of nursing at this point. Not so! Your one-year-old is only about halfway to what is believed to be the biologically normal lower age of weaning. You may be appalled, surprised, relieved, or all three the first time you hear that. You may also recognize that you wouldn't have traded this past year or more for anything, and that you've found a mothering style that suits your family. We've said it before: trust your instincts. And turn the page.

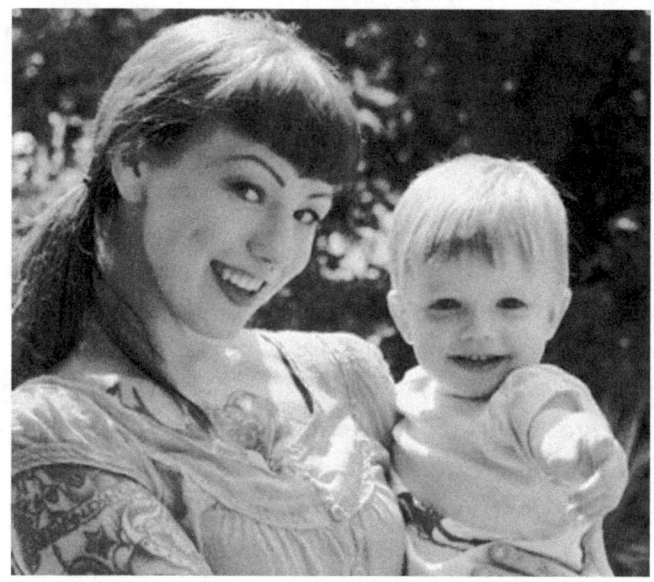

ELEVEN

Nursing Toddlers and Beyond: Moving On

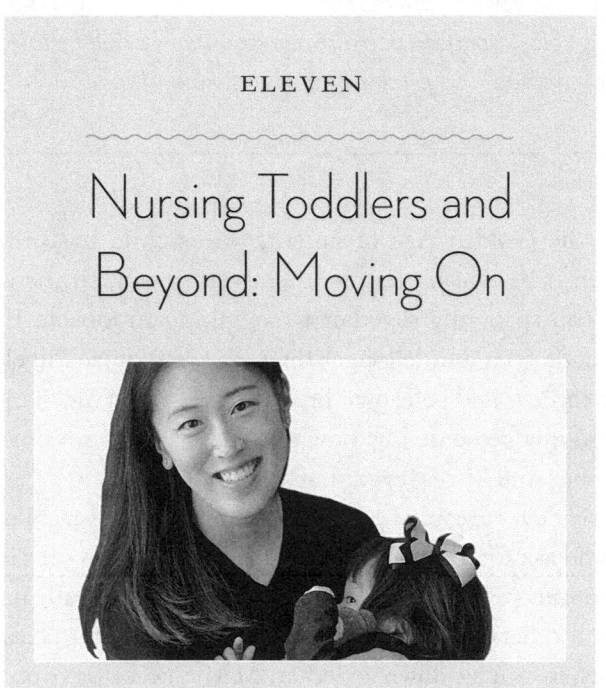

" '*Na*-na Jack Sparrow, Mama,' my two-year-old son said, and I put the action figure to my chest without much thought. Yes, I am still nursing, and not only do I nurse my toddler, I nurse his toys. But as I look down at the action figure's dark hair and braided beard and touch the slightly sneering lips to my nipple, I suddenly feel illicit. Inappropriate. As if I shouldn't tell my husband what I've been doing. In nursing that plastic Johnny Depp, I've surely violated some social norm or standard of propriety.

"From that point on I begin to place limits on what I am willing to nurse. Yes to the tree frog. No to the pink rubber rat. Yes to the hungry-looking little piglet. No to the Shrek Pez dispenser. As I reject nursing a large red monster with sharp-looking teeth, I'm teaching my son about limits: body boundaries, personal space, self-respect.

"Now I sometimes nurse a big orange robot, assorted earthmoving vehicles, Ewoks, squirrel puppets, the occasional pretzel or grape, and more. But I turn down an offer to nurse Luke Skywalker (would I have turned down Han Solo, I wonder?) and also some guy with a half-metal face.

"'Sorry, honey,' I say, 'I don't nurse that kind of guy.'"

—Molly, remembering 2009

THIS CAN BE the Golden Age of nursing. Your child has other nutrition sources, even if he doesn't rely on them very much, so the tie that kept the two of you so tightly together is beginning to loosen. If your night out with friends goes a little longer than expected, it isn't likely to matter; your child's tummy and your own breasts have grown much more flexible. Nursing is solidly cemented by now as a means of communication, food and drink, hugs and kisses, even first aid.

Maybe you never dreamed you'd find yourself nursing a child old enough to walk up and ask for it. But days turn into weeks, weeks turn into months, months turn into years. One day you realize your tiny baby has become a busy, active toddler—and you're nursing someone who takes up part of the couch when you sit down together. Maybe he brings you his favorite stuffed bunny to nurse. Maybe she's begun nursing her dolls. Maybe you haven't gotten here yet, and you're wondering what it will be like. If you're pregnant or your baby is still little, nursing a toddler might seem impossible to imagine. We encourage you to keep an open mind: it's different when it's your own child.

Is It Normal to Nurse Past Eighteen Months?

Absolutely! Kathy Dettwyler is an anthropologist who investigated the normal "weaning window" for the human species: what's the youngest that human children can normally be expected to stop breastfeeding, and what's the oldest? She set society and culture aside and looked just at the biology of a breastfeeding relationship. And she did it by looking at the group of species whose DNA is most like our own. Of course, you can't compare chimpanzees or gorillas directly to humans, but you *can* correlate weaning ages in these apes to certain biological markers: maturity of the immune system, molar eruption, adult size, and gestation. When Dr. Dettwyler looked at the ages at which those and other biological events occur in humans, she found the expected weaning range for humans was between two and a half and seven years. That fits with what we see in many breastfeeding cultures and with families in which children wean on their own.

Is it *Important* to Nurse Past Eighteen Months?

Absolutely! Your child probably wants to, and there are many other good reasons:

- Continued breastfeeding promotes normal jaw development and palate expansion—important for making enough space for the teeth that are still coming in.
- The toddler brain is going through a time of rapid growth that is designed to take place with a lot of tactile and emotional stimulation and a diet that includes a hefty amount of human milk. You naturally touch each other more and interact often when nursing, and other drinks don't stimulate human brain growth.
- Although the total amount of milk your child takes may be less, the level of antibodies and immune factors increases, an important factor when your child is putting rocks in his mouth, kissing dogs, and picking up germs from other kids at nursery school or day care.
- Young children lack mature digestive systems. Breastfeeding keeps them beautifully fed while they continue the transition to solid foods, and keeps them well fed during any illnesses.
- Nursing is a time to reconnect with an on-the-go child. This can be especially helpful if you're working.
- Nursing makes bedtime easier.
- It's the continuation of a relationship that no teddy bear or blanket can touch.
- With all the reasons to continue, "he's too old" isn't a very logical reason to stop. "He's too old because…" is the right sentence to look at. And there isn't usually anything solid that comes after the *because*.

☼ The World Health Organization, having looked at the evidence, recommends that children be breastfed for *at least* two years.

Nursing toddlers are generally pretty clear about how important breastfeeding continues to be for *them*. What about its importance for *you*?

This is an emotionally volatile stage for young children, and breastfeeding provides a valuable mothering tool that can help you soothe, calm, and comfort a child who is having trouble coping with frustrating situations. Nursing provides communication that they can understand when language and logic are still a little beyond them. Mothers of nursing two-year-olds are much more likely to refer to this age of exploration and burgeoning vocabulary as the "Terrific Twos" because they have a way to settle and reconnect with their children that mothers of already weaned children lack. As one mother said, "Sometimes I feel as if a wall goes up between me and my child for one reason or another. When we nurse, I can just feel the wall come down again. I know she feels it, too."

Many mothers continue breastfeeding because it's so central to how they mother their children. It's a whole mothering package—how they interact and manage and connect. Without this powerful parenting tool, mothering is more difficult, and children have one less resource for meeting the difficulties of early childhood. It would take an act of pushing away to stop, and many mothers simply see no reason to do so.

> "My mom is actually quite proud of the fact that I nursed my daughter for a long time, but when she mentions it in conversation to others she always says, 'You know, Lisa nursed Julia for over two years!'"
>
> "In reality, I nursed Julia for over three years, but this is a little too wild for my mom to say in polite conversation. I think it's cute that she's fine with two, though." —Lisa

Nursing Habits: Eighteen Months and Older

By now, you probably have a pretty clear picture of your child's personality. Maybe she's sociable and eager to check out new people and new situations. Or maybe she's sensitive and slow to warm up to anyone new. You probably also have a good sense of the role that breastfeeding plays in her life. For many toddlers, breastfeeding continues to be a major source of nutrition, as well as an important comfort. For others, it is a way to check in and reconnect with Mom either after work or when the toddler takes a break from playing.

How often will your toddler nurse? While the amount of separation you've experienced can be a factor, the child's personality is probably just as important. Many mothers who were at home full-time with all their children remember one who was still nursing frequently at three years old while another was running over for a quick nursing only once or twice a day at age two.

Children with allergies, especially allergies to common foods such as dairy, may continue to breastfeed for nutritional reasons longer than those who are able to tolerate a wider range of foods. That makes sense—your milk continues to be a complete food, and breastfeeding can help keep the allergic child's digestive system healthy.

Your milk supply will continue to dwindle, depending on how often your child nurses. Many mothers of older nurslings have milk supplies that have dropped to where they rarely hear swallows anymore. Yet your child may still cherish his time at breast. Human milk is a wonderful and nourishing food for as long as your child uses it. But it's the *relationship* that matters to the child. Ask any mother of a nursing toddler or preschooler about breastfeeding, and she won't give you a litany of anti-infectives and nutrients. She'll tell you about the many ways that she and her child enjoy the interaction.

Even if your child is nursing fairly infrequently most of the time, expect it to increase if she gets sick. Often a sick toddler will drop all other foods and want to nurse around the clock. She doesn't know it, but she's maximizing the amount of antibodies and immune factors and helping to speed up her recovery. And while your milk supply may be a bit low when she starts this process, by the time your child is well again you'll probably have lots of milk and end up feeling plenty full for a day or two until your supply drops once more.

You can also expect an increase in nursing frequency when your toddler is under stress. Maybe you're moving to a new house, or your child has started day care or moved to a new day care, or you've had another baby.

Those are big and obvious things. But toddlers can be stressed by small things, too, that we might not even notice. A scary encounter with a dog, a day when you were extra busy caring for another of your children, a bad dream, or having visitors over are just a few of the reasons a toddler might want more comforting at the breast. Even mastering a new skill (like learning to walk or jump) can be stressful for a child, disrupting normal sleep patterns and making him want more nursing and cuddling. During these times, breastfeeding is a great way to give your child the reassurance that he needs, while boosting his immune system when it's been weakened by stress. Bottom line: don't expect your road through toddler nursing and on to weaning to be a straight line. Every child is different, and some ups and downs are to be expected.

> Your child may begin to bring you things to nurse, or may want you to nurse his teddy while you nurse him. (Diane nursed a dead worm once at her toddler's request, tucking it under her shirt for a few moments and bringing it out still stiff, still dead. Nursing, it seems, doesn't cure everything.)
>
> Breastfed boys and girls often nurse their dolls, stuffed animals, and toys. Assuming they don't go for their navels, which are easier for them to find, you may be surprised at their ease and accuracy. They learned this from you, and they learned it early. Imagine how much easier breastfeeding will be for them, compared to what it was like for you and your friends. What a short learning curve your daughter will have! And your son will understand how and why to help his partner. *By nursing your child for a normal length of time, you're mending the breastfeeding chain that was broken in the twentieth century.*

The Fun and Foibles of Older Nurslings

Nursing a newborn is almost all physical. You're meeting a variety of needs, yes, but it's all about here and now. It's important to feed a two-month-old as soon as he shows feeding cues so that he gets enough milk, but with a toddler who isn't totally dependent on your milk, nursing can be reasonably negotiated with: "Hang on just a minute." "Wait until we get home." "I'm sorry we can't go to Grandma's today; do you want to nurse while I read to you?" Negotiations and compromise make sense at this age and give you new flexibility. They also mean that you're beginning to help your child separate his needs from his wants. Of course he *can't* wait if he's just hurt himself; of course he *can* wait if you're finishing up the dishes. And so you continue a pattern of perceptive mothering as your child slowly matures. There is more give and take...but there's also more need to consider his feelings and personality. As your baby becomes a toddler, preschooler, and beyond, mothering through breastfeeding increasingly includes understanding his feelings and emotions as much as whether or not he's hungry. Along with that come other changes in your nursing relationship. Here are a few of them.

Still Touching Base

Once toddlers learn they can run, they seem to forget how to walk! Their busyness and high energy mean that some nursings continue to be no more than touching base to make sure you're still there. So be prepared. The child who wants reassurance rather than milk may crawl up, nurse just until your milk releases, and scoot off again, maybe leaving a streak of milk across your jeans in the process.

But there will probably still be a few nursings each day that are long and languid, and are not only beloved by your child but become almost ritualized as your child learns to appreciate pattern and predictability: "No, we always do *this* side first in the morning, *that* side first at night!" In the morning before the day starts is a common time to luxuriate. So is bedtime. These usually become the final touching-base times, when your growing child takes the time to be little again.

Talking with Your Nursling

Nursing a toddler or preschooler gives you a window on the whole world of nursing, because he can talk about it. His comprehension and verbal skills give you more flexibility on when, where, and how you nurse, and his thoughts on the subject are priceless.

FROM THE MOUTHS OF BABES

*Eighteen-month-old, watching her mother's breasts appear above
the bathtub, applauds wildly and cheers!*

Two-year-old in a grocery cart: "Mommy, your nipples are nicer than
nobody else's!"

Three-year-old, planning his future: "When I grow up, I'm going to be
a fireman. I'm going to live at the firehouse. But I'm going to come
home to nurse."

Four-year-old: "Mama, when you nurse me, it's as if you take the love
out of you and put it into me."

Relaxed Physical Ties

Let's face it: one of the joys of nursing a toddler or preschooler is that you
don't have to do it! Not right this minute, not every time. You don't have to
nurse every two hours, or spend forty minutes sitting on the couch. Working mothers aren't usually pumping at this stage. Mothers at home have
enormous flexibility. Your milk supply gradually becomes low enough that
you're comfortable for much of a day without nursing. The foods you eat,
the medicines you take, the way you arrange your day—all of it is much less
connected to your child's needs. Children vary greatly in their need to be
in touch and the people they need to be in touch with, but both of Diane's
children enjoyed an occasional overnight with their beloved in-town grandmother long before they weaned. Grandma didn't nurse, but Grandma had
so much else to offer (including snuggling in *her* bed) that they were happy
to wait until Mommy showed up in the morning. Nursing becomes a comfortable old shoe—flexible, and contoured exactly to the two of you.

Mixed Feelings

Nursing an older child isn't always a garden of delights. Sometimes you
may feel pure joy at being able to relate to your child this way. Other times
you may wonder if it's ever going to end. It's natural to go back and forth in
how you feel about nursing your toddler. All mammals seem to have mixed
feelings in the later stages of nursing, feeling blissful at many feedings, but
annoyed and impatient at others. You're right on track.

"One thing that helped me enjoy nursing my toddlers was my 'blue notebook,' where I would write down cute things they said so I wouldn't forget them. One day it struck me that many of them were about nursing. Reading over the pages reminded me of how special that relationship is."
                                                                —Teresa

"I Want Boobies!"

Here's a tip—if you even *suspect* you might end up nursing into the toddler years, start using a word for breastfeeding or breasts *early on* that you'll feel comfortable hearing your two-year-old yell across the room at a family reunion or in the grocery store. Depending on your comfort level, you may want to avoid things that signal so obviously what your child is asking for.

Many parents fondly remember, long after the toddler years are over, the names their children used. Popular ones are variations on "milkies," "nummies," and "nursies." Sometimes parents or children choose words that have no obvious relationship to breastfeeding, such as "tea," "side," "uzzerside," "cuddles," "eeshies," and "yum-yum." The toddler who used "nite nite" impressed her relatives, who thought she was saying she needed a nap.

The sign language word for milk is a gesture that looks like a person hand-milking a cow, and some parents have taught that to their toddlers as an easy way to signal without alerting others in the room (thenewbornbaby .com/milks-up). Teresa's grandson Xavier made up his own sign for nursing by patting his own little chest.

"I was grocery shopping with my eighteen-month-old son for bananas. While I was in the checkout line, he wanted to nurse, but I had started feeling uncomfortable breastfeeding in public. I tried to distract him until we could get to the car. He kept tugging on my shirt, saying, 'Nanas, nanas.' The woman ahead of me said, 'Why don't you just give him the banana already?' The woman behind me popped her head around to say, 'I don't think it's bananas that he wants!' The woman behind me and I had a good chuckle, and the woman ahead of me looked mortified."
                                                                —Sherrie

Gymnastic Nursing

Most nursing toddlers have mastered breastfeeding without causing Mom any discomfort, even when they engage in "gymnastic nursing"—moving, twisting, and practically standing on their heads to nurse. It can be painful when your toddler turns her head too far to look at something across the room that has caught her attention—without letting go. At those moments you discover just how far your nipple can comfortably stretch! A Japanese print from centuries past shows a mother busy at her dressing table, with toddler attached but looking around, stress lines obvious on her breast. (It seems toddlers have been doing this for a while!) This is an age when reminders to use a "SOFT mouth" or "W-I-D-E mouth" will have more impact, because comprehension and empathy are increasing.

Tandem Nursing

That's the term for nursing your "old baby" and "new baby" together. Many mothers find it an easy way to transition the older child into his new role; it's truly touching to see the two little ones holding hands or patting and stroking each other while they nurse. Other mothers feel three's a crowd. There's no wrong approach to this; look in Chapter 16 for more details and then follow your heart.

Toddler Nursing and Working

In many ways, nursing while you're employed outside the home is easier at this age than when your baby was younger. Your toddler is probably eating and drinking a variety of other foods and is not as dependent on your milk. You may not need to pump anymore, either for your child or for your breasts.

By this age, your toddler will probably have some favorite nursing times, and a more consistent pattern that fits around your work schedule. Sometimes a toddler will be happy nursing in the morning before you go to work, when you pick him up from day care, and before bedtime. Others will want to nurse throughout the evening and maybe during the night as well. Some toddlers stick more or less to their workweek routines even on the weekends, while others seem determined to make up for lost time (and missed nursings!) by asking for the breast frequently when you're around. Remember that ups and downs are normal, and try to be flexible with your toddler if you can. If he's having a bad day, you may find yourself nursing a lot, and that may be just what he needs.

Transitional Objects

Some children have settled on favorite friends in addition to your breasts by now—a blanket, bit of satin, or stuffed animal. *Transitional objects* were once encouraged to help children cope with times when they were separated from their mothers, and they are certainly common today. Most children who nurse for several years have no need to transition their allegiance to something else; by the time they wean, their need for a security blanket has passed altogether. Nursing mothers sometimes say, "*I'm* his blankie." An older nursling, even post-weaning, may enjoy patting her mother's breast or leaning a head against it. Children long since weaned may still take deep breaths of their mother's scent when they come home from school. You may find that you, too, have a fondness for your breasts and body that you didn't have before children. They've served as hearth and home for a good long while!

> "When Jeremy was three, I brought him along on his older brother Dan's school field trip to a restored Iroquois longhouse village. The guide began by discussing with the children the natural resources that the Iroquois tribe had looked for in seeking a new home.
>
> "'What do you need to survive?' she asked the kids. 'What is something that you have to have that you could not live without?'
>
> "Jeremy immediately stuck his hand up in the air and waved it around. The guide pointed to him. 'Yes?'
>
> "'Dits!' he said (his word for nursing).
>
> "'Sorry, can you repeat that?'
>
> "'You know, milk!' Jeremy said.
>
> "'Yes, you would need something to drink. It wouldn't have to be milk, though,' the guide said. 'Now, someone else, what else can you not live without?'

"'No, not something to drink, dits!' said Jeremy, frustrated that she didn't understand. Big brother Dan tugged at Jeremy's T-shirt—he didn't really want Jeremy to go into any more detail about the importance of 'dits.' But it made me smile to think that nursing was number one on Jeremy's list of things he couldn't live without."   —Wanda

Concerns You May Have from Eighteen Months On

Here are some of the topics that often come up at LLL meetings from mothers with children eighteen months and older. If your questions aren't addressed here, you'll probably find them in Chapter 18 or the llli.org forums. And always feel free to call your local LLL Leader!

My Nipples Are Suddenly Sore

Could you be pregnant again? At this stage of lactation, breastfeeding is less effective in preventing conception, even if you haven't had a period yet. If you're pregnant, there's usually no need to wean (see Chapter 16). Your pregnancy can affect your nursing, however. Those sore nipples generally subside, although some discomfort may last throughout the whole pregnancy. Many pregnant mothers (but certainly not all) also describe an antsy feeling that makes nursing anything from mildly unpleasant to downright annoying. This may be your body saying, *One child at a time, please.* But sometimes pregnancies happen before you or your child is ready to wean. Distracting yourself during these antsy times, or finding ways to cut back on nursing at least temporarily, can help. You will normally see a drop in your milk supply as your breasts regroup for a new lactation process. Some children wean because of it, while others don't mind.

See the section on sore nipples in Chapter 10 for more possibilities. If none of these reasons seems to be behind your sudden nipple soreness, your local La Leche League Leader can help you sift through other possibilities.

What Happened to My Milk Supply?

You might have noticed that we've just about dropped the term *breastfeeding* by now. There's still a breast involved, but as the months and years pass, there's less milk because your child nurses less often. But then, the milk matters less and less now anyway. Ask a truly infrequent nurser if there's any milk in there, and he'll probably say, "Mmmm! Yes! Good milk!" Odds are he interprets his nursing experience as simply delicious, and honestly can't sort out for himself how much is love and how much is liquid. Some children nurse for years past their last audible swallow but take great comfort from the experience. So do their mothers, and nursing in those situations is likely to dwindle to nothing so imperceptibly that neither one knows or cares exactly when the last nursing took place. You can read more about weaning in Chapter 16.

> "As my daughter Lisette got older, I would let her know when the person we were about to visit wasn't comfortable with older children nursing. She soon caught on to the concept that nursing was okay with some visitors and not with others. Then one day when a friend came over, she asked her: 'Are you comfortable with older children nursing?' That certainly let the cat out of the bag!"   —Dominique

The Criticism Is Driving Us to Closet Nursing

We don't mean actually nursing in the closet, where your toddler would just throw all the coat hangers around. But many mothers, after their babies reach a certain age, don't want just anyone to know that they're still nursing. They nurse at home, but when they go out they negotiate with their children to wait until they're in a private space again.

This becomes easier and easier to do. Most people just assume that an eighteen-month-old, two-year-old, or three-year-old is long weaned, anyway, so if they don't see you nursing, they're unlikely to ask about it. It becomes more of a challenge if you have a toddler who has trouble with the "wait until we get home" approach. Even those who are fine with this most of the time can become desperate to nurse if they are feeling sick, need a nap, or are having a tough day for whatever reason.

So if you decide to take the closet approach, it helps to have a backup plan or two. If you're shopping and your toddler is frantic to nurse, you can always grab an outfit off the nearest rack and go into a changing room for some privacy. If you're visiting a friend who isn't very comfortable with the idea of a nursing toddler, just say you'd like to go lie down with your child for a while—you think he needs a nap. You don't have to explain that you're planning to nurse him to sleep. As time goes on, though, you may find that you'd rather educate people gently than pretend. Choose an approach that's comfortable for you, knowing that you can change it from one situation to the next.

Many mothers find La Leche League meetings or playgroups with other nursing mothers to be especially helpful—and fun—at this stage; some LLL Groups even form special toddler groups for mothers, or evenings for mothers and partners, whose questions are more about playground nursing etiquette than plugged ducts. As one mother said, "I look forward to those meetings as a monthly breastfeeding oasis in a mostly dry world."

> *"Eric would sometimes wander up to me when there were people at our house and whisper, 'Mommy, are these La Lechegg people?' If I said yes, he'd climb up into my lap to nurse. If I said no, he'd nod philosophically and wander away again."* —Diane

Is It Okay to Limit Some Nursing Behaviors?

Discipline issues related to nursing come up more often as nursing toddlers grow. What if your child is becoming very demanding and insisting on nursing NOW? Should you put some limits on how often and where nursing can happen? Every nursing relationship is different, and you'll be able to draw on your understanding of your child's personality and needs in teaching nursing manners. Maybe your child is overtired and hungry and has "lost it," and breastfeeding right away is just what she needs to get back on an even keel. Maybe she needs a reminder of something you previously agreed on—that you'd nurse at home, for example, but not in the mall. Maybe she's just bored and needs a distraction. Maybe it means you need to rethink the limits you've set. You may have thought it would work to wait until after you drove your daughter home from day care to nurse again, but now she's telling you that she needs to nurse right away and can't wait to get home. Maybe she's had a bad day and needs that extra source of reconnection with you.

Nursing continues to be a place where both of you learn about negotiation, patience, acceptance, exceptions, and compromise—big concepts for a little person. But nursing is a familiar, reassuring relationship in which to learn them.

My Child Is Definitely a Sparkler

If your child was a sparkler in the first few months (as described in Chapter 7), he may still be one. He's the toddler who screams where other toddlers whimper, or who just can't nap, or who continues to give you much shorter breaks than your neighbor's child seems to give, or who still goes from zero to a hundred with very little transition. By now, friends and relatives may be saying that you give in too easily, that you're spoiling your baby, that he needs to learn to soothe himself. But you're the one who knows him best. You can be reassured by the experience of countless mothers: following our instincts rarely steers us wrong.

My Child Is Still an Orchid

So was Conrad. He couldn't sit happily in a stroller; it was too far away from his mother. So she continued to carry him on her hip or in a backpack carrier. When other toddlers in his playgroup played in the center of the room, he sat by his mother, watching and listening. She sensed that all was well with him, that he simply wasn't ready to branch out. One of the playgroup mothers saw him at age eight, boarding a school bus, and said to his mother, "Well, it seems Conrad has turned out to be an ordinary kid after all." "Oh, no, he's more than that," said his mother. "He is..." She searched for the right word. "A *shining* child!" Sensitive children are often the first among their friends to enjoy remarkably independent, unusual experiences, amazing not only the naysaying relatives but their mothers as well. Did we mention how good your instincts are?

> **SOME GOOD BOOKS ON NURSING TODDLERS AND BEYOND**
>
> *Mothering Your Nursing Toddler,* by Norma Jane Bumgarner
> *Adventures in Tandem Nursing: Breastfeeding During Pregnancy and Beyond,* by Hilary Flower
> *Adventures in Gentle Discipline: A Parent-to-Parent Guide,* by Hilary Flower
> *Michele: The Nursing Toddler—A Story About Sharing Love,* by Jane Pinczuk
> *How Weaning Happens,* by Diane Bengson

Raising Children You'll Like as Adults

Discipline books and approaches that give you a cookie-cutter technique to deal with every situation often don't take into consideration different personalities and situations. If you respond in the same way to a sensitive, intense child as to a laid-back, go-with-the-flow toddler, you won't get the same results. As your child's parent, you know him or her better than anyone else. Knowing what your child needs and what's underneath his behavior means that you can provide loving guidance that teaches appropriate behavior within the limits and capabilities of your unique child.

Outside of the guarantee that cookie-cutter approaches don't work for all children, there really aren't any guarantees we can offer. You'll probably find that raising children is a continuing stumble through a landscape where the rules seem to keep changing. "I honestly don't know what to do," one mother confessed to her children during a heated sibling debate. "This one just isn't in the instruction book."

Children are people, with feelings, capabilities, and limitations that vary from child to child, month to month, moment to moment. If we work within those changing strengths and limits and look for the need that drives the behavior, if we show love and consistency, if we respect them as people who are trying their best to adjust to this strange planet they find themselves on with us, *if they know they are loved,* most likely it will all come out fine in the end no matter how much we stumble along the way.

"When my children were small, my sister told me I was over-parenting and that my sons needed to learn to be independent. It just felt right to sleep with my two young boys and nurse them until they gave it up, trying to act as their guide and not as their drill sergeant—listening to my instincts and not to the adults around me. I loved them as babies, I enjoyed them as school-age children, I had fun with them as teenagers, I respected them as adults. By the time they were ten or twelve, I realized I wasn't really parenting anymore. They had a solid central core—that's the best way I can describe it—and I felt as if their father and I were just smoothing any rough edges from then on. Mostly we just enjoyed them. Eventually my sister wrote me a letter, saying, 'I always thought you had a strange way of parenting those boys. But I have to say, they've turned into two wonderful young men.'"   —Tamara

SOME GOOD BOOKS ON RAISING
CHILDREN YOU'LL LIKE AS ADULTS

Kids Are Worth It! Giving Your Child the Gift of Inner Discipline, by Barbara Coloroso

How to Talk So Kids Will Listen, and Listen So Kids Will Talk, by Adele Faber and Elaine Mazlish

Siblings Without Rivalry, by Adele Faber and Elaine Mazlish

Unconditional Parenting, by Alfie Kohn

Hold On to Your Kids, by Gordon Neufeld and Gabor Mate

The No-Cry Discipline Solution: Gentle Ways to Encourage Good Behavior Without Whining, Tantrums, and Tears, by Elizabeth Pantley

The Discipline Book: How to Have a Better-Behaved Child from Birth to Age Ten, by Martha Sears and William Sears

Raising Your Spirited Child, by Mary Sheedy Kurcinka

Living with the Active Alert Child, by Linda S. Budd

Mommy Breastfeeds My Baby Brother, by Mark Repkin

The Successful Child: What Parents Can Do to Help Kids Turn Out Well, by William Sears, Martha Sears, and Elizabeth Pantley

Lisa, an experienced mother of seven very different children, expressed it this way: "I've watched neighbors who didn't really hold their children close at first, who realized, once they had preteens or teens, that things were out of control. They clutched a lot tighter then, but all it caused was more unhappiness. It was too much too late. I've seen my job as holding my children very close at first, and gradually relaxing my hold as they mature, until when they're ready to leave home it's almost as if they've already flown from the nest." Lisa formed a loose, containing circle with her hands as she spoke, raising her arms as she widened the circle. She ended with her arms wide and outstretched, gently releasing what she had contained.

> *"My mother told me that a dear old Swedish nurse once said to her: 'When you have one baby, you need lots of help. When you have the second baby, you can do it on your own. When you have the third baby, you can offer help to others.'"*   —Jan

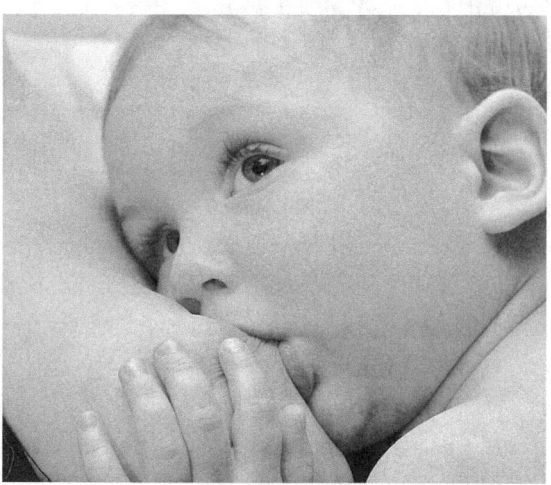

PART III

The Big Questions

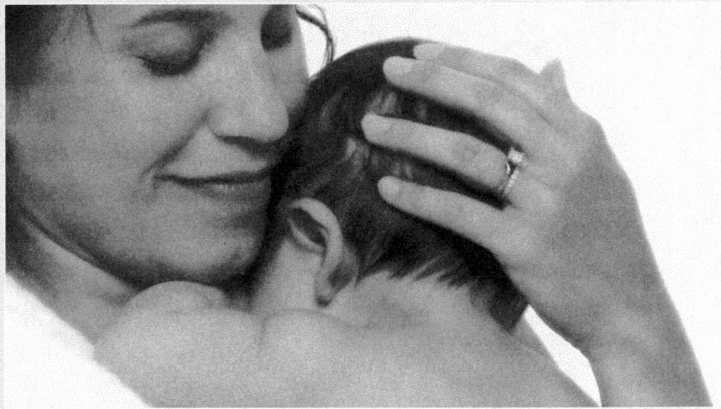

TWELVE

~~~~~~~~~~~~~~~~~~~~~~~~~~~~~

Sleeping Like a Baby

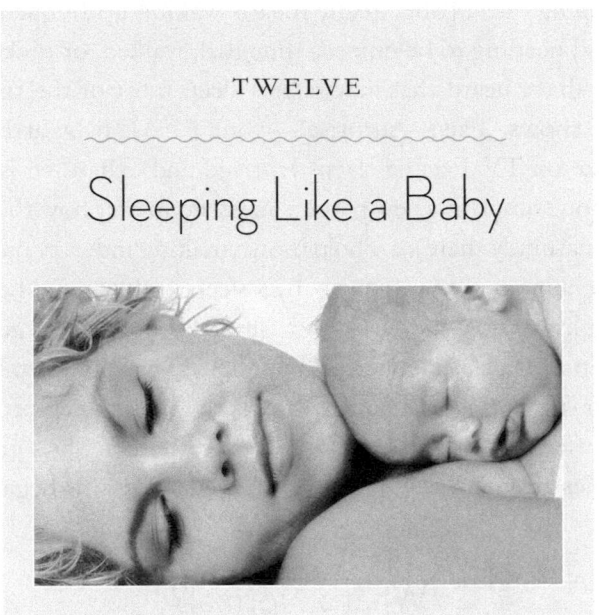

"*Poor little 'Napkin'! Of course you know that 'Napkin' is Louis Napoléon's little baby; perhaps you don't know that his mamma does not nurse him herself. I wonder does she know how much pleasure she loses by not doing it? I wonder does she know how sweet it is to wake in the night, and find a baby's soft little hand on her neck, and his dear little head lying upon her arm? I wonder does she know how beautiful a baby is when it first wakes in the morning, raising its little head... and gazing at you with its lustrous eyes and rosy cheeks, so like a fresh-blown dewy flower? I wonder does she know how delicious it is to give the little hungry rogue his breakfast? No, no; poor Eugenia! Poor empress! She knows nothing of all this. She has had all a mother's pain, and none of a mother's pleasure. She hires a woman to nurse and sleep with little 'Napkin.'"* —Sara Parton, 1857

SLEEPING WITH A baby can be lovely. But if this was the year you were hoping to maximize your rest, having a baby will most likely mess up those plans. "Sleeping like a baby" really means waking up frequently through the night and needing to be nursed, snuggled, walked, or rocked.

You may have heard that new babies sleep most of the time, like the ones in TV shows. Then—surprise!—your REAL baby arrives, and it's not quite like on TV. Feeling sleep-deprived and exhausted is one of the most common complaints new parents have, no matter how they feed their babies, and naturally there's a whole moneymaking industry out there with promises to help you "solve your baby's sleep problems." There are hundreds of books, videos, and websites with tips about how to get your baby to go to sleep alone, sleep longer, and put herself back to sleep if she wakes up. They don't mention that your baby doesn't *have* a sleep problem. Your baby isn't suffering from insomnia or sleep disorders. She's just behaving the way babies around the world have behaved since time began.

What's Normal?

As in so many other areas of life, there's a wide range of normal. In one study, the *average* total amount of sleep in a twenty-four-hour period for a one-month-old baby was about fourteen hours, but some normal, healthy babies slept more than nineteen hours, and others, just as normal and healthy, slept only nine hours out of twenty-four. And where does this sleep happen most easily? With Mama.

There are reasons for this. Our babies are born at an earlier stage of development than many other mammals. Human babies have really large, complex brains and their mothers have a pelvis that is narrow enough for walking on two legs. A developing baby's head has to fit through that narrow pelvis before it grows too big! Our babies are born when their brains are only 25 percent of their final size. A chimpanzee or gorilla, by comparison, is born when its brain is nearly half grown. *Our* babies' brains aren't that well developed until they're about nine months old.

During that time, a baby relies totally on his mother to keep him stable and secure, day and night, just as she did during pregnancy. Without her, his heart rate, breathing, and temperature are less stable. Without her, he is more likely to enter deep sleep in a pattern that's not normal or healthy for infants. He *can* manage without her, but it increases his stress level (which appears to impede his ability to manage stress later in life), and it slows his growth.

At night, babies "expect" to stay safely close to their mothers, waking as needed to nurse or reconnect. Keeping your baby close at night and letting him nurse to sleep meets his physiological and emotional needs. Having a reliable way to encourage a tired baby toward sleep—day or night—is also an incredibly helpful mothering tool. Despite all this, since about 1900 parents in most Western cultures have been advised to make their babies sleep separately and without waking during the night, starting as young as possible, with the idea that it will help them become independent sooner. It hasn't worked very well; genuine independence happens when a baby's needs are fully met, on a timetable that varies from baby to baby. Separate sleep is certainly a threat to breastfeeding—studies have shown that it is linked to decreased breastfeeding and earlier weaning, and is often stressful for both mothers and babies.

> *"Our nights for the first month and a half were really tough. Max and I needed to find our rhythm. As he got older, I learned what soothed him and we got better at nursing. Now he's a dream."* —Kasey

The Sleep-Breastfeeding Connection

What does sleep have to do with breastfeeding? Funny you should ask. Because it turns out that breastfeeding and sleep are connected in some surprising ways.

For example, a British study found that babies who had been randomly assigned to sleep apart from their mothers in the first few days post-birth were about half as likely to be breastfeeding at four months as those who'd been assigned to sleep with their mothers. Babies assigned to sleep in side-cars in those early days were more likely to be nursing at four months than babies sleeping completely separately, but less likely than babies in their mothers' beds.

Why the difference? It could be the amount of nursing. Oxytocin receptors are laid down in the early days of breastfeeding, in response to the frequency of good milk removal, and the babies in bassinets breastfed less often. But surely the mothers whose babies slept in bassinets got more sleep? Not according to the research! Babies in bassinets have to rouse and fuss more to get their mothers' attention, which means they take longer to settle. Mothers have to sit up, hoist the baby out of the box, and lift the baby back into the box (sometimes bumping the baby in the process). So *they're* more awake, too. It just plain takes both sides more time to settle back down. Simply having your baby in one of those separate boxes in the first few days (and feeding less often as a result) can reduce how long you breastfeed, without giving you any more rest.

Dr. James McKenna, a sleep researcher and expert on infant sleep, finds that co-sleeping babies breastfeed more frequently and for longer periods of time at night than babies who sleep alone. But mothers who have their babies in their beds actually get *more* total sleep than those who have their babies in another room, despite spending more time breastfeeding.

IS USING A SIDECAR THE SAME AS CO-SLEEPING?

Yes and no. A sidecar right next to your bed is better for breastfeeding than having your baby sleep across the room. Your baby can hear you moving and breathing, which is important; babies under about six months of age who are near enough to hear their mothers breathing and moving are less prone to sudden infant death syndrome because the sounds stimulate them to breathe. But he has to provide his own warmth, and he doesn't feel as safe without your body curled around him. And in order to nurse he has to rouse both himself and you much more than he'd have to if he were right next to you. Co-sleeping works best when you and your baby are touching.

For some mothers and babies, those night feedings are important for overall milk production. We all have different "storage capacities" in our breasts—while almost all mothers can make enough milk for their babies, the amount we can *store* (and give to our babies in a single feeding) varies a lot. That means some of us need to feed more often than others—and for some of us, skipping a feeding or two during the night means that the baby won't be able to get enough milk overall. Some breastfed babies who have gone through early "sleep training" programs end up with weight gain problems.

Mothers are sometimes told either that they aren't producing enough milk or that the quality of their milk isn't good enough, and that's why their babies wake in the night. Unless your baby is showing other signs of not getting enough milk, the amount of milk is not likely to be the cause of his night waking. And since milk is made directly from blood, "milk quality" is no more suspect than "blood quality."

"When Angela was born, she nursed well and gained weight fairly quickly, but she woke up a lot at night to nurse. When she was three months old, I mentioned this at a Mothers' Morning Out meeting. The organizer suggested I teach her to sleep through the night by putting her to bed at a set time and letting her 'learn to soothe herself.'

"The first few nights were hard. Angela cried more than I'd thought she would. But by the fourth night, Angela had learned to suck her fingers until she fell asleep. I was thrilled with my full night's sleep. Angela also sucked on her fingers quite a lot during the day now, and she cried less overall than she had before.

"Everything seemed fine until her four-month checkup. I was shocked to learn that she had lost an ounce in the past five weeks. The doctor suggested supplementing with formula.

"I decided to call an LLL Leader first. As we talked, I realized that not only was Angela no longer getting any feedings at night, she was requesting fewer feedings in the daytime as well. I began to treat Angela's finger sucking as a feeding cue; I also moved Angela's crib into my bedroom and planned to nurse her once during the night. Actually, she ended up nursing more often than I'd planned—once Angela realized I was close by and the milk was available, she began waking and crying more frequently again. Yes, I was still being wakened at night and was still tired, but I felt more rested because I didn't have to go down the hall. And her weight is back on track. I'm sure the day will come when she no longer needs to nurse at night. Just not yet."   —Vera

So Where Should My Baby Sleep?

In most parts of the world, this isn't even a question—at night babies sleep next to their mothers, period, as they have through most of history. More recently, cribs were invented as separate places for the baby to sleep. These were almost universal in Western countries a few decades ago, when breast-feeding rates were very low, but as breastfeeding began to increase in popu-larity again, so did the age-old idea of the "family bed." No surprise, having your baby close to you at night makes breastfeeding easier.

That doesn't mean your baby needs to be *in* your bed to breastfeed suc-cessfully. But keeping your baby close to you—in a crib in the same room, in a cradle or bassinet beside your bed, in a sidecar attachment to your bed, or actually in your bed—will make it far, far easier for you to be aware of your baby's cues and to respond quickly to breastfeed through the night. It will also mean you get more sleep—you won't have to wake up, walk down a hall, pick up the baby, sit up somewhere to feed him, walk back to the crib, and then back to your bed.

When he's in your bed, you nurse, he falls asleep, and you can just close your eyes and go to sleep. If he wakes a little, he'll be comforted by your breathing (the breathing he listened to for so many months in your womb) and your smell. He can touch you if he needs extra reassurance, wriggling a little closer if he feels he's too far away. Just as babies have always done.

If want your baby on a separate sleep surface, try nursing him on a small towel, pad, or receiving blanket. Once he's asleep, pick him up, pad and all, and transfer both. The warm surface goes right along with him—no cold bedding and strange smell when you lay him elsewhere.

But Is Bed-Sharing Safe?

You might be surprised to know that how safe your baby is in your bed depends in part on how you are feeding the baby. Studies indicate that a formula-feeding mother who sleeps with her baby tends to keep the baby up near or even on the pillows, a suffocation risk, and may or may not sleep facing him. A breastfeeding mother spends most of the night facing her baby. She brings a leg up and her lower elbow forward, creating a protective "fort" for her baby, who sleeps down at breast height where suffocation is actually much less of a risk. James McKenna, infant sleep researcher and author of the book *Sleeping with Your Baby,* calls the mother the "sleep architect" for her baby, helping him maintain a healthy, not-too-deep sleep rhythm from the start, and gradually moving him toward more mature sleep patterns. A sober nursing mother is not a danger to her child. She will *not* roll over on her baby. Partners may not be as aware of their babies when they're sleeping, so in the early months, consider keeping the baby closer to you.

The precautions in the sidebar "Guidelines for Sleeping Safely with Your Baby" may sound daunting. But if you're a non-smoking, breastfeeding mother sleeping on a regular mattress and not taking anything that might make you extra sleepy, you've got most of the potential bed-sharing concerns covered. If there are risk factors that you can't control, you might want to look for other ways to keep your baby close to you at night.

GUIDELINES FOR SLEEPING SAFELY WITH YOUR BABY

Notice that most of this list is about suffocation, not SIDS! The two are often confused. But SIDS has nothing to do with suffocation. The commonsense measures below help protect a baby from furniture and bedding problems.

- Don't have anyone in the bed who has been drinking or taking drugs that can impair alertness.
- Don't have anyone in the bed who smokes, even if he or she doesn't smoke in bed.
- Don't have anyone in the bed who is too exhausted or ill to return to normal consciousness quickly.
- Don't sleep with your baby on a couch or sofa, recliner, armchair, soft or saggy mattress, or waterbed.
- Don't use a thick duvet or comforter (a few layers of blankets are fine).
- Don't put your baby's head on a pillow.
- Make sure the sheets fit snugly.
- Keep pets off the bed.

- Make sure there are no spaces between the mattress and frame or between the bed and the wall where the baby could become trapped.
- Don't have an older child in the bed; it you do, keep an adult between the baby and the older child.
- Don't swaddle the baby.
- Don't leave your baby alone in or on your bed. Even a small baby can wriggle himself off the bed or into a risky position.
- Dress your baby about as warmly as you dress yourself—your body will provide a lot of heat.

Why Not Have Him Start the Night Alone?

Some mothers start the baby in a crib or cradle in "the baby's room," bring him into bed the first time he wakens, then let him stay there until morning. However, the baby who starts the night completely alone *has to rouse himself* in order to sleep with his parents. And rousing is more difficult during the first six months, without the normal sounds and motions of being with his mother. Babies may sleep through the night with this arrangement, never waking for that first nursing and so spending the entire night alone. You might see this as a bonus! But it may be that the baby can't rouse himself on his own, and that's not healthy. Consider having your baby start his night wherever you are—living room, kitchen, wherever—and bring him to bed with you at your bedtime. You'll probably end up nursing him more often...but it just might be the best thing you can do for his health.

SIDS and Infant Sleep

The connection between SIDS (crib death) and co-sleeping is difficult to research, in large part because where babies sleep is so unpredictable, varying from night to night and during the same night. Ask parents if they sleep with their babies, and most will say no. But ask those same parents where their baby wakes up in the morning, and most will say, "In bed with me." James McKenna reports that in Western countries between 44 and 75 percent of breastfeeding mothers sleep with their babies all or part of the

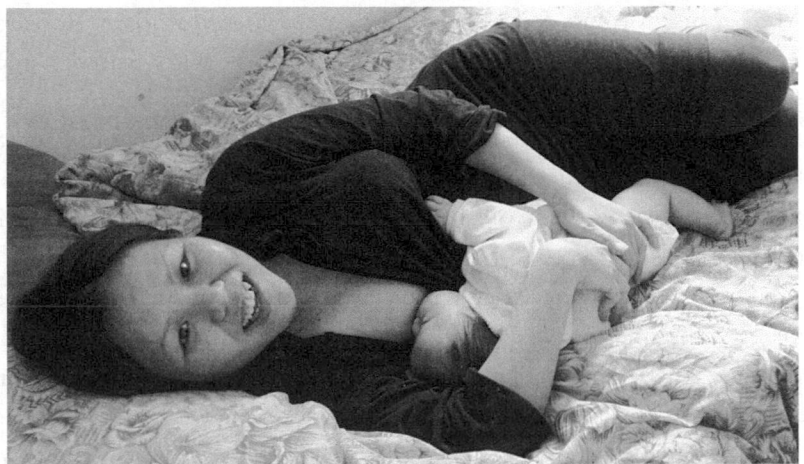

Your "cuddle curl" protects your baby.

night. Bed-sharing just plain works too well not to use it at least part-time! While research is difficult, it's well known that the highest rates of SIDS are in places in which shared sleep is not the cultural norm, and the lowest rates are in places that routinely bed-share.

There is also a tendency today to confuse SIDS risks and suffocation risks. Whenever you see bulky or heavy bedding listed in an article on SIDS, you're seeing a confusion of two completely different issues. *SIDS is not suffocation*, and suffocation risks can be avoided.

Having the baby sleep on his back is perhaps the single best protection against SIDS. That's the position babies naturally assume when they sleep with their mothers. They nurse within their mother's protective "cuddle curl," finish their snack, and roll onto their backs, still within her protective curl.

One study showed that babies who routinely used a pacifier at night were more likely to die of SIDS on a night when they *didn't* have the pacifier. Unfortunately, the results of this study have been interpreted by the American Academy of Pediatrics to mean that all babies should use pacifiers at night. But since pacifiers were invented as a replacement for nursing, they're essentially advocating nursing at night. That makes far more sense than giving a pacifier to a baby who wakes up to eat!

We also know that formula-feeding is linked to an increase in SIDS, maybe because formula-fed babies are less easily roused at night. Researchers tickled both breastfed and formula-fed babies with feathers under their noses while they slept (very low-tech). The formula-fed babies were much less likely to wake up in response to this gentle stimulation, and the researchers speculate that this might be one reason that formula-fed babies are at a higher risk of dying of SIDS: they just don't wake up as easily when something goes wrong.

Having your baby in the same room with you (as long as neither parent smokes) is also helpful in preventing SIDS. The American Academy of Pediatrics now recommends that babies be kept in the parents' room for at least the first six months—peak SIDS time—because it's simply less safe to keep them elsewhere. Your sighs, rustlings, and even snoring are stimulating to your baby, helping to pull him out of any too-long or too-deep sleep.

Unfortunately, some parents, afraid of having the baby in their bed because of what they've heard, have ended up feeding the baby on a recliner or easy chair and falling asleep there. These parents have actually left a safer space in favor of a riskier one!

The reality is, there's no clear research to link bed-sharing to SIDS, and SIDS rates around the world indicate that mothers and babies both do best when they sleep together. See "Guidelines for Sleeping Safely with Your Baby" for details, and make whatever safe sleeping arrangements suit your family best.

Breastfeeding Without a Family Bed

Maybe you have one of the risk factors that makes a family bed less safe: you or your partner smokes, or you have a waterbed, for example. If either of you smokes, it's still safest, for at least the first half year, to keep the baby in your room, where he can be stimulated by the sounds of your breathing and where you can hear and reach him easily.

If you move an older baby to another room, consider using two baby monitors—one so that you can hear the baby, and another so that the baby can hear *your* sounds. You might want to plan ways to get extra naps in during the day; getting up to feed a baby puts a bigger dent in sleep than snuggling closer or reaching out to a nearby bassinet or crib. Some mothers put a bed in the baby's room so they can lie down to nurse, even if they return the baby to a crib.

Nursing Your Baby to Sleep

You may hear the advice that letting your baby fall asleep at the breast creates a "bad habit" because it sets up "undesirable sleep associations" that require you to be there for every nap and bedtime. That's just not true. The natural design is that babies nurse, and often they fall asleep at the breast. You don't "teach" them this, and it's not a bad habit. It's just normal.

Instead, some books suggest that the baby should be taken off the breast while still awake but drowsy, and put down in a crib by himself. When mothers try to follow that instruction, they often find that feedings become stressful. The mother must closely, even tensely, watch the baby so that she can remove him from the breast before he falls asleep—but not so early that he doesn't get all the milk he needs. She has to break the suction and remove the baby, who will, more than likely, cry and protest. After this has happened a few times, babies often learn to anticipate that the feeding is about to be ended abruptly, and they might clamp down or even bite in an attempt to stop the mother from taking away the breast. They may learn to "soothe themselves," but why?

Babies tend to fall asleep when they have a full tummy, feel warm and secure, and feel tired. Breastfeeding provides the full tummy, warmth, and security, and it increases a baby's sleep-inducing hormones! Falling asleep at the breast seems to be part of the basic plan.

When you leave a baby alone in a room, he's not capable of thinking, "Hey, no worries, Mom's just down the hall watching TV." For all he knows, you've packed up and moved to Paris. He also knows that he's helpless to go and find you if he needs food, comfort, or changing. It can be very scary, and the only thing he can do is cry for you.

As children get older, this changes. A toddler understands that when you are out of the room you still exist. She can call you from her bed, and when you answer, "It's okay, I'm just in the kitchen," she is reassured by your voice and explanation. A still-older child won't even need to call you, because she knows you're there and feels safe just being in the same house with you.

Nursing to sleep won't last forever. At first, your little girl will probably fall asleep at the breast most if not all of the time. But as she gets older, you'll find she begins to fall asleep other ways as well. If you want to encourage the process, you can deliberately begin to add other things that help her doze off, like singing a lullaby as you nurse her to sleep. Then you can sing her that same lullaby sometimes without nursing, as you rock her in your arms or pat her back. It's a gradual process.

But a baby? Your baby is built to tank up and zone out. She's growing faster than she ever will again, and sleep helps with growth. Falling asleep after her meal is natural and healthy. It doesn't cause bad habits. All it really causes is … a nap.

Nap Nursing

When your baby drifts off to sleep, you might be tempted to set him down immediately so you can rush off and finish the dishes, but chances are he'll just wake up again as soon as you do. Babies who have just fallen asleep at the breast are usually in a lighter phase of sleep and are easily wakened. If you can hold your baby in your arms for a few more minutes after he drops off the breast and drops off to sleep, you'll see him relax into a still-deeper sleep. At that point, being moved to another location is less likely to wake him up. Another strategy: nurse in a sling, then once your baby is asleep, you can adjust your clothes and do whatever you need to do. Your movements as you walk and move around the house will help keep him asleep and content.

Your older baby is less likely to fall asleep at most nursings. Sometimes he nurses and then lets go on his own and looks around, ready to interact or play, and other times he nurses until he falls asleep. Try nursing him lying down on a blanket or pad on the floor, then gently move away once he's asleep—that way you don't have to move *him* at all.

Many mothers use the "ooze method." They nurse until their child is asleep, and lie there another few minutes. Then, toe by toe, bone by bone, they slink away, holding their breath that their child doesn't wake. Other mothers just enjoy the nap with their child. Some children under eighteen months can enjoy a quiet time alone, falling asleep if and when they get sleepy, but most will want to nurse to sleep.

Naptime and bedtime nursings are often the last ones a child gives up. It makes sense: what better way is there to create the conditions that lead to sleep? Nursing your child to sleep isn't something you need to learn how to do—you almost can't avoid it. Newborns nearly always fall asleep as they nurse, and older nurslings still crave it. Such a simple way to convert the daytime's buzz into quiet and calm. Why not use it while you have it?

Nursing Lying Down

Whether you're looking at smoother daytime naps for the baby or better nighttime sleep for you, it *really* helps to learn to breastfeed lying down. Chapter 4 has a detailed description of how to do it. Some mothers (and babies) find nursing lying down awkward at first, but once you get the hang of it you'll wonder how you managed without it.

SWADDLING

In a word, don't. At least not if your baby is sleeping near you. Swaddling is intended to fool a baby into thinking he's being held. With you nearby to pat him, cuddle him closer, and nurse him, he doesn't need it. And of course swaddling means he can't "hold his own" in bed with you, giving you a poke if you get too close or rolling into a comfortable position after he eats. What most babies want at night isn't a tight wrapping; it's a mother nearby. For more swaddling concerns, see Chapter 5.

Burping the Baby at Night

Most breastfeeding mothers just don't. If yours is one of those babies who are more comfortable at night after burping, try draping the baby over your side while you're still lying on your side, or sitting *him* upright and rubbing or patting his back for a while. *You* don't have to sit up, and he gets a little vertical time to let some air out. You might want to nurse him again on the breast you just used, to help him drift back to sleep.

Too Much Milk?

Occasionally a mother with a generous milk supply and rapid milk release finds that her baby won't easily nurse to sleep. Just as he's relaxing off to sleep with some slow sucking, she'll have another milk release and he's faced with way more milk than he wants at the moment. He may pull off and cry instead of sleeping. You might be able to solve this by following some of the tips on slowing down milk production in Chapter 18 or by switching him back to the less-full breast at this point in the feeding.

Dressing *for* Bed…and Dressing *the* Bed

If your baby sleeps with you, she needs no more than a diaper and a light shirt. You'll probably appreciate a shirt yourself, since there are inevitably more blanket gaps with that extra little person sharing them. Many mothers wear a T-shirt; some cut it short to keep their shoulders warm and their breasts freely accessible. Pajamas or a nightgown with buttons to near your waist also work fine. Some larger-breasted women like to wear a loose sleep bra (to provide support without constriction). In the early days, you may find life easier if you keep a stack of diapers, some wipes, a wastebasket, maybe breast pads or a cloth diaper to tuck into a nightshirt and catch drips, and a change of clothes for both you and the baby at your bedside. Leaks happen whether or not you and your baby share a bed, and a fresh change of clothes can help a soggy insomniac—mother or child—get back to sleep. Depending on your baby's skin sensitivity, you may be able to skip middle-of-the-night diaper changes after the first few weeks, but most mothers like to keep diapers handy just in case.

About the bed: While some women don't leak milk at night, others produce lakes. If leaking at night is a problem for you, waterproof mattress pads, flannel-covered waterproof fabric, or even a section of shower curtain can protect your mattress. Some mothers keep a couple of large bath towels handy, spreading a clean, dry surface as needed and dropping the damp one to the floor until morning. Most mothers find wet spots are more likely to be a problem in the first few weeks, when their supply is high and little legs are too skinny to seal the diaper well. You may also leak again for a while once your baby starts sleeping for a longer stretch at night. But most mothers find that leaking stops being an issue eventually, although the timing varies. Consider any leaking to be a handy way to keep your breast from getting too full. If you didn't leak, you might wake up sooner!

One more valuable piece of nighttime equipment is a night-light, left on where it gives you enough light to nurse by (or change a poopy diaper by), yet is dim enough to sleep by.

"When I was pregnant with my first child, I pondered the best sleeping arrangement for the baby. I had slept in a cradle as a new baby and so had my nieces and nephews. I bought a very nice wooden cradle, excitedly put on the cradle bumpers that had been mine as a baby, purchased a new cradle sheet, attached a mobile, and placed it at the foot of our bed. We bought a bedrail, planning on having our baby sleep in bed sometimes, like if I fell asleep after I nursed her, but mostly in the cradle at the foot of our bed.

"When Elizabeth was born, she spent her first night nursing in the nursery, something we hadn't expected. The next night she was in the bassinet in our hospital room, but not happy there, so we moved her into our double bed so we might be able to get some sleep. We took turns sleeping because we didn't want to hurt her in our sleep and her breathing seemed so stilted, which is apparently perfectly normal for newborns. The third night, we were at home and tried to have her sleep in the cradle, but she wasn't happy, so we moved her to our bed. By the fourth night, we put up the bedrail and just started her in our bed. She has gone to bed there every night since.

"Within a few weeks we were raving to our friends about how easy and fun bed-sharing was. Time in bed with our daughter is a highlight of every day. She wakes up cooing in the morning and has done some hilarious things trying to avoid falling asleep, things I would have missed if she had been in the cradle. It's like having a slumber party every night: we giggle before we go to sleep and she gets to eat in bed! My husband and I have the rest of our lives to share a bed alone, but only a short time to share it with Elizabeth." —Laura

Is This the End of Sex?

What happens to your sex life if you have a baby in your bed at night? Probably the easiest thing is just to leave the baby where he is. You can also move him temporarily to another sleeping surface—a bassinet, cradle, or crib if you have one near the bed, or a blanket on the floor. If your baby's fallen asleep in a car seat, you could bring baby and bucket into the room (although it's not a suitable bed for long periods). The main point is that *the baby doesn't care* what you're doing, so long as *he* feels safe and comfortable. Expect to be interrupted sometimes, though. Some sixth sense often makes babies want their mothers when their mothers are really focused on something else, whether it's sex or sorting socks.

With a toddler or older child who can safely be left alone in your bed, you can just leave the child behind and go to another room for some intimate time together. Every home is full of horizontal (and vertical) surfaces. Get as creative as you need to—maybe even hire a high school student to take your baby for a walk for an hour in the evening and take advantage of that alone time. You'll find a way. That's why so many bed-sharing children have younger siblings!

Musical Beds

Many bed-sharing families go through a whole series of sleeping arrangements during their child-raising years. If your partner has an earlier and more exacting wake-up time, he or she may sleep separately at first—a centuries-long tradition in some cultures. Or an early riser may start the night with mother and baby, then move elsewhere later in the night. Or vice versa.

Some mothers have the baby sleep separately in the same room, then bring him into bed for a leisurely early-morning cuddle and nursing. An older child may start out in his own bed and trot down the hall to his parents when and if he wakens. Or he may crawl in with his older brother across the room. Some families have a daybed or twin mattress on the floor next to the parents' bed for nighttime visitors. Jenna looked forward to school-age Thomas's nocturnal visits, because he'd snuggle in with his dad while she left to snuggle into *his* warm bed, which she felt was the most comfortable one in the house! These musical bed arrangements, which may change many times over the years, have one main goal—to give the most people the most sleep *tonight*.

The simplest early-parenting sleep arrangement is probably to take your own bed off its frame and set the mattress on the floor. "Falling out of bed" is no longer an issue, all the cracks and crevices are gone, you can add a twin mattress to create a wall-to-wall bed if you want, and no one ever needs to know exactly what your sleeping arrangements are.

> "Babies are adaptable! Mengjie has our crazy schedule and goes to bed near midnight sometimes. She gets ten to twelve hours of sleep at night and one or two naps, but they aren't scheduled at all. If I'm asleep, Mengjie will almost always stay asleep. She'll wake up, see me, and go back under after a little nursing."   —Mei Ling

But I'm *Really* Exhausted!

What can you do when you're exhausted and your baby keeps on waking up? Surprisingly, research finds that exclusively breastfeeding women who sleep with their babies get the most sleep of all, even though their babies wake more often. Why? There are probably several reasons in addition to the ones we covered earlier. Mothers who breastfeed exclusively are in a hormonal state that facilitates sleep. We don't have to wake up fully to meet our baby's needs. And since we sleep best when we feel confident that our baby is safe, we don't fret that baby is out of sight. Lily remembers a sense of rightness when someone asked, "How often does the baby wake at night?" and she answered, "I have no idea." Teresa remembers her husband asking if the baby wakened during the night, feeling for a softened breast, and answering, "Apparently."

The reality is that new motherhood usually involves a sleep deficit for a while, regardless of how a baby is fed or where he sleeps. But there are some things that other mothers have found worked for them—maybe some will help you and your baby.

- As much as possible, sleep when the baby sleeps. Turn off the phone and get into bed, even if it's 11:00 a.m. or 7:30 p.m. Learning to nap can be a lifesaver for a tired parent.
- Nurse lying down or laid-black as much as possible. Even if you don't sleep, being horizontal helps enormously.
- Pay attention to your nutrition. Often when we're tired we resort to caffeine and sugary foods to keep up our energy. They may work in the short term but they end up making us even more drained. A healthy, balanced diet will maximize your energy and ability to cope with interrupted sleep.
- Get all the help you can—not so much with tending to the baby, but with everything else (laundry, groceries, housecleaning, cooking, etc.). You may have friends or family who can help out, or your budget may allow for one or more of these services. If the help just isn't available, you may need to let some things go until you're less tired.
- Limit visitors (other than the ones who are helping with laundry, groceries, housecleaning, cooking, etc.). If people do come over, stay in your pajamas or nightgown so they get the message that you aren't really "up and around." It may also encourage you to go back to bed when the baby sleeps.
- Go to a La Leche League meeting and complain! It's a safe place where people *won't* respond with "Well, why don't you just wean?" You'll almost always get useful ideas. You'll *absolutely* get sympathy and reassurance that this stage is temporary, as it certainly is.
- Getting outside with the baby for at least an hour or two every day really seems to make a difference in how well the baby sleeps at night. That fresh air and change of scenery is good for you, too.
- Most babies seem to have their days and nights mixed up at first—they sleep well during the day, then are wide awake at night. Some persist in this unfortunate preference for months. You can encourage them to change by offering to nurse more during the day (babies will often latch even if they are half asleep) and keeping them in the main living areas of your home so they'll be stimulated by noise and activity.
- Or keep that reassuring noise and activity going at night, in the form of white noise—a fan or air conditioner, or a radio set to a quiet station or to very soft static. Some babies wake because of the unaccustomed

stillness of night, after months of their mothers' raucous heartbeat and stomach rumblings!

- ☼ Keep a night-light on so you can see enough to function when your baby wakens, but don't turn on other lights. The gentle message is that night is for sleeping and eating and sleeping again, not for fun and games.

- ☼ Take turns with your partner or another support person in getting extra sleep while the other person tends to the baby. Maybe you could get up with the baby on Saturday, leaving your partner to sleep late, but on Sunday you could sleep in while your partner tucks the baby in a sling to make breakfast for you, brings the baby up for a quick nursing an hour later, and then goes out for a walk with the baby while you keep right on sleeping. (Hey, it's a thought!)

- ☼ Have a "sleep angel." This is a doula or experienced breastfeeding person whom you pay (or who loves you enough) to stay near your room at night *and who expects to be wakened to help you with breastfeeding* or anything else. Sometimes just the panic of being fully in charge of a tiny life keeps us from getting much-needed rest, especially if breastfeeding is still shaky. Knowing that your sleep angel is just a room away, ready to come and help in any way you need at any time you need, can help you relax and get to sleep. In breastfeeding cultures, family has always assumed this role automatically. Sometimes just a night or two with a sleep angel can give you enough sleep to change your outlook.

- ☼ Having one four-or-five-hour period of unbroken sleep may make a world of difference without causing engorgement or a drop in supply. Have a partner or friend watch over you and the baby—a kind of mini sleep angel—for a stretch while you sleep.

- ☼ Ask your partner to help relax your tired muscles by giving you a backrub or a foot massage—or consider seeing a professional massage therapist. Some of your tiredness may be related to aching muscles from carrying your baby around or sitting in less-than-comfortable positions.

- ☼ Remember that our notion of eight straight hours isn't based in either biology or history. Our no-electricity ancestors had a *much* longer night than we have today, and they didn't spend all of it sleeping. They often had a period of sleep, a rather lengthy middle-of-the-night period of wakefulness, and another period of sleep. Lengthen your "night" by going to bed early and staying in bed in the morning, and know that you're sharing your wee-hour wakefulness not only with your ancestors but also with other mothers all over town.

- ⚬ Turn your clock to the wall so you can't see the time. If you're not paying attention to exactly how much sleep you got (or didn't get), you probably won't feel quite as worried or resentful about not getting enough.
- ⚬ Know that this is temporary. On about Day Four, you may feel that life as you know it has sunk into a morass of sleepless chaos. But this is absolutely temporary, and it's absolutely survivable. Get help where you need it, knowing that ending breastfeeding won't help. This is just normal life with a new baby.
- ⚬ If you find that you simply cannot sleep *at all,* check with your doctor. That kind of sleeplessness is neither healthy nor sustainable, and may require treatment.

What About Sleep Training?

Sleep training had its beginnings many decades ago, in an age when we thought Science and Schedules were the way to a trouble-free life. Little babies, of course, need their mothers' presence not only for a sense of security and for physiological stability but also for food. Sometimes the parents who say proudly that their child sleeps through the night have actually trained themselves to sleep through the child's waking—not the safest or healthiest of arrangements. And of course SIDS is more common in babies who sleep alone and without waking during the night. At least one well-known proponent of sleep training, Dr. Richard Ferber, has publicly altered his position on "crying it out" at night in light of more recent research.

Encouraging your baby to sleep for long stretches at night is also a risk to your milk supply, especially if done in the first few weeks, when it is being calibrated. Even after that point, mothers whose breasts have small storage capacities will receive the chemical signal to slow down production when their breasts get full. This is why many mothers who train their babies to sleep through the night discover that they have milk supply issues down the road.

Would Cereal Help?

Parents are sometimes tempted to give the baby some cereal before bedtime to encourage him to sleep longer. When researchers tested this, they found that adding solid foods didn't help babies sleep more—in fact, for some it caused more night waking because of digestive problems or allergies. Parents may have thought it helped because many babies start to sleep longer around the time they start solids, but it's not because of the solids.

Night Nursing and Cavities

If your child suddenly has a few cavities, night weaning will almost certainly be recommended. But is it really necessary?

No. There is no evidence that nighttime nursing causes cavities. Other mammals with teeth nurse day and night, and they don't get cavities. Dr. Brian Palmer studied children's skulls that were thousands of years old—way older than toothpaste—and *he found almost no cavities*. Why would this be? One reason is that human milk does not pool around the teeth during nursing; it is pulled instantly toward the throat and swallowed. Another is that cavity formation is inhibited by the lactoferrin, IgA, IgG, and high pH levels in human milk. Human milk also actively strengthens teeth by depositing calcium and phosphorous on them. The children whose teeth Palmer examined also ate a diet low in carbohydrates and processed sugar. *Many* research studies have shown that *human milk does not cause cavities* unless there is another carbohydrate source.

But nursing children today do sometimes get cavities, even if they have their teeth brushed often and well and haven't had carbohydrates after brushing. The reasons aren't known for sure, but there is evidence that the mother's prenatal diet and antibiotics received during pregnancy can affect the quality of a child's tooth enamel and his resistance to cavities. (In those cases, the permanent teeth are almost always fine.) Our modern diet also has many more cavity-inducing foods. Human milk is no match for the dried fruits, fruit juices, crackers, and those cute little O-shaped cereals that turn into sugars. It's often impossible to get all those sugars off a squirmy child's teeth. There is also a particularly damaging kind of oral bacterium—*Streptococcus mutans*—that's especially hard on tooth enamel in the presence of sugar. Babies can pick up *S. mutans* from adults who carry the strain and who share food, utensils, or mouth kisses with them. It's much more likely to be these factors that caused the cavities, so night weaning almost certainly isn't going to solve the problem.

> *"It is store food which has given us store teeth."*
>
> —Ernest Hooton, 1938

The best way to avoid cavities is to wipe or brush your child's teeth thoroughly at least twice a day. It might help to encourage him to swish with (or at least sip) water after eating. It makes sense not to offer any carbohydrates after bedtime teeth cleaning. But there's no need to keep your child from nursing at night since human milk by itself actually helps protect against cavities.

In extreme cases, some dentists may recommend wiping a child's teeth after each nursing, including during the night (which neither mother nor baby enjoys, as you can imagine). There's absolutely no research that shows this is necessary, but some mothers who have done it think it made a difference, so it might be something to consider if all else fails. Some mothers have found xylitol helpful; ask your dentist about what and how.

SOME GOOD BOOKS ON BABIES AND NIGHTS

The Baby Sleep Book, by William Sears, Martha Sears, Robert Sears, and James Sears
The Family Bed, by Tine Thevinin
Nighttime Parenting, by William Sears
The No-Cry Sleep Solution, by Elizabeth Pantley
Sleeping with Your Baby, by James McKenna
Helping Your Baby to Sleep: Why Gentle Techniques Work Best, by Anni Gethin and Beth MacGregor
Good Nights: The Happy Parents' Guide to the Family Bed (and a Peaceful Night's Sleep!), by Maria Goodavage and Jay Gordon

"By fourteen months, Sarah was mobile enough that napping alone in our big family bed wasn't safe. But a crib wouldn't let me snuggle and nurse her to sleep. We decided on a low toddler bed that she can get in and out of safely. Our naptime routine became a diaper change, turning on the radio, and then nursing. I stay next to her until she is asleep; then I can get up and take care of nearby chores. If she wakes up, I come back and offer to nurse, and she often takes an extended nap. After about six weeks she had learned the routine: I changed her diaper and she went to the radio and pushed buttons until our station turned on, then she climbed into her bed. Later, when I asked if she would like to nap in the big bed or her bed, she pointed to her room and walked to her bed. I feel so happy that she is starting to enjoy her bed."

—Jeanne

I Don't Want Her in Our Bed Forever!

No, of course your sixteen-year-old isn't going to be sleeping in your bed! But the process is two steps forward, one step back, and highly individual. One day, we promise, your baby will sleep four or five hours straight one night. You'll be shocked! Then she might wake over and over from teething. Then the five hours will stretch to six or seven hours without waking up, maybe followed by a short nursing and another two or three hours of sleep. You'll be holding your breath when you tuck her into bed the next time, wondering if it will happen again. It might. Or it might not, but in time her nighttime hours of unbroken sleep will increase, and so will yours. (And when your baby is a teenager, she'll sleep like a rock and you'll find you can't drag her out of bed in the morning.)

If you move your baby or toddler from your room before she asks (as they all do) for her own room, do it gradually and with love. Try out the crib or floor mattress or bed in the new room as a site for naps first. Consider starting a white noise source in your room before the move, and moving the noise source along with the child. Or get a baby monitor and use it backward, piping your nighttime noises into the other room to provide comfort and a sense of continuity. If possible, move the toddler in with an older sibling. Some mothers find a separate room actually cuts into their sleep at first; calls for nighttime company increase temporarily while the little one adjusts. (If you find that nightmares, night terrors, or head banging begins, you may want to return to co-sleeping for a while longer.)

Lots of mothers ease into separate sleep or fewer nighttime nursings by experimenting. You could try bringing your child into bed with you at the first waking, or move her to the new bed after the first nursing. Or try having your partner do the back-to-sleep soothing. Let your little one sleep with your partner but without you, and see how that works as an intermediate step. But here's what makes it compassionate: if your child is unhappy, go back to what was working before and try moving toward separate sleep again a few weeks or months later.

The age of readiness for separate sleep or unbroken sleep varies hugely. One mother *finally* convinced her high-need five-year-old son to try sleeping in his own room. As soon as his two-year-old sister saw the new arrangement, she wanted her own room, too! Like many parents, they found to their surprise that they missed having their children in their bed. And like some parents, they found that important conversations with their teens and even with their adult children still took place with a child lying on their bed. "Mummy, you know what Kristin said today?" "Mom and Dad, what do you think I should do about soccer?" "I've met this boy...." Family beds can be flexible. They can last a lifetime, changing form over and over and over to meet your family's particular and ever-changing dynamics.

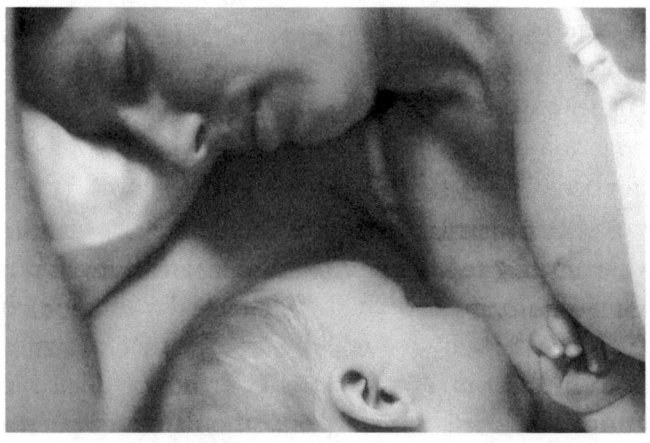

THIRTEEN

The Scoop on Solids

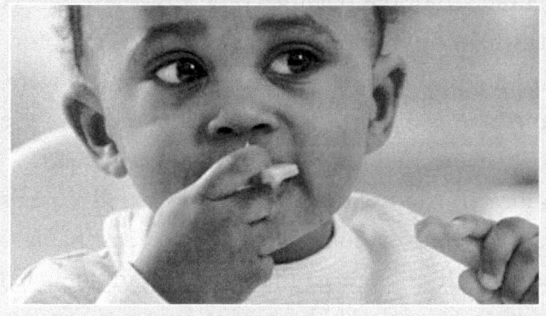

"Matthew rolled over before he was six weeks old, and crawled before he could sit up. At five months, he was sitting on my lap at lunch one day when he tried to put my spoon in his mouth. I thought he might be ready for solids, so I offered him a little of the baked sweet potato from my plate, but he really just wanted the spoon to chew on. About three weeks later, Matthew crawled over to the dog's dish and ate some dog food! My doctor laughed and said this could be a sign that he was ready for solid foods. She was right. That night at supper I passed him over some chunks of cooked-to-mush carrots and he happily ate them and looked around for more.

"His younger sister, Lisa, was completely different. At six months, she smushed some pieces of banana into her hair but not her mouth. Eight months? No! At ten months, my perfectly healthy daughter finally ate a few bites of the food I'd been offering at every meal. My milk

> *was still a major part of her diet for many months to come, but she was started on solids."* —Teresa, remembering 1986

LONG AGO, BEFORE there were baby food manufacturers or even spoons, babies ate what their parents ate. Not the nuts and tough meats, of course, but whatever family foods they could handle. Most likely no one had the time or interest to feed a baby who wasn't already reaching for someone else's food. Long ago, of course, all babies were breastfed.

During the first half of the twentieth century, there was a dramatic shift away from breastfeeding. Mothers were given a recipe for making "formula" for their babies, but let's face it, those formulas were pretty crude. Babies sometimes showed signs of malnutrition after just a few weeks, and doctors realized they needed to provide some supplements.

Their solution? Early solids—highly processed cereals and pureed foods that even tiny babies could keep down reasonably well, and that might be digested well enough to make up for any deficiencies. Feeding cereals and purees to formula-fed babies by six weeks of age soon morphed into *all* mothers being told to start solids within the first six weeks, which is why your Aunt Franny may be suggesting cereal long before your pediatrician—or your baby!—says it's time.

Let's say your baby is four months old. Even though he never seemed all that interested in it before, these days he practically drools as your fork travels from plate to mouth. You're probably hearing from the cheering section that this means he's *so* ready for solids. But is he really?

Here's what some of today's Official Bodies have to say:

- ⚲ *The World Health Organization:* "Infants should be exclusively breastfed for the first six months of life to achieve optimal growth, development and health. Thereafter, to meet their evolving nutritional requirements, infants should receive nutritionally adequate and safe complementary foods while breastfeeding continues for up to two years of age or beyond."
- ⚲ *The American Academy of Pediatrics:* "Introduction of complementary feedings before six months of age generally does not increase total caloric intake or rate of growth and only substitutes foods that lack the protective components of human milk."

- ☼ *The Canadian Paediatric Society:* "Recommends exclusive breastfeeding for the first six months of life for healthy, term infants. Breast milk is the optimal food for infants, and breastfeeding may continue for up to two years and beyond."
- ☼ *The United Kingdom's Minister for Public Health:* "Breastmilk is the best form of nutrition for infants. Exclusive breastfeeding is recommended for the first six months (26 weeks) of an infant's life, as it provides all the nutrients a baby needs. Breastfeeding...should continue beyond the first six months along with appropriate types and amounts of solid foods."
- ☼ *Your Aunt Franny:* "You had orange juice and cereal at a month, and look at you now, you pretty thing! Besides, I want to take a picture of his face with his first food. Let's give him ice cream. What can it hurt?"

Sounds as if Aunt Franny's in the minority. Let's ask one more Official Body—your four-month-old: "Mmmm, shiny! I could sure chew on that fork thing if she'd let me! What's Mama doing? It always smells good when she does that. If Mama does it, it must be important to do. Mmmm, shiny!"

Not exactly the comment of an eager diner—more like someone who covets your utensil. At four months, this makes sense. She's already well fed, so she's really not hungry. It's probably the novelty of the whole "eating thing" that she's finally noticing and is fascinated by. But listen in a few months later: "Ooh, I want, I want, I want. Maybe I can reach from where I'm sitting. Ha! I got my hand in her plate. Mmm, tasty! More!" Now *there's* someone who can choose a food, grab it, put it in her mouth, chew it, swallow it, like it, and reach for more. *There's* someone who's ready for solids, and she didn't need the World Health Organization or your aunt Franny to tell her so.

Maybe you're thinking that other foods would help your baby sleep through the night. Not according to the research. In fact, your baby might sleep *less* well because of the indigestion that too-early solids or formula can cause. Babies sleep through the night when they're able to, which sometimes happens at around six months, but not because of the solids. (And then, of course, they may start waking up again later. Development is often two steps forward, one step back.)

"The more children I had, the less I did to start solids. As with toilet train-ing and sleeping through the night, I learned that this was something that would accomplish itself when the child was ready. Although I duti-fully offered my firstborn mashed banana when she turned six months old, I quickly realized that she was not yet ready, and waited for her to grab food off my plate, which to my surprise actually happened about six weeks later. With my younger boys I just waited and let it happen."
—Dena

So What Makes a Baby Ready for Solids?

Remember how we said that it's Mama's job to provide access and Baby's job to feed? Well, the same applies to all mammal babies when they start solid foods. A mama horse doesn't clip the grass and lay it at her foal's feet. He gets it himself once he's old enough to have a strong set of teeth and the ability to select, chew, and swallow. Mama just finds her own good-tasting grass, which means her baby has good-tasting grass nearby, too. She's pro-viding access, he's feeding. But he didn't until he had the interest, the teeth, the chewing, and the swallowing all figured out. And all of that was *his* job to develop, not *hers*.

The same is true for your baby. His insides are designed to be ready for solid food once his outside has developed enough for him to eat it on his own. If he can't pick up food, get it in his mouth, and chew it without chok-ing, then he's just not ready for solids, and his tummy probably isn't ready, either. He'll acquire all those on-the-outside skills by about six months. And that's when his digestive tract is ready, too.

Sure, you can get food in his mouth sooner. But he'll probably try to push it back out with his tongue. The tongue thrust that decorates his shirt front with strained squash also protects his digestive tract from anything foreign that gets into his mouth. What if you put the food farther back? Now you've bypassed his defenses—something he wouldn't do himself—and while he's more likely to swallow, he's also more likely to choke.

Another natural anti-choking device is your baby's inability to pick up small objects on her own until around eight months, when she develops her pincer grip, using her thumb and forefinger. Until then, her chances of being able to get anything tiny (like a raisin or pea) into her mouth all by herself are pretty slim. The takeaway here is that it's not necessary to do the job for her before she's ready to do it herself!

Why does a baby's digestive tract need to be mature before he starts solids? Two words: allergies and enzymes. Allergies first: If a baby has *anything* besides your milk before the lining of his intestines becomes pretty well sealed against *allergens* (allergy producers) at around six months, some of those substances can slip through the intestinal walls into the bloodstream. Your baby's body reads them as invading forces and produces antibodies against them. Problems such as eczema can result. Allergic responses to early solids don't happen in all babies, and the allergies aren't always life-long, but they happen often enough that it's a really good reason to hold off on solids until that intestinal wall is good and secure, at about six months.

Enzymes are what we use to break down foods for digestion, but babies aren't born with the enzyme levels they'll need as adults. Why should they be? They're eating the most digestible food in the world—their mothers' milk. Give a baby something else before he starts producing adult-type enzymes at around six months, and you're more likely to see upset tummies, diarrhea, smelly gas, and a baby who *swallows* food but can't *use* it well. It might even come out in the diaper looking pretty much unchanged.

A baby's system is less likely to have an allergic reaction to foods by around six months. His digestive enzymes are up and running at around six months. He's able to eat food all by himself at around six months. It's pretty clear that this is when human babies are designed to start eating solids.

By letting your baby wait to eat table foods, you won't have to bother with any of the baby cereals, which are really just processed starches with very little nutritional value. The main reason people recommend baby cereal is that it's fortified with iron. But most breastfed babies don't need nearly that much iron. Too much iron can increase not just constipation but infection and even microscopic bleeding (see the section on vitamins and minerals in Chapter 8).

Signs That *Don't* Mean Baby Is Ready for Solids

There are a lot of signs that may make it seem to you or your friends and family like your baby is ready for solids. But do they really mean that? Not usually. Here are the most common red herrings.

Growth Spurts

Does your three-month-old baby suddenly seem much hungrier? Breast-fed babies don't need larger and larger amounts of milk for at least the first six months or so. Instead, their intestines become more efficient, their metabolism slows, and at around four months their rate of growth naturally slows. Unlike formula-fed babies, breastfed babies don't need larger and larger amounts of milk.

Instead, you may be seeing a *growth spurt*. These tend to happen around three weeks, six weeks, three months, and six months. Suddenly your baby may want to nurse all the time and your breasts may feel constantly empty. But it's not because you don't have enough milk. It's because your baby's taking milk faster than you can make it. Your milk supply will gear up accordingly. Growth spurts tend to last for three days or so and then your baby settles back down to eating the same amount as before, sometimes leaving you with full breasts that take another few days to settle down. (If you feel your milk supply is truly faltering, check out Chapter 18, "Tech Support," for suggestions.)

Efficiency Experts

Is your baby finished in five minutes where at first he took forty? That's normal, too. Many babies get much more efficient at removing milk and don't nurse as long when they're older. *SLURP* and they're done.

Distractibility

Around four to five months, babies start noticing the big, bright world outside their mothers' arms and suddenly can't concentrate on nursing. This doesn't mean that they're less interested in breastfeeding or are outgrowing it. They're finally developed enough to be really aware of their world, but they haven't developed enough to take in both the world and milk at the same time. It's just the Four-Month Fussies, and it doesn't last. Pretty soon your baby will be old enough to plug into both his surroundings and your breast at the same time. (Until then, he may nurse more often at night, when life is less exciting.) To help your baby settle down and nurse during this stage, try breastfeeding in a soothing, darkened room, maybe lying down, either in silence or with quiet, relaxing music.

Starting Solids the Easy Way

Your baby can join the dinner table fun, even if she's not quite ready for solids. Beginning whenever she can sit on her own, whether or not she's truly ready for solids, you can bring her high chair up to the table next to you, or sit her on your lap at the table. Give her a spoon and maybe water in a sippy cup, and let her play Dinnertime. Is she looking enviously at your plate? Put some baby-suitable food in front of her and see what she does. Babies who aren't ready for solids may play with food, maybe even taste it, but they won't get serious about eating it.

Then the day comes when that food in front of her makes it into her mouth and down the hatch! You don't have to control the amount. She'll take care of that, just as she does when she nurses. And one of the cool things about waiting until she does it herself is that there's usually much less mess, partly because she's more skilled, and partly because she really wants to do it.

Unless she comes from an allergic family, you don't have to make a big deal about waiting a few days between each new food to watch for allergies (see the sidebar "Foods to Avoid in Baby's First Year"). She's a big girl now—that intestinal wall is solid—and odds are she's not going to have a problem. If she does show signs of a reaction (rashes on her face or bottom, for instance), she may have a true sensitivity to a particular food. Just offer one kind of food every few days to find the culprit. (In fact, the occasional sensitive mother gets a rash from her baby's saliva once she starts solids. If this happens, try wiping your breast with a damp cloth after nursings.) To help head off problems for either of you, don't give her anything you know you or anyone else in the family is allergic to.

You may be told to avoid fruits because they can make your child favor sweet foods. Don't worry; *nothing* tastes sweeter than your milk!

Once you know your baby is willing and able to feed himself, you can try spoon-feeding if you like. Use a baby spoon or even a regular table spoon to give him tiny bits of any appropriate food you're eating. Try holding the spoon sideways and touching his mouth, signaling him almost the way you might with your breast. He'll "lip" it off the spoon if he's interested, or turn his head away if he isn't. Or offer a bit on your finger and watch his expression when he tastes the food. But remember that no baby needs to be fed with a spoon or finger. Starting solids is something they can do themselves, enjoy doing themselves, and control best by themselves.

The sour face? That's going to be common with every new food for some babies. It isn't necessarily that they don't like it; they've just never tasted it so strongly before. But they *have* tasted it! Formula always tastes the same, but your milk has always had faint echoes of whatever you eat, so these first tastes of family foods will probably seem familiar to your baby. In fact, research shows that formula-fed babies don't accept new tastes as willingly.

Your baby will signal you that his meal is over when he starts fingers-painting with his food. When food smeared exceeds food swallowed, you can end the meal with a cheerful "All done!" and clean up.

SOME SIMPLE STARTER FOODS

Fruits—*Slightly Mushy or Baby-Fist-Sized Chunks to Hold*
Apple—peeled, grated, or lightly cooked
Avocado
Banana
Blueberries—frozen or raw
Melon
Pear

Meats—Cooked (Shredded or Slivered) Versions to Gnaw On
>   Chicken—remove the bone, or offer a cooked drumstick with just a
>   little meat still on the bone
>   Ground beef, pork, or lamb; a bone from beef, pork, or lamb with
>   fat and most meat removed
>   Fish—serve small pieces of flaky well-cooked fish; watch for bones

Vegetables—Cooked Till Limp or Cooked and Mashed
>   Beans—very soft or mashed
>   Carrots—ditto
>   Hummus—Hmmm…maybe offer it on your finger!
>   Peas—frozen or cooked; removing skins helps digestion
>   String beans
>   Sweet potato—big chunk or mashed with water or your milk
>   White potato—big chunk or mashed with water or your milk

Grains (Avoid Wheat in Allergic Families)
>   Whole-grain breads (stale for gnawing)
>   Whole-wheat breadsticks
>   Rice cakes
>   Sticky rice

Proteins and Fats for the Vegan/Vegetarian Baby
>   Seed butters (such as tahini) as dips or spreads
>   Beans and lentils, very soft or mashed
>   Seitan
>   Avocados
>   Nut butters (for non-allergic families)

Note: If you are raising your baby vegan, don't forget his need for supplementary vitamin B_{12}; talk to your doctor if you have any concerns.

If a food is traditional for babies in your family, and if your baby is old enough, go for it!

FOODS TO AVOID IN BABY'S FIRST YEAR

Allergy, Rash, and Food Sensitivity Risks

Berries containing small, hard seeds, such as strawberries, raspberries, and blackberries

Citrus fruits, including oranges, lemons, and grapefruit

Corn products

Cow milk and dairy products (maybe the most common allergens)

Egg whites (yolks generally are okay)

Kiwi

Peanuts and peanut butter

Shellfish

Wheat and wheat products

Choking Risks—Not Suitable for Babies and Toddlers

Hot dogs, even small slices

Nuts

Popcorn

Raw carrots and similar hard foods

Other Problem Foods to Avoid

Dried fruits (including raisins, dates, and figs—too sticky for them to deal with easily)

Honey or corn syrup (may contain botulism spores, which you can handle but a baby under one can't)

Foods high in saturated fat, such as fried foods (unhealthy, hard to digest)

Foods high in salt (unhealthy)

Foods that contain sugar or artificial sweeteners (unhealthy)

Balancing Solids and Breastfeeding

You can relax about this if you let your baby lead the way. There isn't usually much impact on your milk supply at first, because most babies start by eating very little. "Servings" may be tiny—one or two bites each. Over time, they take more and more solids, keeping your milk supply the same but increasing their total calories. Then gradually, usually well after a year, they begin to favor solids over your milk. First it's your milk with solids for the joy of it; eventually it's solids with your milk for the joy of it. And they do it all by themselves. Pretty simple, eh?

To make sure your baby is getting as much of your milk as he needs when you're beginning solids, it generally helps to nurse him before you both sit down to eat (if you get a chance). This will take the edge off his hunger and put him in a better mood for the meal. When you're both finished eating, offer to nurse again. He may fall asleep at your breast and take a nap, or he may not, and that's fine. When he's older, you can just do what feels right—feed him before, after, either, or neither. Some meals will replace feedings, and some feedings will happen instead of meals. No calculator needed!

She Wants to Eat off My Plate!

Smart baby! She knows not to trust her own judgment yet. Maybe babies are programmed, for their own safety, to want only what they see the grown-ups eating. You can try putting her food on your plate first, offering it to her when she wants it.

What About Salt and Spices?

We've grown accustomed to much more salt than we need. Leave the salt off when you fix your baby's food. Babies can enjoy surprisingly spicy and flavorful foods, but, to quote an earlier edition of this book, start out with "plenty of fanfare but very little condiment"!

Whole Foods Are Ideal

La Leche League has always recommended a well-balanced and varied diet of foods in as close to their natural state as possible. Fresh foods are usually better than frozen, and frozen foods are preferable to canned. By concentrating on unprocessed foods, you and you your baby will get all the known nutrients in their natural proportions. You may even get micronutrients that science hasn't discovered yet.

> *"When I realized that Graham was going to eat how we ate, I knew I had to change. It wasn't easy, learning to cook and think about food in a totally different way while taking care of a baby. And how were we going to afford organic food? Now Graham is two and I can look back at my consternation and smile. Today we eat an organic whole-foods diet, local when we can, and I regularly cook things I had never heard of eighteen months ago. I planted my first garden this year, and he helped! I can't wait to harvest and cook stuff together. Who knew an eight-pound addition to the family could be so transformational?"*
>
> —Amy

Consider Organics

Certified organic fruits and vegetables are grown without any (or only a few approved) pesticides. Certified organic meat contains no hormones or antibiotics. And the farming is usually more environmentally friendly. But organic food can be also be expensive.

If organic foods are tough for your budget, consider at least buying organic versions of the thin-skinned fruits and vegetables that are more likely to have high pesticide residues, such as peaches, nectarines, apples, pears, strawberries, cherries, bell peppers, spinach, and lettuce. Fruits with thick skins or rinds, such as bananas, oranges, avocados, pineapples, and mangoes, are more protected from pesticide residue. Onions and asparagus also tend to have fewer pesticides. More information on the pesticide load of fruits and vegetables can be found at foodnews.org. They even have an iPhone app!

BANANA STICKS

Did you know that inside every peeled banana half are three baby-sized bananas waiting to be let out? Gently squeeze the sides near the cut end until you see the banana start to break into three sections, and separate the sections carefully—just right for a tiny fist!

A FEW GOOD RESOURCES FOR INTRODUCING SOLIDS

Baby-Led Weaning: Helping Your Baby to Love Good Food, by Gill Rapley and Tracey Murkett

Whole Foods for Babies and Toddlers, by Margaret Kenda

Feeding the Kids: The Flexible, No-Battles, Healthy Eating System for the Whole Family, by Pamela Gould and Eleanor P. Taylor with Dr. Katherine Cason

Whole Foods for the Whole Family, by Roberta Johnson

My Child Won't Eat! How to Prevent and Solve the Problem, by Dr. Carlos Gonzalez

Child of Mine: Feeding with Love and Good Sense, by Ellyn Satter

rapleyweaning.com (here *weaning* means adding anything else to a breastfed baby's diet, *not* ending breastfeeding)

borstvoeding.com/voedselintroductie/blw/engels.html

Pamphlets from your local LLL Group

Chewing for Your Baby?

Lois moved to Alaska before her first child was born. When her daughter was six months old, she absentmindedly chewed a bit of salmon for her at a party and fed it to her. An indigenous Upik woman sidled up to them and asked shyly, "Do you chew for your baby?" It was something all the Upik women did; they didn't think outsiders would.

Chewing for your baby is probably as old as humanity, and many of us have used it to make a less appropriate food more baby-worthy. It even adds some digestive enzymes. Is there any harm in it? If you're HIV-positive, we're still waiting for studies to know for sure. The only other harm would be from bacteria in your own mouth. And by now your child's mouth is probably well colonized, for good or ill, by whatever the family had to offer. But if you've had serious tooth decay problems yourself, you might want to steer clear of this original baby food grinder to avoid giving your baby the bacteria that make cavities more likely.

Is There a Window of Opportunity for Introducing Solids?

Babies don't come with an instruction book, so it's really unlikely that a child will flunk solids because his mother missed that page. It *is* true that some children have real difficulty with chewing and swallowing and need a specialist's help. Maybe the notion of a window of opportunity first came from children who didn't start solids "on time" and who went on to have difficulties. But of course, these children were late in starting because they *couldn't* start earlier.

There's another type of window of opportunity that has been examined in research studies—that perhaps gluten (present in wheat, rye, and barley) must be introduced between four and seven months of age to avoid having problems with gluten later on. The babies in those studies were not necessarily exclusively or even mostly breastfed, however. Their intestinal tracts had already been altered by the too-early introduction of other foods or liquids. Does this affect the studies' results? Who knows! Consider the studies something to ponder, especially in allergy-prone or colitis-prone families, but not something to take seriously until better studies come along.

"If dinner was potentially staining (tomato sauce), we let the kids eat topless. Bath time immediately followed dinner if necessary." —Cathy

He Feeds Himself and It's Still Messy!

Babies don't know messes are work to clean up—they just know they're fun! After all, this is not Queen Victoria you've invited to tea.

Here are some ways to keep the mess down and the enjoyment up:

- ☼ Use a high chair without the tray, to have a family dinner table. Abbie's family screwed two small cup hooks to the underside of the table and tied a loop of twine to each arm of the high chair. With the chair hooked to the table at meals, her baby couldn't push himself over backward. (This may not be an issue with high chairs that have wider bases.)
- ☼ In warm weather, outdoor meals are ideal. You can just hose down the high chair afterward.
- ☼ Use a plastic tablecloth under your baby's place at the table as well as on

the table, and you won't have to look back at the carpet years later and say, "Yep, that's where Michael sat."

- Keep his cup at your own place. He'll learn to reach for it when he wants a drink, and there'll be less spillage. But do offer water. He may still be on a mostly liquid diet, but we all enjoy a beverage with our meals (and cups are such fun!). If you use a sippy cup, consider removing the valve. Maybe more spills, but easier for your baby to manage, and better for learning how liquids work, which means less spilling in the future.

- Keep a washcloth handy to mop up spills, hands, and face. But don't be too overzealous. Imagine having your own dinner interrupted six times by a cold, wet cloth across your mouth.

- If you don't use a dining table, your baby can sit with you on the couch or floor and cruise the coffee table during dinnertime once he's older. Later, you might find yourself using a table after all because it creates a space where everyone is facing one another. It literally brings families together. Research indicates that a family dinner is linked to improved children's grades, reduced risk of obesity, and even reduced risk of substance abuse in the years ahead.

- Remember that dogs can be excellent floor cleaners when there are children at the table.

Why Can't I Just Hold His Hands Down and Feed Him?

Some parenting books suggest that you keep control of the feedings, partly to help your child understand who's in control and partly to keep things neater. These books overlook our basic biology, though. We naturally feed ourselves from infancy on. When a baby is learning about solids, he learns with all his senses, not just taste. Feeling, turning over, examining, and squeezing are all part of the learning process. Imagine being blindfolded and having someone else put a brand-new taste and texture in your mouth. Yes, your baby can see his food, but the sight means nothing to him. You would ache to take that blindfold off and investigate the new food thoroughly. So does he.

Will letting him feed himself lead to a healthier attitude toward food, in this era plagued by obesity and eating disorders? Maybe. There are numerous reports of children whose parents controlled their meals and who rebelled in the only way they could—by refusing food, sometimes to the point of ill health. Nancy Williams, a marriage and family therapist in California, shared the following with us: "When hold-their-hands no-mess parent-controlled infant feeding got big out here I predicted what I would see in the future. I am sad to have been right. I see a high number of adolescent girls with bulimia and anorexia whose parents used controlled feeding. I think the problem is that they have no control over their eating as infants and they grow up with this distorted sense of lack of power, particularly around food. The experience of eating itself is not satisfying because it is not driven by normal hunger and satiety."

An interesting study found that most three-year-olds who are given just a little too much food to eat left the extra behind; most five-year-olds eat the extra. They have learned, over time, to ignore their internal cues. Directed feeding, whether it's "clean your plate" or preventing exploration and self-feeding, may not be in a child's long-term best interests.

You've given your baby an excellent start toward a healthy diet by following his appetite cues during breastfeeding. A little mess as he learns the textures, tastes, and delights of solid foods is just another part of that healthy start.

What if I'm Working?

If you're working full- or part-time, you may want to wait until you're with your baby to offer solids the first time, so you can enjoy the experience and make sure he's truly ready. At first, offering solids only when you're both home will be enough. When your baby is ready to eat regularly, talk to your caregiver about what to offer and how much, sharing your interest in letting your baby feed himself (she may really like that idea—less time and trouble for her). Instead of buying baby foods, you can provide leftover finger foods from your own dinner when you pack his lunch.

> "One trick I used with my oldest in day care was to mash up carrots and other cooked veggies and freeze them in ice cube trays so I could send them along for lunch."
> —Serena

What if He's Not Interested?

Not a big deal! Your milk is all he needs for many months to come, providing a nice wide comfort zone. It's a complete blend of protein, fat, carbohydrates, vitamins, minerals, electrolytes, and fluids, not to mention anti-infective, anti-inflammatory, and immune-system-boosting factors. Your "late starter" or "long-term dabbler" isn't missing any developmental milestones. In fact, she may sense that her body is more sensitive, and the lack of interest may protect her from foods that could create sensitivities. Or she may still need to develop her chew-and-swallow skills. She just needs a few more weeks or months. And if there's a particular food she doesn't like? She'll probably be happy to try it again later.

He Eats Anything I Give Him—Is He Going to Wean?

Some babies think solids are the greatest thing since, well, sliced bread. Make sure you have plenty of opportunities to nurse for comfort as well as food, and he probably won't throw you over for cooked carrots. Should you limit his solids? Not if he's self-feeding nutritious foods. But watch the sweets and junk foods. Your Eager Eater won't know they exist if they're never on the menu.

SAMPLE DIET OF A TYPICAL WELL-NOURISHED TODDLER
(not to be taken seriously!)

Early morning: Wake up, nurse.

Breakfast: Two bites of scrambled egg; dump the rest on the floor. One bite of toast.

Late morning: Nurse three more times between breakfast and lunch. Several pieces of carpet lint.

Lunch: Half tube of Pulsating Pink lipstick. One handful dry dog food (any flavor). One ice cube.

After lunch: Nurse, nap.

Afternoon snack: One rock or uncooked bean, thrust up left nostril.

Dinner: Pour juice over mashed potatoes. Two shreds of chicken, one green bean. Nurse.

Bedtime snack: Throw a piece of toast on the kitchen floor.
Late evening: Nurse to sleep.

He Hardly Eats a Thing!

Most toddlers go through a phase when they seem to live on air. That's completely normal. Most of his fuel will come from you for a good many months to come. Starting solids is usually a slow process. And then there's the issue of slowing growth. If your baby kept gaining at the typical infant rate, the most petite lass would be a sumo wrestler in no time. Toddlers often grow very slowly for a while, and slow growth in a small body means not very much food required. Take a look at the "Sample Diet of a Typical Well-Nourished Toddler" above, and you'll probably feel better about your own child's diet.

Baby-led is mama-simple. Wait until he's around six months old, and follow your baby. Less mess, less worry, less money, less checking, and much more fun for everyone.

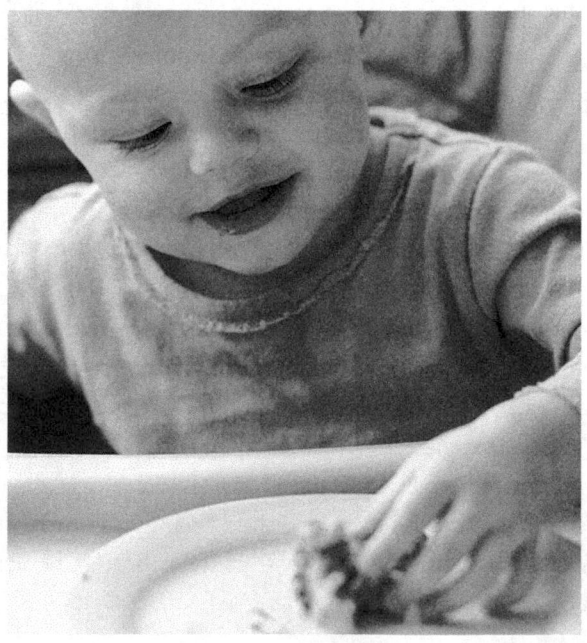

FOURTEEN

When You Can't Be with Your Baby

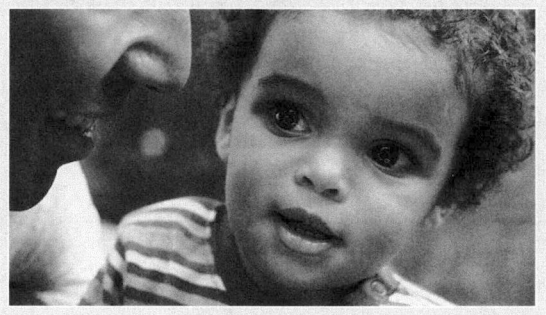

"When Anna was born, I was in the United States Army, a clarinet player in a highly selective ensemble. Yet, as soon as I held Anna in my arms, I knew that I never wanted to leave her. Not even for an hour! She was so tiny, so sweet…and happiest in my arms and at my breast. I felt incomplete without her; our connection was obviously what Nature intended.

"Until she was six months old I went directly to her after my morning rehearsal, pumping once in the four hours we were separated. At six months, she could have a serving of fruit or cereal mixed with my expressed milk, which afforded me more flexibility. I brought my baby and a caregiver to concerts and on overnight trips. I demanded the time and space to express milk when my duties required me to be separated from Anna longer than the time between feedings. I did my best to ensure that my baby was fed and secure while I performed at a level acceptable to the ensemble I was part of.

"I was fortunate that my commander was married to a La Leche League Leader and supported my efforts. He knew that I would be a more productive member of his unit if my baby was cared for. The hierarchy in the Army is very defined, and in the eyes of some, I overstepped propriety in order to meet my baby's needs. But to me, breastfeeding was Anna's need and right, and I would do whatever it took to meet that need for her. I made Anna's needs the framework around which to fit my work, instead of finding ways to make my baby fit into my job.

"I discovered that it was possible to meet the needs of my baby and give my work the attention it deserved, but this took a great toll on me physically. When could I sleep? I felt resentment about being spread so thin. But I also discovered that while a baby's needs are immediate, they are not permanent. The intensity of her needs evolved and could be satisfied in other ways as they became less immediate.

"I am still amazed that my career did not fall apart when I could not give it my full attention. I worked hard to regain any ground I lost when my babies were so dependent, and I learned to accept that my children's needs waxed and waned. The years spent juggling have been worth it. Because we stayed physically close to facilitate breastfeeding, we developed an emotional bond that stayed constant after breastfeeding ended. I never imagined that becoming a mother would change how I saw myself, that my achievements in music would pale in comparison to my achievements as a mother."

—Cassandra, remembering 1999

EACH MAMMAL'S MILK gives clues about how often those mothers and babies need to be together. Some, like rabbits and bats, make milk that's very high in fat and protein. They feed their babies, hide them away, and go off for the day (or night) to find food while the babies slowly digest their milk. Many hours later, the mothers return and feed the babies again.

Human milk isn't designed for that kind of mothering. Because our milk is relatively low in fat and protein, our babies need to refuel often. And our breasts are designed so that they need to be emptied often while the baby is small or they start to get uncomfortably full and milk production drops. By adjusting his nursing patterns, the human baby can also adjust the milk to meet his changing needs—a process that works well only if he can feed as often as he wants to. That's our basic biology.

But some mothers, out of necessity or choice, are separated from their babies at times—maybe for an hour here and there, or for hours every day, maybe even for a few days or more. Can breastfeeding continue? In most cases, yes, with a little extra effort. All of biology is bendable, but only so far, which is what this chapter is about: bending biology where it can bend, and bending *to* it where it can't.

Returning to Work

All the reasons that you chose breastfeeding are still important, and some are even more important now. For example, babies in day care are exposed to germs from many different families and have a significantly higher risk of infections and illness than babies who are with their mothers full-time. The antibodies in your milk help your baby fight those germs and recover quickly if he does become ill. What mothers often find matters even more than health issues, though, is the continued connection that breastfeeding fosters. Breastfeeding keeps mothering hormones circulating in your system. Knowing that your baby is drinking your milk helps you take care of him even when you're apart. And at the end of a long workday, breastfeeding provides the most normal, secure way for your child to grow into his expanding and sometimes scary world.

It can be a scary world for you, too, leaving your baby, adding questions about breastfeeding, wondering how it all will work. Planning will help you control your situation so that your situation doesn't control *you*.

Planning Your Maternity Leave

The longer you can be full-time with your baby, the easier it is to get breastfeeding established and keep providing milk while you are separated. Governments around the world that see children as one of their biggest future assets offer maternity leaves that allow mothers and babies many months of a solid, healthy start together. Canadian mothers are usually able to combine maternity leave with parental leave to give them a full year with their babies if they choose. New Zealand mothers are given six months. In Sweden—brace yourself—mothers and fathers *each* have 240 days of parental leave paid at 80 to 90 percent of their full salary, and fathers can give the mothers up to 180 of their days. If they have twins or more, they get an extra 180 days for each additional child. Policies like these allow mothers to get breastfeeding going well, and maybe have a baby taking solid foods well by the time they return to work. The work of going back to work is definitely harder in the few remaining countries where maternity leaves are still counted in weeks (a typical U.S. leave is a scant six weeks). But if that's your situation, it's still doable.

A big question is when to *start* maternity leave. Research shows that having a longer leave *after* the baby is born increases breastfeeding success. But research also shows that women who start their leave a few weeks *before* the baby's birth are less likely to have a Cesarean section or other complications. Norway improved its mother-baby health when it began providing three weeks of pre-birth leave, one more reason that an ample maternity leave protects the health of mothers and babies.

Even if the law or your employer doesn't provide for more than a few weeks of maternity leave, you may be able to get an extension. This will usually be unpaid, but planning ahead may make it possible to stretch out the time you have with your baby. Some mothers ask for an "early inheritance" from their parents to allow them to spend a few more weeks or months with their baby before starting back. It can be one of the most valuable baby gifts a grandparent can give!

Planning Your Baby's Care

Picking the right caregiver for your baby depends on your work schedule, your budget, the options available in your location, and your priorities in terms of setting and type of care. You might be lucky enough to have family members who can help out, or an on-site day care at work. Maybe you and your partner can work partly or fully from home, or work different shifts, to minimize the time your baby spends in outside care.

Babies' stress levels are lower when they're cared for by someone who loves them—a parent, grandparent, or other person very close to the family. That's a quality of care that a day care center simply can't provide.

If you don't have a family member to help or a day care option at work, consider finding a place closer to work than to home. That will mean a shorter period of time away from your baby. (When you're bursting with milk, that half-hour commute can seem VERY long.)

Let potential caregivers know that you'll be leaving your milk for your baby, and ask about their handling and storage arrangements. We still occasionally hear of mothers being told that it will cost them extra if they want to bring in their own milk, or that their milk can't be stored in the same fridge as formula. If your day care tells you this, you can download the U.S. Centers for Disease Control (CDC) document "Proper Handling and Storage of Human Milk" at cdc.gov/breastfeeding/recommendations/handling_breastmilk.htm. It clarifies the safety of human milk and reassures care providers that no special precautions are needed.

You might also want to ask about the facility's feeding schedules. Breastfeeding works best when babies are fed in response to their cues, of course. But most day care providers use a schedule, and some are more rigid than others. Asking for a more flexible approach can feel uncomfortable; it may help to remember that you're being an advocate for your child. Scheduling is most likely to be a problem if your baby gulps down an entire bottle of your hard-earned milk close to the time when you come to pick him up. It's really frustrating to have full and aching breasts out of sync with a full and disinterested baby! It helps a lot if the schedule can be arranged so that your baby is ready to nurse when you arrive. (If you don't routinely breastfeed before you and your baby head home, be sure to call ahead on those days when you'll need to, so they don't give a bottle too close to pickup time. And if you do routinely breastfeed before going home with him, be sure to call if you're going to be late!)

Nursing your baby when you pick her up not only is a great way to reconnect after many hours apart but also gives you a chance to pick up some of the germs and bacteria in the center, so that you can start producing antibodies for your baby against those specific germs. If there are objections, you can ask for a private spot you can use. There's certainly no need to wait to nurse. Day care providers can seem intimidating. They may be older; they seem wiser and more experienced. But you're paying for a service, and your baby's needs come first. You have a right to request whatever you need!

You may want to talk to your caregiver about *how* the feedings from a bottle are given. There are ways to feed from a bottle that help support breastfeeding and also reduce the risk of overfeeding and ear infections (see Chapter 18). There's also a tear sheet in Chapter 20 describing a bottle-feeding method that supports breastfeeding.

QUALITY BABY DAY CARE?

A baby's stress hormone (cortisol) levels rise when he's with caregivers with whom he has no secure and positive attachment *and who have no emotional investment in him*. To minimize your baby's stress, look for a place that has:

- A low staff turnover, so that your child isn't constantly exposed to newcomers.
- A low child-to-staff ratio. (In some places, five infants to one caregiver is the maximum allowed; that still means your child is a quintuplet!)
- Minimal structure. Even though "day care as enrichment and education" is a popular concept, babies and small children need love and focused adult attention, not education.
- A setting that will store, use, and respect your milk.
- Caregivers who are warm and affectionate, not rushed and rigid.
- A setting that allows older children time outside.

Planning Your Milk Supply

The first few weeks back at work are a time for getting your routine worked out. Already having a stash of stored milk helps. Expressing more milk than your baby needs will really get your milk supply built up, too, so that you'll have a cushion to fall back on—an insurance policy in case of difficulties. The easiest way to do this is to pump once or twice a day right after your baby nurses, beginning a few weeks before you start work or once you feel breastfeeding is running smoothly for both of you, and freezing whatever milk you pump. Even if you pump just once after the first feeding in the morning when your supply is greatest, you'll soon build up a freezer stock-pile. For *lots* more information on pumping, be sure to see Chapter 15.

Don't worry if you don't get much milk at first. You're pumping *in addition to* feeding, so there's not likely to be much left over. At first you're just telling your body to make more. You should begin to see the results in a couple of days. And when you're pumping at work *instead of* breastfeeding, you'll get even more.

So what is a "full feeding" and how much milk will you need to send in each day? Breastfed babies normally take about 2–4 ounces (60–120 ml) of milk at any really substantial feeding. (This amount doesn't increase much for breastfed babies from about six weeks on, because their metabolism and growth slow down over time and their ability to use the milk improves. Formula-fed babies lack this improved efficiency and require more and more formula as they grow.) If you are away for nine hours (workday and commuting time), assume that your baby will probably need about six 2-ounce (60 ml) containers each day. You'll probably want to send more than that at first so the caregiver has a freezer stash on hand, then adjust up or down as needed. Using small containers until you have a better feel for how much your baby needs means the sitter won't be throwing out any unused "liquid gold."

If you aren't able to express enough milk on a particular day, or if your baby routinely drinks a bit more than you pump during the workday, pumping on the weekend can put you ahead again. A freezer well stocked with extra milk makes your days much less stressed.

If you run into any challenges during your maternity leave—sore nipples or plugged ducts, for example—don't hesitate to get help quickly, while you're still home. This is the time to line up your support (see Chapter 2) and conncct with your local La Leche League Group, if one is available. It can be really, really helpful to talk with other working mothers in your area who know the breastfeeding-friendly day care providers and who may have ideas that helped them keep breastfeeding going.

Planning Your Expression Schedule

When you first start expressing your milk, you may feel you're stealing milk that your baby expected to have at the next nursing. Remember that your baby *will* get the milk, just not right away!

There are two common approaches to starting your stash, with a lot of options in between. One idea is to put the pump near where you often nurse, and do a few minutes of pumping after several nursings each day. Another approach is to put the pump someplace that you pass often, and do just a few minutes' pumping whenever you go by. You can let the equipment and milk stand, with a towel over them, and store the milk and clean the parts twice a day. You'll find guidelines for storing milk in Chapter 15. At the end of the day, make up single-feeding containers and freeze.

How will it work at work? In a nine-hour separation from your baby, you can expect to need to pump two or three times. (Which is it, two or three? That depends on your baby and on your breasts' storage capacity, which you won't learn right away. Plan for three pumping sessions at first. If you find you need to pump only twice a day, expect to need an extra session occasionally during growth spurts and other unusual times.)

Here's a workday approach that works for many: Nurse first thing in the morning, with another short nursing right before leaving the house or at day care. If you have time, express for a few minutes as soon as you get to work. The next chances to express are usually mid-morning, lunch, and mid-afternoon. Nurse your baby when you pick him up before you leave day care, and then whenever he likes in the evening and again before bedtime. Nurse at least once during the night, too, if he wakes up for it. (And he almost certainly will, at least at first, because he's been missing you and wants to reconnect.) Night nursing can help you maintain your milk production and gives you extra time with your baby.

At home, of course, you and your baby nurse for interaction, love, fun, sleep, waking, food, beverage, and treating bumps and bruises and scary things. It's these "conversational" nursings that keep a milk supply—and a nursing relationship—in good shape. At work, you'll pump just to supply milk and your baby will take a bottle just for food. It won't be the same for either of you, but it will hold things together until you're *back* together at the end of the day and nursing normally again.

This is real life, of course, so your pumping schedule won't be set in stone. Neither will how much you get when you pump. As one experienced mother said, "Put in your pumping time, and don't fret about the amount you got. It's *going* to vary. If you see a change over time, that's when to take action. But not after one bad session. Bad sessions happen."

It's important to make sure that you breastfeed as much as you can when you're with your baby. Your nursing relationship is founded on your baby nursing, not bottle-feeding, and you both need that time together. And there's a very real risk—especially with young babies—that bottles given more often or more willingly than nursing will result in your baby refusing the breast. So even though you may have bottles of your milk ready to go in the refrigerator, it can create problems if you have someone else give one to the baby while you make dinner or take care of something else. Your baby needs you and you need your baby. Many short nursings are worth more to your milk supply than a few forty-minutes-on-the-couch sessions. And it's actually easier and more efficient to offer several little unscheduled snacks instead of a single larger one at a specific feeding time.

> *"Pumping actually was helpful for my work in many ways. It gave me a much-needed break, and I often read articles and information I wouldn't normally have read during work hours. And when I would come home and my son's babysitter said that Theo drank all of the milk I had pumped the day before, I would feel so proud and excited that I could be giving that to him and still be working."* —Chana

Customizing Work and School Arrangements

Through all of history, women have been creative about combining motherhood and work. These are some of the many variations that other mothers have found. One or more of them may feel right for you.

- 💡 Reduce your hours or job-share. In some cases, once day care costs are factored in, the shorter hours actually mean better income. If you're in school, you could take courses on a part-time basis or take some of them online.
- 💡 Work the same number of hours but on a more flexible schedule. If you have a long commute, for example, maybe you could do your work in four longer days rather than five so you'd have less total time away from the baby and an extra day to hang out together and keep up your milk supply. Taking the middle day (such as Wednesday) off can help, so you're away only two days in a row.

- ⚲ Do some or all of your work at home. The Internet and other electronic connections have opened up work-at-home possibilities for many women. A caregiver in your home could help out as needed. Some work-from-home mothers have found that a hands-free headset (especially with a mute button) means they can handle business and baby simultaneously.

- ⚲ Bring your baby with you. Jennifer was a golf course manager with a private office. She set up a napping spot and fenced-in play area in the office, and had a nanny to take care of the baby while she worked in the clubhouse and out on the course. She found she could often nurse or hold her son while reviewing paperwork or working online in her office. Amber shifted her workday by an hour and had her husband, who did the main child care, bring their daughter in to spend the last two hours of the workday with her, when the office was nearly empty and their daughter was happy to sleep and nurse in her mother's lap. Sophia didn't want to ask her employer for special treatment; to her total surprise, her boss approached *her* about bringing her baby to work! Meredith is a university teaching assistant and baby Ella is the assistant's assistant, watching the class (and nursing as needed) from her sling.

- ⚲ Consider a career shift. Kim left her office job after Jaimie was born and opened a store selling cloth diapers and other environmentally friendly baby items. Since it was her own store, and her customers loved babies, keeping Jaimie with her was never a problem. Now she has two employees who happily bring their babies to work as well. Tania had been working in human resources; after son Jason was born she created her own business, checking references for busy employers—something she could do from home.

Can't change your work or school schedule? Maybe you can customize your breastfeeding arrangements.

- ⚲ Go to your baby at lunchtime, or have your baby brought to you. A day care setting near your office can help make this possible. Marianne (see below) was able to pump enough at home to cover her baby's needs during her part-time job.

- ⚲ Some mothers don't pump at all, using formula when they're at work and breastfeeding at home. This is certainly better for both mother and baby than weaning completely to formula. But it is the least desirable choice because the baby is exposed to the risks of formula-feeding and the mother is likely to have problems keeping her milk supply going. Maximizing the amount of breastfeeding when you're together will help make this work.

☼ Return to work on a Thursday or Friday to minimize the initial separation. It will be like a trial run with a two-day vacation before Monday rolls around. If you can, take the next two Wednesdays off. You'll work no more than two days in a row for a full two and a half weeks, allowing you and your baby a much gentler transition into the work world.

> *"I worked twenty hours a week and arranged a four-day-a-week schedule. It meant a longer day for me, but it meant I could get away with not pumping at work. Instead, I pumped at night and sometimes in the morning. Why did I spread my twenty hours out over four days instead of five? Well, by the time I returned to work, my son was five months old and I was hooked on LLL meetings. So I didn't work on Wednesdays because that's when the meetings were held!"* —Marianne

Talking to Your Boss About Expressing Milk at Work

Most women feel at least a little uncomfortable talking to the boss about expressing milk at work. It can feel pretty personal and at some point the word (gasp) "breast" might come up. But it doesn't necessarily have to be a major conversation. You just need to clear the use of a clean and private place a few times each day. You'll also need to make sure it's okay to take a couple of twenty-minute breaks each day (this is about the same amount of time most smokers take) in addition to your lunch break (which could be another opportunity to pump). If taking the breaks is an issue, offer to work a bit later to make up the time. If you have the right kind of job, you can simply work while you pump and avoid the break issue altogether; that's one reason hands-free pumping (see Chapter 15) was invented!

It's to your boss's advantage to have you breastfeed. You're likely to need more days off work if you fed formula. Your own health risks are increased by formula-feeding, too. Studies have shown that breastfeeding mothers—and other employees—feel more positive about companies that support them in continuing to breastfeed. So it's definitely worth it to give you that private space and a few breaks.

Some mothers worry about bringing all this up before the baby's born. But that's much easier than having to figure it all out when you come back to work. You'll probably find it helpful to talk to other women in the office who've breastfed. They'll have some been-there-done-that ideas and tips, and can help you get whatever you need. Your human resources department may be able to help with suggestions from past employees as well. If there just aren't any private spaces available, you might be able to borrow someone else's office or an empty meeting room. And more than one woman has simply turned her back to the door or rigged a removable curtain and rod across a cubicle opening. Not ideal, but these are all approaches that have worked for other moms. A "Baby's Lunch in Progress" sign can let co-workers know that they shouldn't barge in. Last-ditch options: your car or the bathroom (the latter might need an extension cord if there's no outlet, and isn't a legal option in all countries).

If it's hard to talk to your boss in person, maybe a note or e-mail would be a little easier. You can take your time in writing it, point out the reasons breastfeeding is important, and run it past a few friends to be sure the wording says what you want it to. Explain why you'll be doing it and what you'll need, rather than asking permission. You're well within your legal rights almost everywhere in the world.

> "When my daughter was eight months old, my job as a U.S. Army musician required that I spend more than six hours at a football stadium, separated from her. I was a Staff Sergeant, which means I had no clout when it came to interfacing with officers. The Chief of Primary Care at our health care facility for the stadium was a Colonel, which means he was a VERY HIGH RANKING, educated, experienced individual who had a lot of power in the Army.
>
> "I contacted him to request a clean, private place to use my breast pump. He told me I was lucky to breastfeed as long as I did and the responsibility to keep it up rested on me, the individual, not the institution. This from a respected medical professional!
>
> "I told him (bear in mind the difference in rank) I was sorry he felt

> *that he could not design a workplace that was conducive to my continued breastfeeding, especially considering that he, a medical doctor, should be well aware that current recommendations suggest a child not be weaned until at least after the first birthday.*
>
> *"Knowledge is power. There was a freshly painted cubicle with an electrical outlet and a locking door at the football stadium that weekend.*
> —Cassandra

Storing Milk Expressed at Work

A refrigerator, or an insulated thermos or cooler with ice packs, will keep your milk consistently cold at work. If you have a standard workweek, you can even give that day's milk directly to the sitter for the next day when you pick your baby up, so she can use it the following day. Milk pumped on Friday can be stored in the refrigerator for use on Monday.

Variable Schedules

Elena is a pilot whose schedule was different every week, with a different destination and often an overnight stay each time. In between, though, she often had five or seven days in a row at home. She found she wasn't always able to store and bring home her milk, but if her supply dropped a bit she could make it up again on her longer at-home stretches. Your job may also have these variations, or may involve overnight travel at times. In some cases, you may be able to bring a caregiver for your baby with you. He or she can stay at the hotel during the day while you're working and then you'll be able to feed the baby at night. Keeping a stockpile in the freezer can help even out any low spots in your production.

Military Mothers

Being both mother and military can be one of the most challenging work environments, especially if you're on active duty. Maternity leave, sometimes called "convalescent leave," is often short, schedules and pumping don't always mix, and sending your carefully collected milk home for your baby may not be possible. Your first weigh-in and fitness test after the baby is born can be very stressful, often requiring intense exercise and diligent dieting.

Deployment deferment after birth varies widely by country and branch but is generally short compared to a baby's needs. Despite these significant obstacles, many mothers have found ways to make breastfeeding work. Some military policies require that mothers be given a space to pump, although that may mean a space that's not completely private or sound proof. Temporary or partial weaning may be necessary; in other situations, you may be able to keep up your supply by pumping even if you aren't able to get the milk to your baby. The intense exercising and dieting required for the first postpartum weigh-in and fitness test probably won't affect your milk (see the section on exercise and dieting in Chapter 8), and breastfeeding may even help you lose weight. But if it's all just too much, many services allow for separation due to parental hardship both during the pregnancy and after birth.

For more information, read *Breastfeeding in Combat Boots: A Survival Guide to Breastfeeding Successfully While Serving in the Military* by Robyn Roche-Paull, a retired La Leche League Leader who provided milk for her child while in the U.S. Navy. There's also great information on her website, breastfeedingin combatboots.com.

Introducing Bottles

If you return to work when your baby is older, a cup and some solid food may be all he needs. But if you're going to be separated from a young baby regularly, you'll probably be using bottles. They're the most common, convenient, and usually easiest way to feed a small baby away from the breast, and they're what most day care providers expect.

First of all, there's no magic window of opportunity for starting. Just wait until breastfeeding is well established and going smoothly for both you and the baby. It generally makes sense to start offering a bottle about two weeks before you have to go back to work or school.

Don't be too surprised if your baby won't take the bottle from you. Those are his adored breasts; why would he want second-best as long as you're around? So try going out for an hour or so and having your partner, Grandma, or an experienced friend give it a try. If that doesn't help, see "If Your Baby Won't Take a Bottle."

Your baby won't starve while you're at work. Your baby can get those daytime feedings in during the evening and nighttime hours instead if he prefers, in a pattern called "reverse cycling." At one LLL meeting, mothers described how their babies sometimes slept eight or nine hours at night, then moved to concerns that their babies might not be eating often enough while they were at work. Hey, if a baby can go that long at night, he can go that long during the day. But he really, really, really can't do *both*! Night nursings are a big help to every working mother's milk supply, especially if your baby doesn't eat much while you're at work. For easier nights, see hints on sharing sleep in Chapter 12.

IF YOUR BABY WON'T TAKE A BOTTLE

First of all, be patient and creative. Something almost always works.

Basic Approaches

- Have someone other than the mother offer.
- Offer the bottle as just one more interesting thing, when the baby isn't really hungry. Let him explore it and find out for himself that there's—cool!—something he recognizes in it. Squeezing a drop onto the tip for him to taste may help.
- Dance and sing while you offer the bottle; make it part of a dinner show.
- Offer the bottle when he's really sleepy, either just waking up or just drifting off, when he's running more on instinct than on intellect.
- Try different types of bottle nipples to see if there is one the baby will accept.
- Offer a plain cup or sippy cup. Nobody said milk has to come from a bottle!

Make Bottle-Feeding More Like Nursing

- Warm the milk (but not in a microwave, which can create hot spots).
- Hold the baby close, mimicking a nursing position.
- Use lots of cuddling and cooing.

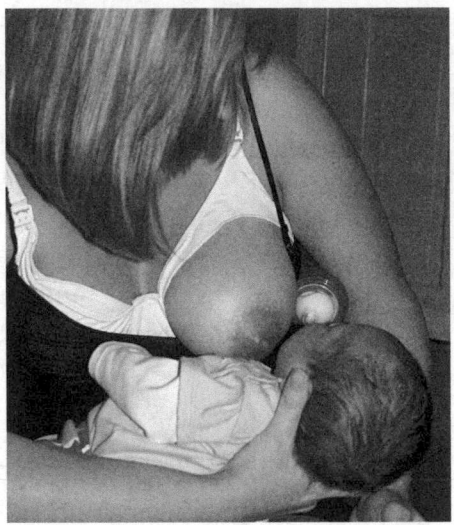

Bottle under arm to feed in a breastfeeding position.

- Wrap up in something of the mother's. One father wore his wife's robe when he offered. It worked! (This is just to get things started; your day care provider won't have to borrow your clothes.)
- See if yours is a baby who'll learn bottle-feeding better from Mother herself than from someone else.
- Offer the bottle tucked underneath an adult arm so the baby feeds from it in a breastfeeding position, with the bottle nipple very close to where your nipple would be.

Make Bottle-Feeding Different from Nursing
- Hold the baby in a totally different position, facing away from you, or in an infant seat.
- Offer the bottle in a new setting—in the sitter's home or walking or in the car after a drive.
- Chill the bottle and milk.
- If your baby is older, have fun in a shared bathtub with a water-filled bottle. Sprinkle it over each other, laugh, suck on it, be goofy with it. Make it a game.
- Offer a "milk slushy"—partly frozen milk from a spoon. Nobody said it had to be a liquid!

- If the baby has begun solids, put water or diluted juice in the bottle, then water or juice with just a little milk in it, and gradually increase the amount of milk.

Remember that the first weeks back at work are likely to be tough, no matter how well you and your baby prepare. It's a part of bending biology.

Help! The Sitter (not necessarily the baby) Wants More Milk!

Here are some things to investigate before you put your pumping into overdrive.

Could It Be the Setting?

Your baby might be starting to get more milk than he needs at day care. Here's a list of ways that sitters can avoid giving your baby too much milk:

- Watch the baby, not the bottle, to know when the feeding is over. Milk remaining in the bottle can be used for the next feeding.
- Share the "Bottle-Feeding a Breastfed Baby" tear sheet in Chapter 20.
- Remember that breastfed babies don't need more and more and more, even though formula-fed babies do.
- Use "newborn" or "slow flow" bottle nipples to slow down the flow.
- Offer a pacifier if he's well fed but still needing to suck.
- Never cut the nipple opening to speed up the feeding.
- Offer attention and holding as well as food. Your baby might have learned that he gets held when he's fed (how clever of him to figure out that that's what it takes). Caregivers may be willing to use a soft carrier some of the time to give your baby the body contact that means almost as much to him as food.

Could It Be a Growth Spurt?

Maybe your baby really does needs more milk for a while. Sometimes this happens during growth spurts. If you were home together, you'd just nurse more often. At work, try to pump an extra time or two during the day while the growth spurt lasts. Some mothers add an extra pumping at home or even in the night, knowing that it's temporary. Or dip into your freezer stash and rebuild it as you go. If it's happening because he's starting to nurse less often at night, then your extra pumping sessions may be more permanent.

More Pumping than Breastfeeding?

A working and breastfeeding relationship goes far more smoothly when it's founded on plenty of nursing instead of plenty of pumping. You may have fallen out of the habit of those little "just because" nursings that aren't about food, but those casual, quick nursings are what keep a milk supply robust. Many mothers find they can easily double the number of nursings when they stop thinking of them as meals and remember that they're really about connection. All that connection adds up to a stronger milk supply.

None of the Above?

It could be the pump; check Chapter 15 for some troubleshooting tips. Has your period recently come back? Is there any chance that you're pregnant? Any new medications—maybe birth control or decongestants? Call your La Leche League Leader, who can also recommend a board certified lactation consultant if needed. Sometimes it takes more than one head to figure out what's going on. You can also check *The Breastfeeding Mother's Guide to Making More Milk* by Diana West and Lisa Marasco, which goes over low-supply causes and solutions in far more detail than we can cover here. Their website, lowmilksupply.org, can give you a running start.

Missing Your Baby, Your Baby Missing You

Going back to work can be a stressful time, especially if you live where maternity leaves are measured in weeks rather than months or years. No matter how well you have all your resources lined up, no matter how much you've missed your job or the income or your co-workers, separating from this little person who has turned your life upside down and your heart inside out may be one of the hardest things you've ever done.

The research-based reality is that neither one of you is built, physiologically or emotionally, for long and regular separations. Growing research from a number of different countries shows that a baby who is separated from his mother for the hours that full-time outside work requires has elevated cortisol levels—a clear sign of stress. It isn't always easy to tell how a baby is doing; the baby who seems quiet and content in the child care center may actually have higher levels of stress hormones than the one who cries and protests.

In general, the cortisol levels of children in day care are dramatically elevated for about the first three years of life, significantly elevated for the next three, and normal by about age six. Studies that have looked at the first seven years find a trend toward increased aggression, anxiety, and attachment difficulty in children who were in day care through their early years.

Are you overheated yet? Let's take a step back and look at this from another direction. The focus in the United States and some other countries has been on making "quality day care" affordable. But babies define quality differently than politicians do. For babies, quality is all about being nurtured by people they are securely attached to. The research tells us that *any* early day care is stressful and less than ideal for babies, and few have asked the mothers what *they* want! If money were no consideration, a study from England indicates that most mothers would not go back to work as soon as they do. While some mothers want to return fairly early, and certainly have the right to, most would love to wait longer.

This has been really tough stuff to write about, and we know it's really tough stuff to read. You won't find talk of cortisol levels in most books on going back to work. But this is the real world, and the real world is now. Health insurance needs, money problems, and workplace requirements not only exist but are given more weight than research findings. So what's a mother on a short maternity leave to do?

Here are some ideas from other working mothers for helping their babies through the workday:

- ֍ Take the time to help your baby get to know your caregiver before you begin leaving him. If it is a day care center, try to spend some time—maybe a week or two—there *with* your baby before you start work, so that it is a familiar place when he's first left there *without* you.
- ֍ Leave some items with your baby that have your comforting scent on them—a T-shirt you have slept in, maybe. Try to arrive at the day care early enough to be there for a while and help make the transition a

smooth one. Maybe you can nurse your baby one more time. Or hold him while the day care provider talks to him or plays peek-a-boo. It's hard on both you and your baby to rush in and drop off a crying, protesting infant.

- ☼ Babies sometimes protest being picked up as much as they do being dropped off at day care. Be patient with this, and take some time to help your baby through the transition. Don't rush in and scoop him up; sit beside him or near him and give him time to be ready to come to you.
- ☼ Ask the caregiver for a daily update on your baby's behaviors. This will help you be more sensitive and responsive to him—for example, if you know that he didn't nap well that day or that he ate more than usual, you can adjust the evening plans to fit his needs better.
- ☼ Don't be surprised if your baby starts waking up more at night, even if he or she has been sleeping longer stretches before you returned to work. Many babies realize that during the night you're at home, and they naturally want to be with you then. If your baby is not eating well during the day, these nighttime feedings can be crucial to getting enough calories—and to maintaining your milk production as well. Keeping your baby close to you at night (in your bed, in a co-sleeper arrangement attached to your bed, or in a crib set up right next to your bed) will make your nights easier.
- ☼ Babies who don't breastfeed during the night often do "marathon nursings" in the evening, when they seem to nurse on-and-off continuously for several hours. Again, this is a way of reconnecting, maintaining your milk, and getting both nutrition and immunities.
- ☼ Consider using a sling or soft carrier when you and your baby are together. It will allow you to get some housework and cooking done while keeping your baby reassured and comforted by your presence. That on-your-chest contact is even good for your milk-making potential, boosting your level of prolactin, the milk-making hormone. Many carriers are designed so that you can nurse while wearing them.

In the future, when you have the time, money, and energy, do what you can to support legislation that supports mothers and children, so that our daughters aren't faced with our dilemmas. For the present, your efforts to continue your normal nursing relationship when you're together can help modify the stresses of day care. Finding other working and breastfeeding mothers to talk with, cry with, brainstorm with, and share support with can be an invaluable help. We can all use a little help from our friends!

BOOKS AND WEBSITES THAT WORKING MOTHERS HAVE FOUND HELPFUL

Hirkani's Daughters: Women Who Scale Modern Mountains to Combine Breastfeeding and Working, by Jennifer Hicks

The Milk Memos: How Real Moms Learned to Mix Business with Babies—and How You Can, Too, by Cate Colburn-Smith and Andrea Serrette

Nursing Mother, Working Mother, by Gale Pryor and Kathleen Huggins

Sequencing, by Arlene Rossen Cardozo

Working Without Weaning: A Working Mother's Guide to Breastfeeding, by Kirsten Berggren

llli.org/NB/NBworking.html

workandpump.com

breastfeeding.com/workingmom.shtml

womenshealth.gov/breastfeeding/living/work.cfm

womenshealth.gov/breastfeeding/programs/business-case

Changing Your Mind

Stacy was an enthusiastic reporter who couldn't imagine not being out on the streets, researching and writing stories—until her son was born. She had made arrangements with a licensed child care provider and thought she had everything worked out... until the first morning when she showed up at the day care center with her baby and her stash of pumped milk. She left her son there, drove to work, typed out a resignation letter on her computer, handed it in, and went back to pick up her baby and take him home. "I wasn't quite sure how we were going to manage, but I knew I couldn't leave my baby," she said.

Diana, who had been five months pregnant with her first son, Alex, when she graduated from college, had planned to start graduate school a few months after he was born. She'd already been accepted and had a class schedule. But as the date neared, she felt an increasingly awful feeling in the pit of her stomach, and she finally realized that being with her baby now meant more to her than her dream of a graduate degree. She was afraid to bring it up with her husband, but when she finally did he told her he had been feeling the same way—wanting her to stay home with Alex—but hadn't known how to tell her.

Cindy found a lovely day care center while she was pregnant. "It was bright and clean, all done up in primary colors. The staff were young and upbeat and intelligent. I thought it was great. Then I went back after Julie was born and it looked like a refugee camp! I had known I was going to have a baby. But I hadn't known it'd be *Julie*." Cindy found ways to delay going back to work until her daughter was in preschool.

It's okay to change your mind about going back and decide to stay home with your baby. And there may come a time down the road when you change your mind again and return to work or begin a new career. A lot of motherhood in the years ahead is going to be about changing your mind to fit your changing world and your family's changing needs.

THE ZEN OF INFLUENZA

"While I was pregnant, we assumed I'd return to my magazine editor job. But motherhood took me by storm. I spent my leave rocking him and staring at his tiny features while tears slid down my face at the thought of leaving him for eight hours a day.

"So I didn't. I went back to the office for one very long Monday, turned in my notice on Tuesday, and have been home ever since. It's the thing I wanted most in the world.

"And it's the hardest thing I've ever done.

"There is richness—deep, glorious richness—in being home with my child, but for my mind, programmed to run at a hectic pace, slowing down has been one of the biggest challenges of my life. After the flurry of new-baby activity slowed, there came the day when no one came and no one called. To my surprise, I felt groundless, unmoored. I had the thing I most wanted, and I had absolutely no idea what to do with it.

"But I was used to running, so I ran. I joined a playgroup, went hiking, went to the library. I called a friend with a baby and made plans to meet. Before I knew it, my mornings were a mad dash to find something, anything, to do.

"And then, at seven months, came the flu. We stayed home, and our friends stayed away. By Wednesday, claustrophobia set in. Couldn't we go somewhere, anywhere? The thermometers—both the one outside the window and the one taking Graham's temperature—said no. The walls came closer. By Friday, I had a hunch I had something to learn. I stopped pacing, took a deep breath, and came face-to-face with the fear behind the running: maybe "just me" wasn't enough for Graham's growing brain.

"But I sat and waited. And fortunately, Graham seemed to know what to do. He gripped the leg of my pants with one chubby hand and handed me a toy. For him, there's just right now, a fistful of Mommy's pants, and a wooden block. Maybe I could do this after all.

"That whole afternoon, I stayed put. The phone rang and I didn't answer it. My laptop called and I gently closed its lid. I watched my baby. And here is what I saw: I saw the way my brave, sick child looks when he comes up for air after an enormous sneeze, eyes and nose streaming, and smiles. At me. Sneezing is funny, and we alone are in on the joke. The rest of the world might be hearing history's best PowerPoint presentation, but I have a meeting with sneeze humor and a tiny boy whose bleary eyes are dancing with mine. The world stood still, and I knew I'd been running straight away from the thing I wanted the most.

"Now when the walls close in and I'm tempted to run, I sit still instead. Always, I'm rewarded.

"And as I sit, I hold on tightly to two things I know are true: no one can do this job like I can, and this time will never come again. There will be morning coffees and new offices and important-sounding challenges in my future. But never again will my baby be seven months old with his first-ever flu, and never again will he and I sit on the floor sharing his first sneeze-inflicted giggle. There are more ways than one to miss your child's babyhood, and this time, we have the flu to thank for bringing us home."

—Laura

Sequencing

The decision to go back to work or not doesn't have to be a permanent one. You can take time away from your career for now and go back in a few years when the kids are older. Even in today's fast-paced world, where technology changes so rapidly, there are often ways to stay involved in your field while still spending most of your time with your children.

A groundbreaking book called *Sequencing* by Arlene Rossen Cardozo introduced a concept in the mid-1990s that's still useful today. She explains how some women can use their skills in new ways and, like Donna (see her story below), have a good income during the childrearing years. This concept inspired a new organization called Mothers & More (mothersandmore .org), which believes that women deserve recognition and support for their right to choose if and how to combine parenting and paid employment. Both Dr. Cardozo's book and the Mothers & More organization may be great resources if you decide to shift your focus toward being with your kids for now.

"When I was pregnant with my first son, Noah, I developed a very painful pregnancy condition. I had to go on disability and was told that my job as a social worker would not be waiting for me when I was 'well again' after the baby was born.

"I stayed home with our baby for those first precious twelve months. But when the bills crept up and my husband lost his job, I had to go back to work. In order to continue breastfeeding Noah while bringing in an income, I completely changed careers, and this hippy-dippy nature girl became an independent consultant for a beauty products company, giving facials and makeovers and selling skin care products from home. I worked only about ten to fifteen hours a week and made more than before. Putting breastfeeding first led me to consider this creative work option.

"When you have a commitment to do the best for your child, you explore what you never before thought you would consider in life. My professional social work career, though I loved it and was extremely good at it, was no longer serving my family and the lifestyle we wanted. We wanted a change, so we focused on how we could make our breast-

> *feeding relationship the goal of our changes rather than an excuse for giving up or a problem to complain about. I am so glad we did!"*
>
> —Donna

Don't Miss Out on This Precious Time

Mothers and babies need time to be together in the early days and weeks. This is a special season in both your lives that lasts only a very short time. You're discovering each other and beginning one of the deepest and most meaningful relationships you will ever have. Housework, meals, and other responsibilities, which will always be there, don't matter as much as getting to know your newborn and developing a strong breastfeeding relationship, which will happen only now. And it takes time. There are not very many mothers who really feel on top of their role before about six weeks after the birth. You have a lot on your plate right now, and much of it is about just learning to be this baby's mother.

So try not to spend too much time stressing about how you'll manage the future. Stressing won't help and just takes time away from what matters now. You and your baby will find your way together. Just like the first few weeks after he was born, returning to work or school is a transition that can feel overwhelming. But breastfeeding will help you through it and keep you together.

Some mothers, consciously or not, harden themselves to the reality of an early return to work and try not to "melt into their babies" during their maternity leaves. While it's understandable to try to protect your heart, most mothers are far, far happier in the long run if they give their heart freely to their baby, even though it makes the transition tough at the start. Try not to let the demands of your job determine the depth of your relationship. You'll both find ways to survive an early return to work, and a strong relationship with your child will outlast any job you'll ever have.

Find some other working mothers to talk with. Consider them your first pumping experience, and pump them for information! They can give you reassurance and a reality dose that will help you feel you're getting your working-mother feet under you. When you learn what works for you, pass it on! Mothers on the llli.org forums are eager to hear your ideas.

Understand that the early days or first couple of weeks at work will be rocky, no matter how old your child is. There's no way around that completely. But it will pass, just as the traumas of your first few weeks of motherhood did. You'll find your own rhythm. You'll find your own style. And you'll find it together.

Other Separations

Maybe you can't be with your baby because of a vacation, out-of-town wedding, or hospitalization. You're not looking at a long-term, repeating separation from your baby. Still, the fact that you'll be away for more than a workday makes it stressful, and too long a separation can jeopardize breastfeeding itself.

Vacations, Trips, Weddings

First of all, do you really want or need to go? Many women have found that the relaxing vacation they'd anticipated was actually pretty stressful, because they missed their baby and worried about their milk production.

Could you arrange to take the baby with you? Maybe a relative, friend, or babysitter could look after the baby while you're at the wedding reception or out for dinner, for example, and the rest of the time you could enjoy some relaxed time as a family.

What you wear will affect how easily—and where—you can breastfeed when you bring your baby along. Companies such as Motherwear (motherwear.com) and Expressiva (expressiva.com) make gorgeous nursing evening outfits, and many two-piece outfits already work. Make or buy a sling in a fabric that complements your outfit, and you and your baby will be the star of any event!

What if you really do need or want to leave your baby behind? Chapter 15 has lots of ideas on pumping and storing milk. With enough lead time, you can provide your own milk, or maybe get donor milk to make up the difference. It's well worth trying, because even a little formula introduced into the diet of a fully breastfed baby increases his risk of health problems, now and in the future. Consider formula your last option—a possibility, but worth working really hard to avoid. And while you're away, it will help to pump your milk regularly and thoroughly to keep up your supply, even if you don't have a way to store it and bring it home.

Hospitalizations

What if you need to be in the hospital? Can you delay the procedure a few months? If not, there may be a policy allowing your baby to stay with you so long as the baby has a second caregiver with him. Depending on your situation and hospital policy, it may be possible to arrange to miss only a couple of feedings at most. You can ask to have a breast pump available (and make sure that it includes the user's kit) or arrange to bring your own pump or kit from home. If it's not possible to have your baby with you full-time in the hospital, you may want to begin pumping a couple of weeks in advance to increase your supply and build up some stored containers of milk in the freezer. Then plan to continue expressing while you're separated from the baby, and arrange for your milk to be given to your baby.

Unless your baby is premature or seriously ill, there's no need to stop breastfeeding (or pump and throw your milk away) just because you've had anesthesia. As soon as you are awake, the anesthesia is essentially out of your blood, so it's essentially out of your milk. Likewise, it's rarely, rarely necessary to stop breastfeeding just because you have to take a medication. Almost all medications, with the exception of a few, such as certain radioactive drugs and chemotherapy, are safe for breastfeeding. The single best resource for information about a particular drug is *Medications and Mothers' Milk* by Dr. Thomas Hale, updated every other year. Your LLL Leader should have access to a copy. Information in the *Physician's Desk Reference,* often called the PDR, is *not* reliable. It's provided not by pharmacologists but by the drug companies themselves, and they often take the route of least liability by saying that their drug is not compatible with breastfeeding, whether or not it is.

No matter what hospital unit you find yourself on, you can ask to talk to a lactation consultant from the maternity unit. She can be a wonderful ally for you. And a local La Leche League Leader, may know some things about hospital policy, helpful nurses, and even layout that can be helpful to you.

Coming Back to Your Baby

Sometimes after a separation of more than a day, a baby will refuse to nurse and even seem to reject his mother. He didn't know where you'd gone, his trust in you has been bruised, and he's letting you know he's not happy about it. Most of these breast refusals are temporary. Some reacquainting time, maybe a warm bath together, some shared sleep, and his hurt feelings are soothed. If breast refusal continues, see the information on nursing strikes in Chapter 18 or talk to an LLL Leader for ideas.

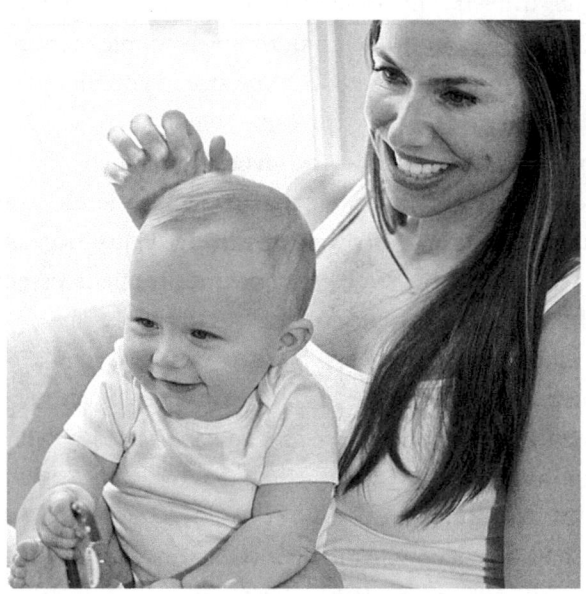

FIFTEEN

Milk to Go

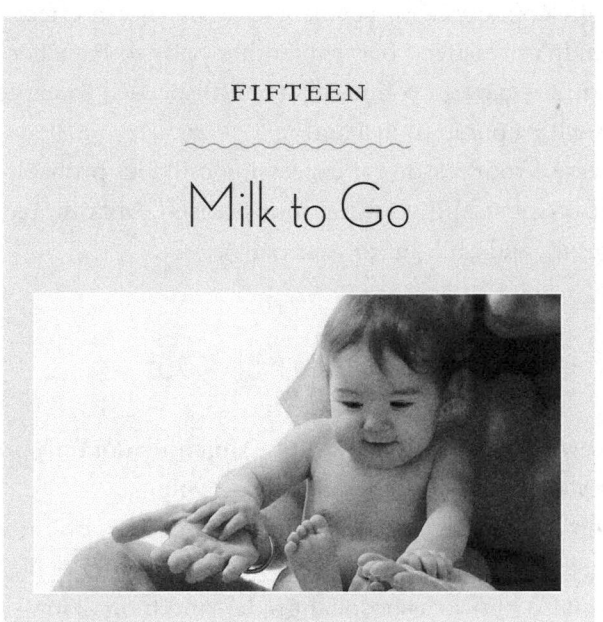

"Sebastian was born eight weeks early, and they whisked him off to the nursery after only a couple of minutes. My doula helped me hand-express some milk into a sterile container, reminding me that if Sebastian had been full-term, I would have put him to the breast right away. I didn't get a lot of milk, but it was reassuring to see that I had something to give him. I kept on hand-expressing for the next few days, and when my milk came in I switched to using the hospital's electric pump. The nurses gave him my milk through a tube. I pumped every three hours around the clock until he had grown enough to breast-feed. During his whole hospital stay, he never had anything except my milk."

—Esmaralda, remembering 2001

ANNA HAD TO go back to work when her baby was two months old. Bethany's baby was born three months early. Carrie had sore nipples and a reduced milk supply because her baby couldn't nurse effectively at first. And Dara didn't breastfeed but wanted her baby to have her milk. What do these mothers have in common? They all needed to express milk for their babies with a pump or by hand.

Regardless of your reason for expressing milk, it's probably going to be a three-part process: Milk Out (of your breasts), Milk Stored (until your baby receives it), and Milk In (to your baby).

Part One: Milk Out

When you can't be with your baby, expressing milk not only provides food for him but also keeps your milk production going.

Most women today start by looking at pumps. Go online or to a baby store and you'll find plenty: manual or electric, single or double, hands-free, rental-grade (also known as hospital-grade), and more. How do you know what kind to buy? Do you need a pump at all?

Hand Expression

Back in the days before pumps were available, women hand-expressed their milk when they couldn't be with their babies; in many parts of the world, they still do. We're so used to the technological approach that we often forget the simple strategy of hand expression. But it has its benefits. It's free,

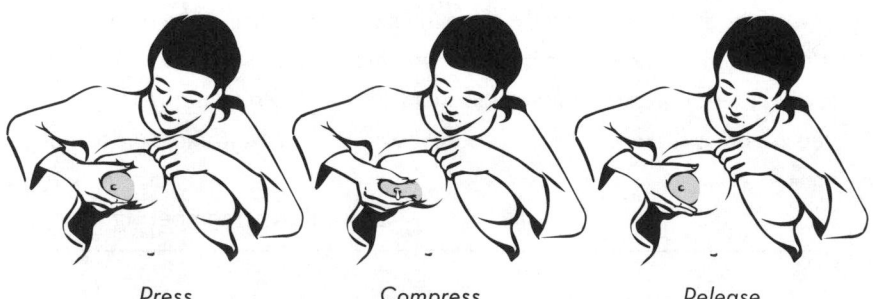

Press. *Compress.* *Release.*

it's highly portable since your hands are always with you, and you don't have to worry about finding an electrical outlet.

On the other hand (pun intended), hand expression does take some practice, and no two women use exactly the same method. You need to get to know your own breasts and the best places to apply pressure to get the milk to flow. At least at first, it will probably take longer to hand-express your milk than it would to use a pump. And not all women feel comfortable doing it, although once you get the hang of it, it can quickly become second nature. One busy working mother could hold a coffee cup under each breast with her fingers, express with her thumbs, and be done in five minutes! At the very least, it's worth learning the techniques because there are times when almost every mother wants to express a little milk, like those nights when the baby sleeps extra long. A minute at the bathroom sink, and you can stumble back to bed feeling comfortable.

How to Hand-Express

The basic idea in *any* milk expression is to stimulate a milk release, then move the milk through the ducts to the nipple pores and out. To practice, you may want to put a big bowl in your lap and have a towel handy. That way you don't need to aim carefully, and you can mop up any drips. Begin by "waking up your breasts" with a combination of breast massage, breast shaking, and nipple tugs or rolls. Jane Morton, MD, a pediatrician, researcher, and professor in California, teaches a technique that is easy to remember: Press, Compress, Release:

1. Start by holding your breast with your fingers and thumb cupped around your breast in a C shape, near but not touching the areola. Then:
2. **PRESS** your fingers and thumb back toward your chest.
3. **COMPRESS** the breast between your fingers and thumb, moving them slightly toward the nipple without lifting them from the breast.
4. **RELEASE** without removing your hand from the breast.
5. **REPEAT,** moving your hand to a different place around the breast after every few compressions or whenever milk flow stops, so that you compress all the milk ducts.

This is just a starting point. Even if you're doing it fabulously, you won't usually get milk right away, but then neither does your expertly nursing baby. (That's a good thing—this delay keeps you from spurting milk every time someone brushes against you.) It takes some time to locate your personal "sweet spots" and figure out the technique that's best for you. When you get a spray of milk from at least one nipple pore (instead of drops or a dribble), you've found what works. What's most effective for one woman may not be so for another; it's a process of trial and error.

Express into any container you like. A flexible bowl lets you form a spout for pouring into another container; you can use a pump flange or regular funnel attached to a bottle or bag; or, like the coffee cup mother, you can learn to aim carefully.

Breast Pumps

A pump has advantages over hand expression in some circumstances. There's very little to learn, you can multi-task, and you needn't focus on what you're doing. To pick the best pump for your situation, it helps to understand how they work and how they're different. An effective pump mimics (as closely as it can) the sucking action of your baby. A baby's suck isn't continuous. It stops and starts in a suck-release-suck-release rhythm, or *cycle*. Babies also have a suck strength that's enough to draw out the milk without causing tissue damage. A pump has to balance this cycling and suction in a very precise way. If the suction is too strong or the cycles are too long, it can bruise or wound your nipples. If the suction is too weak or the cycles too short, it may not collect milk well.

Rental-Grade (or Hospital-Grade) Electric Pumps

These workhorses are built to last for many years and many users. They're expensive enough that they're usually rented rather than sold. This type of pump has one or more cycle speeds that match the average baby's suck cycle. Some are even programmed to cycle quickly at first to stimulate a milk release, like your baby's small, rapid sucks when he first latches. And many have a range of suction levels so that you can tailor both speed and suction strength to work more effectively for you. They're closed systems, meaning that the working parts don't come in contact with the pumped milk. Each user must purchase a personal kit of parts (tubing, flanges, valves, etc.) to attach to the motor. You can express milk from both breasts at the same time with no loss of suction or speed, which saves time and usually stimulates better milk production. Rental-grade pumps almost always remove milk more thoroughly and effectively than any other kind of pump.

Consumer-Grade Electric Pumps

If you browse the pumps at your local baby products store or on a website, you'll probably see claims that they're as good as rental-grade pumps. Don't believe it! But the better-quality consumer-grade pumps are usually good enough *when you have an established milk supply* and are not pumping exclusively. (Some mothers *are* able to maintain a full supply with these pumps even without breastfeeding. If you go that route, monitor your milk production and be prepared to switch to a rental-grade pump if you find your supply slowly dropping.)

There are many different pumps in this category, from expensive, high-quality pumps that can maintain adequate suction and cycling patterns for the months that you might be pumping at work (and for your second or third baby, too) to less expensive but lower-quality pumps that can withdraw enough milk for an occasional feeding but can't maintain a milk supply. The higher-end versions allow double pumping without sacrificing suction or speed, and may have a setting that mimics that fast suck at the start. Consumer-grade pumps are designed to be used by only one person.

Many consumer-grade brands include a battery option. This can be handy, especially when electricity isn't available, but pumps drain batteries quickly—expensive and problematic if they go dead in the middle of pumping.

Consumer-grade pumps keep getting better, but some of the newest features don't have much of a track record, and it can be hard to sort the good from the bad. Before you spend money on a new style of pump, talk to your friends about what worked for them and consider talking to an LLL Leader or International Board Certified Lactation Consultant (IBCLC) to see what they recommend.

If you're looking for a working mother's pump, steer clear of inexpensive electric or battery-operated "discount store" quality pumps. They just don't have the power to combine suction and cycling in a way that will remove milk adequately several times a day, week after week.

WHAT ABOUT *USED* PUMPS?

Used consumer-grade pumps are all over eBay and Craigslist. Maybe your co-worker or friend wants to give you the pump she doesn't need anymore. The trouble is, consumer-grade pumps aren't built to last much more than a year or so, the average length of time that a mother might be pumping for one baby. When they start to wear out, they don't just suddenly stop working. The suction and cycling mechanisms veeerrrry slowly break down, and eventually you realize you aren't pumping as much milk and the suction doesn't feel as strong (or is too strong). Consumer-grade pumps aren't closed systems like rental-grade pumps, so milk or moisture may have entered the mechanical parts, where bacteria, mold, and viruses can grow. Is this a genuine risk? The companies all say so, of course, but there just isn't good research either way. Some of the potential bacteria and viruses—HIV, for instance—die within hours or days. Some of them don't cause illness in humans. And some, like tuberculosis bacteria, can hang around for a very long time. Our best advice is to consider the source, use your best judgment, and at least buy a new pump kit.

If the pump you see for sale is rental-grade, it might be stolen. A legitimate seller will give you the serial number so you can contact the manufacturer, who keeps a list of serial numbers of stolen pumps.

Manual Pumps

If you're pumping only occasionally, maybe to have some milk stored in case of an emergency or for infrequent short separations, this type of pump will probably work just fine for you. Some mothers have even bought two, so they can double-pump without electricity.

HOMEMADE HANDS-FREE PUMPING

You can buy a hands-free pumping bra (LLLI sells one) or kit. But here are three ways to make them.

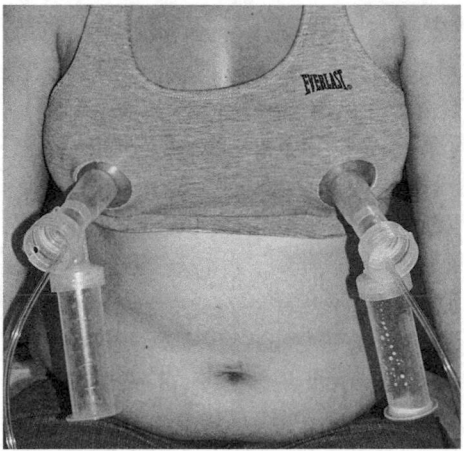

Homemade hands-free pumping bra.

1. Buy an inexpensive sports bra that zips up the front and fits snugly over your nursing bra. Put the sports bra on with your nursing bra's flaps down and adjust your breasts normally. Using small scissors, cut increasingly larger holes in the fabric of the sports bra at your nipples until the holes are big enough for you to work the flanges through but small enough to hold the flanges firmly and evenly against your breasts. Voilà!
2. Skip the nursing bra and just use any sports bra. Cut holes out of the fabric at your nipples for the flange.
3. Visit kellymom.com/bf/pumping/hands-free-pumping.html for the "rubber band method."

Choosing Breast Flanges

Sometimes mothers find pumping painful even though they are using a good-quality pump. If you don't already have a nipple injury that's causing pain, the most likely problem is a mismatch between the size of the *breast flanges* (also called *breast shields*) and your breasts. The flanges are the funnel-shaped pieces that touch your breasts. Friction from a too-small flange can lead to pain and swelling on the nipple and areola, and can even abrade the skin after a while. If a flange is too large, too much tissue will be pulled in, which can also cause swelling.

The standard size (24–26 mm) that comes with most pumping kits may be too small for you. Some pump manufacturers include the next size up (27–29 mm) in their kits, or make them available as accessories, and there are even larger sizes. A few women find that they are more comfortable with a 21 mm flange or flange insert.

To know if you're using the right size flange for your nipples, you can take a look at what happens to your nipple and areola *when you pump*. You should see the nipple moving easily in the tunnel, pulling your areola slightly with it. Look at your nipple immediately after you pump. It will almost certainly be bigger, but it shouldn't seem darker or truly swollen, and it should be comfortable both while you pump and afterward. You can always use a little edible oil (such as olive oil, but not possible allergens such as peanut or corn oil) to cut down on the friction, but if a flange really fits the way it should, you won't need any lubrication. Some lactation consultants find that condensation in the pump tubing can indicate that the flanges are too small. With the right size flange, you may even find that you get more milk, because the pump is finally accessing the right part of your breast. Let comfort and milk flow be your guide.

It may take a few trips to the store or to your breastfeeding helper to get the right size flange for you, but it's well worth the small extra expense to get it right. You may even find that eventually you go back to a size you had tried earlier and rejected, since breasts and nipples can change over time. And any leftover flanges can be recycled for use as kitchen funnels (one of us still uses hers decades later) or bathtub toys.

Some companies also make specialty flanges. One type has a soft funnel section for better comfort and stimulation. Another type has an adjustable or angled "neck" to allow women to lean back while they pump without leaking milk. This can be great if you find yourself constantly rocking forward to tip collected milk into the bottles.

How Often?

If you're expressing your milk instead of nursing and your baby is only a few days old, it's best to put in eight to twelve pumping sessions each day (with at least one of them during the night) for the first few weeks to establish a full milk supply. Of course, the reality is that it's hard to get in twelve pumping sessions with a new baby or other children. Some thoughts from others who've been there:

- 💡 *Aim for ten, work for eight, never go under six.*
- 💡 *Don't think "every three hours" or you won't get eight in. Three hours will stretch to three and a half, and by the end of the day you've done five, with no way to catch up. Instead, think—and do—eight.*
- 💡 *Cluster-pump. Don't worry about evenly spacing the sessions—babies don't!*
- 💡 *Put eight or ten pieces of candy next to the pump and eat one at each pumping. By the end of the day, they should be gone.*
- 💡 *If you want to keep a chart, don't make it rocket science. Have a sheet with all the hours of the day on it, and circle the hours when you pump.* (There is a sample pumping chart in the Tear-Sheet Toolkit in the back of the book.)
- 💡 *If one day doesn't go well, understand what went wrong and try harder the next day.*
- 💡 *Find eight half-hour TV programs that you really like spaced throughout the day and pump while you watch.*

Once your milk supply is well established, how often you have to pump will depend on your particular body. Some women find they can get by on six or sometimes even four pumpings a day after the first few months. Remember that we make milk the fastest when our breasts are the emptiest, and that the back pressure of unremoved milk can slow the rate and drop the amount we produce. So breasts with really good storage capacity (and no, that can't be judged by looking at them) can go longer between pumping, and breasts with a great supply but limited storage will have to have milk taken out more often.

How to Pump

These seem to be the steps that most women find helpful:

- 💡 Find one or two comfortable places in the house or at work that are accessible to whatever other needs you have (baby, other children, files, computer, headset, TV).
- 💡 Coat the inside of the flanges with oil if desired.

- ☀ Open your clothing and bra.
- ☀ "Wake up your breasts" with massage, shaking, lifting, stroking to encourage milk flow.
- ☀ Tug or roll your nipples to encourage milk release.
- ☀ Center the flanges on your nipples, top to bottom and side to side (the angle may be different on each breast).
- ☀ Pumping should be as comfortable as nursing. The flanges don't need to be pressed uncomfortably hard to your breast and you don't have to lean forward to pump. Use pillows, a stool, or whatever you need for comfort.
- ☀ Turn the pump on at your "starting setting," which may be faster and gentler than your "keep it flowing" setting.
- ☀ Your first milk release will start to flow or spray, then subside after a few minutes. Keep pumping, and after a few minutes you'll probably see a second milk release, and possibly a third. Keep pumping, until your breasts feel soft (unless you're engorged). Sometimes it's worth pumping a bit longer to see if you can get yet another milk release; you'll learn what works for you.
- ☀ As you pump, try breast compressions to increase your milk flow (see Chapter 6).
- ☀ Take a break midway and massage your breasts to help increase milk yield.
- ☀ Try pumping one side while your baby nurses at the other. It can encourage more milk releases.
- ☀ Single-pumping (first one side and then the other) allows you to use breast compression and massage while you pump but may not yield as much milk (although some women with very low supplies get more this way) and often takes longer. If you single-pump, do each side for five minutes, then repeat.
- ☀ A pumping session that replaces a nursing will probably last no more than fifteen minutes if you're double-pumping or about twenty minutes if you're single-pumping. Don't watch the clock to know when you're pumping session is over—feel your breasts to see if they're lighter and softer. If you can't tell, begin by pumping for fifteen to twenty minutes, paying attention to how your breasts feel. When you know your breasts better, you'll know when to stop.

- After you've finished pumping, tip the flange down and spend a minute hand-expressing a bit more into it. This will strip out the last remaining milk that the pump couldn't get, further increasing your output (and thus your supply).
- Unless you're pumping for a premature or ill baby, just rinse the flanges and set them aside for the next pumping, washing them up at the end of the day. Hot, soapy water is fine for healthy, full-term babies. If your baby is hospitalized, follow the hospital's guidelines for expressing and storing your milk.

Many women get their double-pumping routine down to a total of ten minutes, including setup and cleanup. But it does take practice and learning your body's quirks. If you're starting with a really low supply, you'll find additional thoughts in Chapter 18. There's also a helpful video about maximizing your milk collection developed by Dr. Jane Morton at newborns.stanford.edu/Breastfeeding/MaxProduction.html.

Creative Techniques

Use your imagination to find ways to make pumping fit more easily into your life. More than one mother has put her battery-operated pump in a sling or backpack and made herself a hands-free pumping bra (see the sidebar "Homemade Hands-Free Pumping") so that she can move about and care for her baby while she pumps. One mother double-pumped by bracing one forearm against a flange and holding the other flange with two fingers and using both hands to work the piston and cylinder—no electricity needed. You can use furniture, body parts, clothing, anything that works for you to make pumping easier. And pass along your ideas when you hit on some that work well!

When to Pump While You're with Your Baby

If you're pumping when you're with your baby because you're trying to build up your milk supply, get milk to supplement with, or create a freezer stash, you'll need to think about the best time to pump while still continuing to breastfeed.

Most moms pump after breastfeeding, to get milk that the baby leaves.

If your baby is not removing milk efficiently or nursing long enough, pumping at this time can be really important in order to drain your breasts thoroughly and keep up your supply. If you're pumping for milk to supplement, it will probably work best to use whatever you pump at the next feeding (see Chapter 18 for the best ways to give supplement). If your baby is nursing well, you may not get very much when you pump after a feeding, but that's okay—you're telling your breasts to make more milk. If your supply is low, your baby may be too unsettled after nursing for you to pump. Try offering him the rest of his meal by supplementing, with a little dessert at the breast if you can because he loves it so much, and then pump.

Another option is to pump between breastfeeding sessions or in the middle of your baby's nap. You'll probably get more milk because your breasts have had a chance to replenish some of what baby took at the last feeding. If your baby wakes up and wants to nurse soon after you pump, there might be less milk available in your breasts, but he'll be getting the pumped milk soon, and the pumping will have helped to boost your supply.

Whether or not to pump at night depends on your situation and need for sleep. Is your baby nursing effectively? You might want to nurse just at night. On the other hand, your milk supply is somewhat higher at night in response to higher prolactin levels, which would be a reason to add a pumping. On the other hand, sleep deprivation can decrease milk production. If you have to have an aggressive pumping schedule, pump in addition to nursing IF you happen to wake up during the night, but don't worry about it if you don't. Some mothers drink a large glass of water before bed to encourage night waking.

For pumping while separated from your baby, see Chapter 14.

Troubleshooting Milk Supply and Pumping Problems

Whenever a group of mothers who pump get together, pretty soon the conversation turns to milk. The issue is usually not being able to pump enough, either over the long term (commonly around two to three months) or from the beginning of the week to the end. Let's look at common problems and solutions in order of likelihood.

Problem: Getting Less Milk Each Time You Pump

Could It Be Your Pump?

- Are all the parts (electrical, tubes, valves, etc.) plugged in and properly connected?
- Are any parts frayed, worn, clogged, or soggy? Discs and membranes can tear, tubing can get pinched and broken, dried milk can prevent a valve from sealing, membranes can get wet. Start at the flange end and look carefully at every part all the way back to the motor.
- What about the suction and cycling speed? Take it to a rental station, whether or not you rented it, and ask to have the levels checked. You can find local rental stations by checking the manufacturer's website.

Could It Be How You're Pumping?

- Have you have been pumping as often or for as long as you used to?
- Are you waiting until your breasts feel full before you pump? A full breast slows down milk production, which means your milk supply will gradually diminish.
- Are you so busy that you've had to miss a pumping session here and there or cut them short too often? Try a hands-free arrangement (see "Homemade Hands-Free Pumping") to free up your hands so you can multi-task while you pump. Schedule pumping time on your daily calendar. But if you really can't pump any more than you're doing now, know that any amount of pumping you can do is great. Tomorrow is another day.
- Are you having trouble releasing your milk to the pump? If you've bonded to your baby and not the pump, that's as it should be. A baby uses both cuteness and sucking in wonderful combinations to remove milk. Try smelling something your baby has worn while you pump. Some moms keep photos or videos of their babies on their phones, iPods, or computers to look at while they pump. If you find it too upsetting to think so much about your baby, just concentrate on the massage, compression, and hand expression techniques mentioned above to increase your ability to release milk. Taking a hot shower or using warm wet compresses on the breast just before pumping or hand-expressing may also help the milk flow more easily.
- Are you pumping less milk because your baby's older? If your baby is

nursing less overall, then your milk supply will naturally be lower and your baby won't need as much milk.

> "When my second baby was nursing, I sang nursery rhymes for my three-year-old daughter, Emily, to dance to—it was a way of entertaining her with my hands still on the baby. When I needed to express milk for the baby, I found singing the songs, especially making the mistakes Emily would usually make, really helped the milk release."   —Sarah

Problem: Pumping Hurts

Pumping should be really comfortable, but not all pumps and arrangements work for everyone. Possible solutions:

- Start with rapid, light suction. Babies generally start with gentle sucks first. Try doing the same with the suction on your pump to ease your nipples into the process.
- Use lower suction overall. A pump provides the most milk when it's set at the upper end of fully comfortable. That is *not* the same as *un*comfortable! Think of a drinking straw that's been sucked on so hard that it flattens out and no liquid can flow. With uncomfortably high suction, your milk ducts can do the same.
- Change the flange size. If your nipple or the skin around it rubs in the tunnel, or if your nipple is swollen or darker after pumping, you may need a different size flange, as discussed earlier in this chapter.
- Add lubrication. Coating the interior of the flange or your breast with a bit of olive or vegetable (not corn or nut) oil may provide just enough lubrication to make pumping comfortable.
- Upgrade your pump. Rental-grade pumps work best for almost everyone.
- Adjust the sucking speed. Nipples need intermittent breaks in suction.
- Make sure the pump is set up correctly for the way you're using it. For instance, using the double-pumping setting while single-pumping can cause soreness.
- Check for infection. Yeast and bacterial infections can make pumping painful.

- Check for allergic reactions. You may be having a rare skin reaction to the type of plastic used to make the flange.

If none of these ideas helps, call an LLL Leader, another pumping mother, the place where you bought the pump, or the pump company's hotline. For more been-there-done-that pumping tips and empathy, visit the llli.org forums.

Part Two: Milk Storage

Your fresh milk is not the same as cow milk, goat milk, or formula. It has living cells in it that actively fight pathogens. Even frozen, human milk has all the nutritional properties babies need and, depending on the length of time it's been frozen, it still offers anti-infective qualities that no formula or other milk product can beat. So it's worth storing your expressed milk in a way that maximizes these nutritional and anti-infective qualities.

What to Store Milk In

Milk to be given later to healthy full-term babies can be expressed into any clean container, but most mothers use either bottles or disposable bags made just for human milk collection and freezing.

To avoid possible toxins, use containers that are not made with the endocrine disruptor bisphenol-A (BPA), identified with a number 3 or 7 recycling symbol. A safer alternative is polypropylene, which is soft, semi-cloudy, and has the number 5 recycling symbol and/or the letters PP on the bottom of the container. You can avoid the potential dangers of plastic completely by using glass bottles. Don't use disposable bottle liners or plastic bags that aren't made specifically for human milk collection and storage. Other kinds are less durable and tend to leak, and some types of plastic can even destroy nutrients in your milk.

To save your sanity, you can put the date on the bag or bottle that you pump your milk into. If your baby goes to day care, you'll probably also need to write your baby's name on the label. A tip learned the hard way: if you use bags, it's much easier to write the date on an *empty* container, not a full one. And be sure to use waterproof ink!

How to Store Your Milk

Once your milk is in your chosen containers, you'll be doing one of three things: giving it straight to your baby, putting it in the refrigerator, or freezing it.

Your expressed milk will stay fresh for a long time (see below), but the fresher it is when your baby gets it, the more of the important nutritional and immunological qualities he'll receive. Refrigerated milk has more anti-infective properties than frozen milk. And milk that has been frozen for two weeks has more anti-infective properties than milk that has been frozen for two months. It's best to refrigerate or chill your milk right after expressing it if it can't be given to your baby in the next few hours. But remember that even long-frozen milk is far superior to formula.

For a reality check, take a look at "Real-World Milk Handling" below.

Milk Straight to Your Baby

Your milk will stay fresh for at least four to eight hours at room temperature, approximately 77°F (22°C). The hotter the day, the shorter the time, but there's no need to jump right out of your seat to put it in the fridge, assuming you have a healthy, full-term baby.

If you pump in the morning before work, you can bring that milk to the sitter for the first morning feeding. It won't have to be refrigerated and will have the highest level of nutrition and germ protection.

If the baby doesn't finish the bottle, it can be refrigerated promptly and given to him at his next feeding. There's usually some backwash of bacteria from his saliva in the bottle, which reduces the number of hours a partly used container can sit out unrefrigerated. How long? It hasn't been researched, so we can't give you numbers. But refrigerating until the next feeding should be fine. If your milk was fresh, living cells will dive right in to clean up any germs. Even milk that was frozen, thawed, and partially used will grow bacteria more slowly than formula would.

Milk to the Refrigerator

You can combine the milk from several pumping sessions in one container as long as you chill the newly expressed milk separately before you put it into the container, so that you're adding cold to cold. Freshly pumped milk can stay refrigerated for at least three to eight days. If you're working, that means that you can usually avoid sending frozen milk to the sitter. Any unneeded milk can be frozen for use later as needed.

Warming Refrigerated Milk

The best way to warm your chilled milk before serving it to your baby is to hold the container under warm running water for several minutes. Or immerse the container in a pan of water that has been heated—though not truly hot—on the stove. Don't heat the milk directly on the stove because it can get too hot. And *don't* use a microwave because it can cause hot spots in the milk, which you may not notice but which could burn your baby badly.

Don't worry if the milk has separated into two layers during its time in the refrigerator. This is normal. All freshly expressed milk separates, even fresh cow milk (most milk in stores is homogenized to prevent separation). The top layer is the cream and the lower is the whey. Just swirl it gently to redistribute the cream before giving it to baby. One of the valuable components of our milk is the long-chain fatty acids. If you shake your milk to mix it, you'll actually break up some of those chains. That's not harmful, but it's not as valuable. So stick to swirling and don't worry if the milk doesn't look totally mixed.

Also, don't worry about the color of your milk. It can change after you eat certain foods, but that doesn't harm the milk at all. Just tell yourself, "If I were nursing, I wouldn't be seeing this!"

Milk to the Freezer

Milk expands as it freezes, so don't fill containers all the way to the top if you plan to freeze them. In fact, you might find it makes the most sense to fill each container with only 2 ounces (60 ml) of milk. Two to 4 ounces (60 to 120 ml) is what your baby is likely to want in a single feeding, so less of your precious milk is likely to be wasted if you collect it in these amounts. You can add refrigerated milk to previously frozen milk: think "add cold to cold." Store your milk in the middle of the freezer, as far away from the freezer door and sides as you can, since temperatures can fluctuate there.

If you decide to freeze your milk in bags designed for it, consider storing them double-bagged (the outer bag needn't be designed to hold human milk) and horizontal to save space, or store them upright inside a sealable container to reduce long-term freezer burn or a freezer taste. Use the oldest frozen milk first to keep it from getting too old.

POWER OUTAGES

If you have the awful luck to have a power outage or freezer failure, your milk is probably okay for up to two days if the freezer is full of food or one day if it is half full (grouping foods together will help them stay frozen longer). If your freezer is a compartment inside a refrigerator, it may defrost faster. Adding any available ice to the freezer will help the milk stay frozen longer. If it's below freezing outside, you can store your milk in snow or in deep shade, but don't leave it exposed to the sun because it could thaw even though the air temperature is cold. As long as it has a frozen core, it's okay to refreeze it.

Thawing Frozen Milk

It's safest to thaw your milk in the refrigerator overnight or hold it under cool running water, gradually increasing the water temperature to heat it to a comfortable feeding temperature, which is usually what feels warm, but not hot, on your wrist. Or heat thawed milk as described under "Warming Refrigerated Milk." But maybe you don't need to heat it at all—just like big kids, some babies are happy to drink cold milk.

SOAPY SMELL?

Some women have milk that smells or tastes soapy after thawing or even standing for a bit. These women are thought to have a high level of lipase enzymes that break down the fats in milk. The milk is *absolutely safe* and most babies will still drink it. You can deactivate the lipase before freezing the milk by heating freshly expressed milk to scalding (bubbling around the edges, but not boiling), then quickly cooling and freezing it. This reduces some of the anti-infective elements somewhat, but formula is still far higher in risk and far lower in value.

Storing Thawed Milk

Previously frozen milk that has been thawed can be kept in the refrigerator for up to twenty-four hours. If it hasn't been used by that time, it should be discarded or refrozen.

DO YOU HAVE TO STERILIZE PUMP PARTS AND BOTTLES?

Fresh human milk kills almost all bacteria, viruses, and fungi that it comes in contact with, so you don't have to sterilize pump and bottle parts. Washing them thoroughly with hot, soapy water is usually all they need. If you have a dishwasher, run the pump flange and connector and bottles through it whenever it's convenient.

Don't sterilize the pump parts that *don't* come in contact with your milk; tubes, diaphragms, or pistons can melt under high heat. If they have to be washed (which is unlikely), you can do it by hand. To dry tubes quickly, stand in an empty space away from people, pets, and furniture and whip them in circles. Centrifugal force will send the water out the ends. If there's a small amount of moisture left, hook the tubing to your pump, turn the pump on, and whoosh the tubing dry.

Storage Duration of Fresh Human Milk for Use with Healthy Full-Term Infants

Where	Temperature	Time	Comments
Room temperature	66° to 78°F (19° to 26°C)	4–8 hours	Containers should be covered and kept as cool as possible; covering the container with a damp towel may keep milk cooler.

Where	Temperature	Time	Comments
Insulated cooler bag	5° to 39°F (–15° to 4°C)	24 hours	Keep ice packs in constant contact with milk containers; limit opening cooler bag.
Refrigerator	39°F (4°C)	3–8 days	Collect in a very clean way to minimize spoilage. Store milk in the back of the main body of the refrigerator.
Freezer compartment of refrigerator	5°F (–15°C)	2 weeks	Store milk away from sides and toward the back of the freezer, where temperature is most constant. Milk stored for longer than these ranges is usually safe, but some of the fats in the milk break down over time.
Freezer compartment of refrigerator with separate doors	0°F (–18°C)	3–6 months	
Deep freezer	–4°F (–20°C)	6–12 months	

REAL-WORLD MILK HANDLING

There's very little research on the day-to-day problems of milk handling, so the printed guidelines tend to err on the side of caution and ignore many of the real-world questions you may have. Here are some answers based on common sense, since we don't have research, and based on the fact that your breastfed baby has, essentially, your immune system.

- It's okay to reheat leftover milk that was refrigerated after a previous feeding.

- In general, what works for your own food handling and storage works for your exclusively breastfed baby.
- You can pump and put the whole pumping kit (flanges attached to containers) in the fridge until the next pumping session. The cold flanges also feel pretty good on your breasts when you go to pump the next time!! Clean the whole setup at the end of the day.
- More than one mother of a healthy, full-term baby has used the sniff test on her milk to see if it's still fresh. (Sour milk isn't a health hazard, though it might upset intestines briefly.) The sniff test doesn't detect germs, but can tell you if milk has soured, which is, of course, the result of germs (as opposed to a soapy smell, which is the result of lipase). And more than one mother has tasted her milk as well.
- There are lots of little ways to push the envelope, but don't combine too many of them. If milk stood at room temperature for six hours, was partially consumed, then refrigerated for a day, then frozen, then went through a freezer failure and was refrozen, um, *we'd* throw it out.

> *"The trick to using glass bottles for freezing milk seems to be to screw the lid on lightly to allow for expansion. I've also heard of using canning jars."* —Jeannette

What About Traveling?

With today's increased security, it may be necessary to prove to airline personnel that your pump isn't a detonation device. Bringing the instruction book should help. And don't be surprised if you're asked to drink a bit of the milk to prove it isn't poison (U.S. regulations no longer require this, but some airports might still ask you to do it).

Putting your milk along with some frozen ice packs in a small cooler or insulated bag should get you where you're going. Milk can also be shipped home if it's packed in dry ice. Wrap the frozen containers in newspaper, scatter chipped dry ice around the outside of the grouped containers, and seal the package tightly. It should last this way for several days. If your milk is even slightly frozen when it arrives, it can be refrozen.

If you're traveling away from your baby and you can neither save nor ship your milk, then you'll have to discard it, knowing that it isn't going to waste because every bit you pump makes it possible for your baby to have that same amount when you're back together.

So, you've pumped it, you've stored it. Now for the last step: getting the milk into your baby!

Part Three: Milk In

This part of the process is covered in detail in "Supplementation" in Chapter 18. The method you use will depend on your baby's age, the reason for supplementing, and the amount of supplement needed.

Putting the Parts Together

Expressing milk may not be much fun, and it doesn't empty the breast as thoroughly as a well-nursing baby. But it can be extremely important in getting you and your baby through breastfeeding difficulties, making working and breastfeeding simpler, or giving your baby his normal food when breastfeeding isn't possible. With a little care, it can be used to support, not replace, the age-old relationship that you share with your baby.

SIXTEEN

Everybody Weans

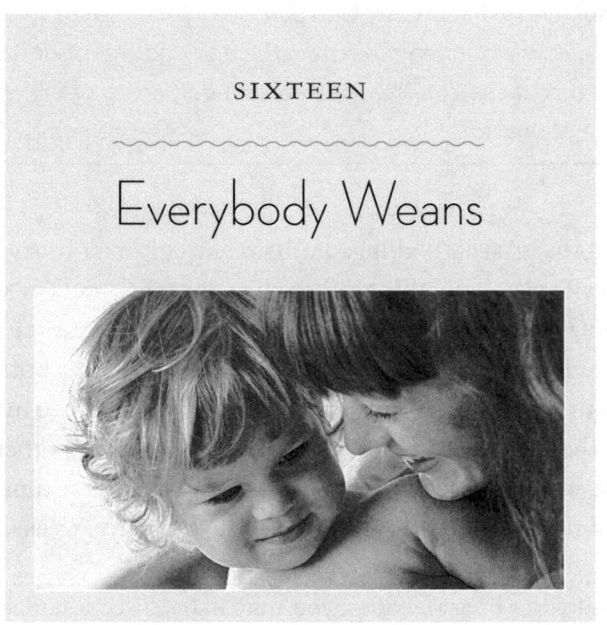

"When I was pregnant the first time, I made up my mind to breastfeed for six months. But by the time David was six months old, everything was going so smoothly that it seemed a pity to quit—and I didn't want to have to go out and buy formula. Maybe I'd keep going for another three months. At nine months, he was enthusiastically eating solids but still nursing quite often, and again weaning seemed like more trouble than it was worth.

"When I found out that I was pregnant again, I thought, 'Well, I'll have to wean now.' My doctor reassured me that it wasn't necessary, and I was so tired during early pregnancy that continuing to breastfeed just seemed easier. After the new baby was born, I was too busy to contemplate weaning, and I was glad I still had this easy way to soothe and comfort David.

"But when he was about two and a half, he began to lose interest.

His favorite nursing had always been first thing in the morning. One warm summer day he woke up and started to nurse, then let go and asked, pointing to my breast, 'Can you make juice?' 'No,' I said. Clearly disappointed, he climbed down from the bed and led me downstairs to pour him a cold cup of juice. That was the beginning of the end of our nursing relationship."   —Ann, remembering 1977

WEANING MEANS DIFFERENT things in different cultures. In some cultures, the first swallow of something other than mother's milk is weaning, so using formula or starting solids is weaning. In others, weaning means ending breastfeeding completely. We think weaning involves both. From the first time your baby eats or drinks something other than your milk—maybe even from the first time your baby sucks on something other than your breast—the weaning process has begun. It ends the last time your child nurses. And that means weaning can take several days, weeks, months, or years.

If you're loving breastfeeding, you may hate to see it end; if you're not having such a great time, you might be looking forward to it ending. One thing's for sure: breastfeeding *does* come to an end eventually, for *everyone*.

When should this end happen? Ending breastfeeding is a very personal decision, and only you and your child know what's best for you, so we won't tell you that you *should* nurse for any specific length of time. What we *can* tell you is that your baby has a biological and emotional need for breastfeeding for at least the first couple of years of his life, and frequently longer. Your own experience is almost certainly going to be different from what you planned. Breastfeeding is more than a feeding method—it's a relationship, and relationships play out differently for everyone.

How Long Will My Baby Breastfeed?

If given the opportunity, most babies will breastfeed until they naturally outgrow the need, which appears to be sometime between two and a half and seven years. This educated guess is based on biological markers or milestones in higher primates, including the length of gestation, age of first permanent molar eruption, and relationship of young to adult body size, as compared to the same markers in humans. Do those ages sound surprising? That's understandable. Some cultures, including much of North America, expect babies to wean around their first birthday or earlier. But our society's expectation isn't in step with our biology. Young children do best with the sucking, reassurance, nutrition, and boost in immunities that breastfeeding provides throughout their early years.

There is so much research showing this that the United Nations Children's Fund (UNICEF), the World Health Organization (WHO), and the Canadian Paediatric Society all recommend breastfeeding for *at least* the first two years of life, and beyond for as long as mutually desired. But past a certain age (which varies from family to family), mothers tend to keep it more private and out of the public eye. You probably know a lot more nursing toddlers than you think!

One of the usual criticisms of "extended" (normal-length) breastfeeding that mothers hear or worry about is that it could make a baby more needy, clingy, or dependent. But personality differences aside, research indicates that the opposite is true: children who are *not* nursed past infancy tend to be somewhat less secure and less independent than their peers who breastfed longer.

What's the Advantage to Me of Continued Nursing?

Whether your nursing child bumps his knee or has his feelings hurt by his big brother, his tears and tantrums often melt away with just a little nursing. Illnesses are milder and easier to deal with. You have on tap a highly effective pain reliever with no negative side effects!

The hormones and enzymes that are released by nursing help gentle a child into sleep. Traveling is more complicated if bottles and formula and a special teddy or blanket replace the simplicity of breastfeeding. With breastfeeding, your child feels instantly secure no matter where he is because his "home base"—your familiar and comforting breasts—is still there.

When a breastfeeding child is sick, nursing again provides comfort, and your milk may be all that he can keep down. No manufactured "electrolyte replacement fluid" also has nutrition *and* anti-infectives *and* growth hormone that help children get better faster. (After Mei Ling's child weaned, she said, "He got sick last week, and I didn't know what to do! Nursing is what I *do* when my kids are sick. I felt so helpless!") Nursing is an all-purpose mothering tool that makes a whole lot of parenting—from tantrums to flu—a whole lot easier.

And of course breastfed children tend to be very healthy, right through the phase in which they seem to put everything in their mouths but eat hardly anything. In their book *Facts for Life,* UNICEF, UNESCO, and the World Health Organization state, "Babies fall ill frequently as they begin to crawl, walk, play, drink and eat foods other than breastmilk. A sick child needs plenty of breastmilk. Breastmilk is a nutritious, easily digestible food when a child loses appetite for other foods. Breastfeeding can comfort a child who is upset."

Does the idea of a nursing toddler still seem strange? A lot of mothers (including many LLL Leaders) couldn't fathom nursing a toddler or older child when they were first getting started nursing; they got there one nursing at a time. So if you're just at the beginning stages, there's really no need to worry about it now. Just know that there's no reason to stop before you and your baby are ready, and the longer you breastfeed the better it is for both of you.

Weaning at Nature's Pace

This is typically a matter of two steps forward, one step back. When weaning happens on its own, mothers often don't know for sure the last time they nursed. Your baby starts solids. Maybe he falls on them with shouts of glee; maybe he just finger-paints with them for another six months. At some point, he begins to take more solids and nurse less often than he used to. His diapers aren't as much fun to change, because his stools are, well, pretty adult. Then he gets a cold and ramps up the nursing. The increased milk makes his stools looser and maybe even yellow again. It doesn't last, and after a while he prefers a story again to nursing. Getting your child to sleep may take longer before it gets shorter, if he now says he wants both a story *and* nursing. Then one day he's so busy playing with friends that he forgets for an entire day. Or he starts sleeping through the night, just when you were sure it would never happen.

Telling your child "Just a minute while I finish the dishes" is part of weaning. We respond quickly and without question to a newborn; we're slower and more likely to negotiate with an older child, all part of gradually putting on the brakes. Impatience may creep in: "It was irritating when my toddler fiddled with my other nipple even though I thought it was cute when the baby did it." A gradual spacing of nursings and decrease in nursing time is all part of the normal process.

Eventually, your nursing relationship winds down to one or two short nursings a day (plus nursing to ease the pain of skinned knees and bruised feelings). It may continue to taper off from there, or your little one may announce calmly that, thanks, he'd rather have grapes! Children naturally have a tremendous desire to move on to the next stage of development: once they can walk they stop crawling. As the wider world opens up to them, they gradually close the door on babyhood. So *even if you never lift a finger, even if you never ever ask him to wait, Your Child Will Wean,* just as surely as his teeth will come in. Doing nothing works just fine.

What if I Want to Wean Now?

Most mothers have times when they think about weaning. Here are some common reasons and possible ways to work through them. (We're not trying to talk you out of it; we're just helping you explore the situation in case weaning isn't what meets your combined needs best.)

I Want My Body Back

That's a common feeling. But because we have a cultural expectation of nursing for about a year, or less than half the normal duration, we begin to feel that normal sense of "nursing impatience" abnormally early. Remember that early weaning will leave you without the single most effective mothering tool you will ever have: an easy way to calm and settle your child.

Early weaning does give you your breasts back, but life may not be quite as easy as you'd hoped. Your baby will still want to be held, and carried, and cuddled—maybe even more than before you weaned. Tantrums and illness may increase as a result of weaning. Sleep times—your child's and yours—may be more problematic. Weaning doesn't make your child need you less; it just gives you one less tool to use to meet his needs.

"When Scott was almost three, we spent a week with his cousins. He loved it! He ate with them, played with them, even threw us over at night and slept with them. He was too excited and busy to nurse (I was very pregnant and had little milk at that point anyway). As soon as we got home, he led me to our favorite nursing chair, climbed up, touched his lips to my nipple, shrugged, and said, 'No milk for me.' And that was that. I think he honestly forgot how.

"When my second son, Eric, was about two and a half, I was hospitalized an hour from home. I saw him once a week for six weeks, and we nursed once a week for six weeks. Same situation as his brother's, in a way—between two and a half and three years old, a week between nursings, and very little milk. But he went on to nurse for several more years.

"Why such a difference? Partly mothering, I think. I was more relaxed about everything with Eric, and nursing was more relaxed, too. But partly personality. They're different boys. I like to think that each got what he needed and moved on when he was ready."   —Diane

Wouldn't Life Be Easier Without Breastfeeding?

There are times when *many* breastfeeding mothers think that weaning would make life so much easier. But then there's the reality. Your baby still needs to be fed and nurtured. If he's under a year old, you will be dealing with the expense and bother of mixing, heating, feeding, and cleaning several bottles of formula a day. When you go out, you'll have to be sure to take enough bottles, formula, and water with you for the length of time you'll be away, and then carry the used, often smelly bottles around until you get back home. If your outing lasts longer than you expected, you may run out of feeding supplies.

Maybe it's not the way you're feeding your baby that's the problem. Maybe you're just worn out. You've been giving and giving...you need to fill up your "mothering reservoir." We can't keep going indefinitely without taking care of ourselves. Here are a few ways to squeeze more time out of an already full day in order to refill your reservoir:

- Go to a playgroup or visit an LLL meeting to connect with other nursing moms. These get-togethers are often the glue that holds a mother together!
- Do you have a friend who also has a baby or toddler? Try getting together at each other's homes to do housework and baby care together. Sharing your day with someone else makes everything easier.
- Read books in five-minute spurts. Or listen to one on a podcast or CD while you nurse the baby to sleep or wash dishes.
- Record your favorite TV show, and watch it a few minutes at a time.
- Have your partner take the baby out for a while. Or your partner can stay home while *you* go out. Or you can just have "Mommy's night in," doing something fun at home while your partner cares for the baby in another room.
- Get out of the house and take your child with you. Children aren't the only ones who benefit from the openness of leaves, flowers, and sky when those four walls start to close in.
- Take a nice, hot bath with lots of bath oils and candles. Bath time for Mommy is a cherished ritual in some households. Bath time for baby is also a cherished ritual, but your baby's bath time needn't count as *your* bath time!
- Try putting a laptop on the kitchen counter so you can sneak in some online time standing up while your child is busy at your feet with the measuring cups.
- Bring a book and lie down with your nursling for naptimes. If you can stay awake, you might get in a whole hour of reading. If not, the snooze is a bonus!
- Start a morning or weekend routine in which your partner and baby have breakfast together alone. It can be a warmly remembered time for everyone.
- At the very least, a good long nap can make everything look a whole lot brighter.

Breastfeeding's Just Not Working Out

Has breastfeeding been a nightmare for you? Milk supply problems, breast or nipple problems, a balky baby? This isn't the way it's *supposed* to be. You deserve to have the breastfeeding experience that you wanted, and you *definitely* deserve to be enjoying your baby!

Chapter 18 has lots of good information and resources for solving breastfeeding problems, and LLL has many other helpful resources and books. But how much *personal* help have you had working through these problems? There are many breastfeeding helpers out there who would be very happy to work with you to try to fix what's not working. LLL Leaders are available for phone help; many provide help at monthly meetings; some may even come to your home. There is never a fee. If the problem is beyond their expertise, they may be able to refer you to an International Board Certified Lactation Consultant (IBCLC) who has experience in resolving more difficult situations. (There may be a fee for the IBCLC, but anything she charges will be a whole lot less expensive than formula and its related illnesses.) You may even benefit from a referral to a specialist. There are people out there who can help you, *even if you think you have already tried everything there is to try.*

That's a trap we sometimes fall into—thinking we've already explored every avenue. But experienced breastfeeding helpers have tools, tips, and education that they've developed over many years to resolve problems like yours—help that isn't in books or on websites. It's like the difference between reading a travel book before taking a trip and going with someone who lives there. The resident has a wealth of information and insights that the book can't begin to cover.

Remember that breastfeeding helpers vary. Some are more up to date than others, or have better diagnostic skills, or are just a better fit. If the help you're getting isn't helping, *try someone else.* You can find another LLL Leader in your area at llli.org >> Find Local Support, and there are lists of board-certified lactation consultants by area at ilca.org >> Find a Lactation Consultant. And ask your local friends or online at the llli.org forums.

If you've really reached the end of your rope and you've decided that you just can't do it anymore, you know what's right for you. That's how good parenting works. Sometimes you can't find enough information and support to fix the problems. Give yourself a truly warm hug for your efforts (and here's a big one from us, too!). You'll find information about how to wean just a bit later in this chapter. And know that any amount of milk or nursing that you provided is a lifetime gift to both of you.

Just because this breastfeeding experience was tough doesn't mean future ones will be. LLL named its magazine *New Beginnings* for this very reason—because each new baby is a new beginning. If you had a milk supply problem, you'll likely have more milk the next time because pregnancy and nursing both help with future supply. If your baby had difficulties, your next baby most likely won't have those same issues. If your birth or hospital experience didn't go well, you've learned much more for next time. In fact, your next breastfeeding experience very well might help heal some of the emotional pain from this one. LLL will be there for you anytime you want us.

I'm Pregnant

Pregnancy rarely *requires* that you wean. About three-quarters of nursing mothers have some nipple tenderness or pain in early pregnancy, and more than half begin to feel fidgety and impatient when they nurse during pregnancy. Most find that their milk supply drops significantly as well. These all seem to be Nature's way of putting the needs of the new baby first, though nursing while pregnant does not hurt the fetus. Some mothers opt to work through the fidgetiness or nipple soreness; others choose to wean; others wean and resume nursing later on—feelings and responses are all over the map. Follow your heart; every situation is different.

If you'd like to explore the world of *tandem nursing*—nursing both an older child and a younger one—check out Hilary Flower's *Adventures in Tandem Nursing: Breastfeeding During Pregnancy and Beyond.*

There may be cases in which it's important to wean in order to maintain a pregnancy, but they're extremely rare. The concern is that the oxytocin released with nursing will stimulate uterine contractions and start labor prematurely. But were you cautioned against orgasm, which releases even more oxytocin? Women with a history of premature labor *may* be advised to avoid sex, orgasm, and nursing during the pregnancy, but the sex prohibition is usually to avoid mechanical disturbance of the cervix. After all, even extreme happiness causes oxytocin release. We're designed so that our uterus can't detect oxytocin well (because it doesn't develop many oxytocin receptors) until hours before the baby is born.

I Want to Get Pregnant, But It's Not Happening

This can be a tough one. Many of today's older mothers hear a loud ticking sound from their biological clocks. But frequent nursing is a powerful fertility suppressor, as part of a well-designed system: when a baby grows older and starts nursing less often, that's a signal that he's finally able to share his mother with a younger sibling. Through most of history, this coincided roughly with the mother's own recovery from the birth. The World Health Organization's review of the research finds that it takes a good two years for a woman's body to recover fully from pregnancy and childbirth, and for mother and the current baby *both* to be ready for a new pregnancy; survival rates for both are greater with more than two years between children. The high-need or fragile child who nurses more frequently than average keeps his mother infertile a bit longer, to make sure his own needs are fully met.

Most women find that fertility returns around the time that their periods return regularly (although they can ovulate before the first period). If your periods *haven't* returned and you want to get pregnant soon, you could consider night weaning, not pumping during the day, or just generally cutting back, to see if that starts them up. Often a break of six hours on one or several nights is enough to kick-start fertility.

One situation that can affect your fertility even when you're having regular periods is a short *luteal phase*—the time from the day after ovulation until your period starts—even if your total cycle is long enough. Charting your cycles can tell you when you ovulate and the length of your luteal cycle. Short luteal phases are associated with high levels of prolactin, which can be caused by several things, including breastfeeding. For this reason, some doctors recommend weaning. Instead, you might ask your doctor about progesterone supplements to correct the short luteal phase.

I'm Going Back to Work or School

Does it seem like breastfeeding will be too difficult to manage when you go back to work or school? No opportunities to pump? A workplace or school environment hostile to nursing moms? We have ideas and strategies in Chapters 14 and 15 that might help.

Fortunately, breastfeeding is flexible. It really doesn't have to be all or nothing. If you can't pump during the day, you can still breastfeed when you're with your baby, which will help fill in the nutritional and immunological holes in formula, and help you reconnect at the end of your workday. Your milk supply will decrease after a few days; just express enough milk at work to stay comfortable. (And if you change your mind and want to increase your supply again, just nurse more!)

I Need to Wean for Medical Reasons

It's very rare for a medical procedure or surgery to require even temporary weaning. If you're told to wean even briefly, it can be well worth getting more information before taking a step that can have far-reaching effects.

As mentioned in Chapter 14, there's no need to stop breastfeeding (or to pump and throw your milk away) if you have general anesthesia. As soon as you're awake, the anesthesia is essentially out of your blood supply, so it's essentially out of your milk. Anesthetics that don't put you to sleep are minimal enough that if your healthy, full-term baby drinks some, it won't matter (if drinking it worked, that's how they'd have *you* do it!). Local anesthetics affect only that area and don't appear in your milk in large amounts. These guidelines are for normal-term and older infants. Babies who are premature or ill may need some time before breastfeeding again; check with an LLL Leader or other trained breastfeeding helper.

There are *very few* medications that don't work with breastfeeding. The main exceptions are certain radioactive drugs, chemotherapy, and a very few long-lasting drugs. A great resource to find out specific information about a particular drug is *Medications and Mothers' Milk* by Dr. Thomas Hale, updated every two years. Your LLL Leader may have a copy, or at least access to the information. In fact, it's such a valuable resource, and the list of problem drugs is so short, that we suggest you find someone who has a copy before taking *anyone's* word that breastfeeding isn't compatible with your drug or procedure! For more information and strategies, see Chapter 18. If you absolutely have to wean suddenly because of medication you need, see "Weaning Your Baby Abruptly" later in this chapter.

If you're being asked to wean due to a chronic illness, you should know that a surprising number of illnesses are either improved or unaffected by breastfeeding. For instance, diabetic mothers often find their insulin needs are lower while they're breastfeeding. And mothers with limited mobility or vision can find nursing the baby (especially in laid-back positions—see Chapter 4) far easier than dealing with bottles.

I Just Can't Take the Criticism!

Maybe your friends or family approved of your breastfeeding a *baby*, but now that he's no longer a little infant, they don't see any point. Maybe they've never been around an older nursling. Maybe they've never been comfortable with this whole breastfeeding thing. Maybe they're blaming normal baby or toddler behavior on breastfeeding. But this is *your* baby, *your* breastfeeding relationship. Weaning will change your life and your child's, not theirs.

If you're not ready to stop, don't feel you have to. Telling them that you truly appreciate their concern and that you know they're saying this because they care tends to defuse the tension; people like to think you see them positively. Humor can disarm them, too, and of course you can gently tell them that you've studied the issues and made an informed decision. If none of that appeases them, you may just have to agree to disagree.

Showing that you're confident will go a long way toward discouraging "helpful" suggestions. Groups such as LLL are a great place to learn how others cope with criticism. Other mothers will reinforce the importance of breastfeeding far beyond the first few months of life, and give you a safe place to vent. Knowing you're not alone and being reassured that your instincts are solid will help you feel stronger in the face of any further criticism.

WHAT CAN YOU SAY WHEN THEY ASK
WHEN YOU'RE GOING TO WEAN?

Well, not *now*—it's only three o'clock.
But we're just getting *good* at this!
You know, I had no idea when I started how important this would be

to both of us. There just isn't any good reason for us to stop. It's
so nice to know that the research supports us, too.

He's teething right now and it's the one thing that makes him feel
better. Maybe later.

Oh, his dad nursed until he was five, so who knows?

You'll have to take that up with the baby.

I love it, and so does he. Besides, it's so good for him, why should
we stop?

Not for a while.

*"Even before Jeffrey turned one, well-meaning friends, relatives, and
even my husband were asking, 'Are you still nursing?' The pressure
wore me down, and I began to feel guilty about something that should
have been special and natural. We started closet nursing. I tried not to
nurse in front of my husband, and I lied to him when he asked how many
times I had nursed Jeffrey that day. I told friends and relatives that we
were finished.*

*"Jeffrey began to notice when anyone talked in a negative way
about nursing and thought maybe something was wrong. Daddy told
him he was 'a big boy now and shouldn't be nursing anymore.'*

*"I began discouraging Jeffrey from nursing two months before his
second birthday. I still remember the confusion we both felt. Yet I was
told, 'You've got to do it. Let him cry it out. It's time.' Jeffrey gave it up
without much trouble, as if to say, 'Okay, Mom, if that's what you want.'
Perhaps he was glad to see the conflict finally ending.*

*"When he had really stopped nursing and the engorgement was
gone, I remember thinking, 'Wow, I finally stopped nursing! No one
thought I could do it, but I did. Now my body belongs to me again. But
where's the fanfare? Where are the congratulations from the families?
Where are those feelings of satisfaction?' There was just me and Jeffrey giving up and giving in and feeling hollow inside. I let pressure
prematurely end one of the most meaningful experiences I have had
with my son. I felt used by everyone, and that is when I got mad. Mad
at myself for not being self-confident enough. Mad because I spent
so much of that short period of time feeling guilty and embarrassed. I
was so disappointed that my husband had not been supportive when*

> *I desperately needed someone on my side, when people criticized me for always giving in to Jeffrey, insisting I couldn't have any milk left anyway.*
>
> *"Since then I have attended a local LLL meeting and met other women who support breastfeeding beyond six months or one year. If I ever have another child, I'm ready to relax and nurse, nurse, nurse without guilt, despite what anyone says. All I'll have to do is to look into that baby's face, and I won't hear the comments of those who disagree."*
>
> —Lynette

I Don't Want to Wean but My *Baby* Does

Some mothers find, to their surprise and disappointment, that their baby seems ready to wean before they are. A common goal today is at least a year; a common age at which "he weaned himself" is nine or ten months. But if the normal human minimum age for weaning is more than twice that, what's going on? One possibility is what Dr. Michael Latham of Cornell University calls "Triple Nipple Syndrome": breast, pacifier, and bottle. If a baby has learned that a breast is just food and a pacifier or a bottle is for comfort, he can decide that it's not worth the bother of negotiating for the breast. Even babies who aren't given alternative sucking sources may wean early if breastfeeding is offered reluctantly or according to a schedule. They may settle for freely offered nursings like nap and bedtime, and gradually phase even those out as the mother's supply declines.

If you want to avoid Triple Nipple Syndrome but you need to use bottles because your baby needs supplements or is in day care, these ideas may help:

- 🔅 If your supply is low and your baby is supplemented at home routinely, make the bottle-feedings strictly business and the nursings a time of cuddles and cozying.
- 🔅 Try offering the bottle before breastfeeding, as described in Chapter 18.
- 🔅 Avoid pacifiers. They were designed to replace a breast, and they often do. A breastfed baby normally gets plenty of sucking from his meals

and snacks. If you want a pacifier for quieting a baby in the car, consider keeping it in the car.

- ☼ Remember that nursing is at least as much about communication as it is food, and feel free to use it as your ancestors always did: for every reason under the sun.

What if your baby is weaning even without bottles or pacifiers being in the mix? It's worth taking a look at how things are going overall. See if any of these suggestions might work for you.

- ☼ Take time to relax together—in the bathtub, at naptime, outside, or in other settings where nursing can happen as part of a happy, sharing time.
- ☼ Let breastfeeding be a source of giggles and silliness as well as a restaurant.
- ☼ Use breastfeeding as an all-purpose mothering tool—to keep him quiet when you're on the phone, to distract him if he shows too much interest in the stereo, because the vacuum cleaner scared him, to soothe him after Aunt Franny gets a little too friendly.
- ☼ Go to an LLL meeting and watch other mothers interact with their babies. When and why are they nursing? Being part of a playgroup of breastfeeding mothers can help because it answers—often without words—questions you didn't know you had. And seeing other little ones nurse may encourage your child to ask.

There's nothing sacred or rule-bound about when to nurse a baby. It's those little "just because" nursings that keep your relationship strong. Many mothers with more than one child find that each nursing relationship tends to last longer than the one before, which suggests that our culture really does inhibit us and we tend to relax into mothering over time.

My Baby Is Suddenly Refusing My Breast

If your baby has *suddenly* stopped nursing, especially if it's before the end of the first year, it could be a "nursing strike." This does *not* mean he wants to wean. Something has made him not want to breastfeed right now, and it can usually be worked through with time and patience (and a few tips and tricks). Common causes include earaches and stuffy noses. See Chapter 18 for details on how to survive a nursing strike.

My Baby Has Never Taken My Breast Well

There are many reasons this can happen. A skilled breastfeeding helper can usually help, but not always. That doesn't mean that your baby has to lose the benefit of your milk. Would continuing to pump, at least for a while longer, be an option? Many mothers find it very satisfying to be able to give their babies their milk, and they and their babies are healthier for it. We have more information about exclusively pumping in Chapter 17.

What if Normal-Length Breastfeeding Won't Work for Us?

Breastfeeding is "dose-dependent," meaning every bit of milk that your baby gets and every day he is cuddled at your breast is just that much better for both of you. Breastfeeding your baby for even a day is the best baby gift he could receive. Here's a breakdown of how breastfeeding helps you and your baby at each stage. These are just the basic health effects—the emotional value is dose-dependent, too!

If You Breastfeed Your Baby for Just a Few Days...

he will have received your colostrum, or early milk—his first and easiest "immunization" that also gets his digestive system working smoothly. Breastfeeding is how your baby is built to start life, and it helps your uterus recover from the birth. Given how little it takes to offer it, and how very much your baby stands to gain, it just makes good sense to breastfeed for at least a day or two, even if you bottle-feed after that.

If You Breastfeed Your Baby for Four to Six Weeks...

you will have eased your baby through the most hazardous part of his infancy. Newborns who are not breastfed are much more likely to get sick or be hospitalized, and have many more digestive problems than breastfed babies. After four to six weeks, you'll probably have worked through any early nursing concerns, too. Make a *serious* goal of nursing for a month, contact LLL if you have any questions, and you'll be in a better position to decide whether you want to continue.

If You Start Weaning at Three or Four Months...

her digestive system will have matured a great deal, and she will be much better able to tolerate all the foreign substances in formula. Giving nothing but your milk for the first four months gives strong protection against ear infections for at least six months. If there is a family history of allergies, though, you'll greatly reduce her risk by waiting a few more months before adding *anything at all* to her diet of your milk.

If You Breastfeed Your Baby for Six Months...

without adding any other food or drink, your baby will be much less likely to suffer an allergic reaction to formula or other foods. The American Academy of Pediatrics, the Canadian Paediatric Society, the United Kingdom Ministry of Health, and the World Health Organization all recommend waiting until about six months to start solids. Breastfeeding for *fewer* than six months is linked to poorer health throughout a baby's first year of life, increases a little one's risk of ear infections and childhood cancers, and increases the mother's risk of breast cancer. A bonus if you're not ready for another baby: exclusive, frequent breastfeeding during the first six months, if your periods have not returned, provides at least 98 percent effective protection against pregnancy.

If You Breastfeed Your Baby for Nine Months...

he'll have the food he's designed for—your milk—through the fastest and most important brain and body development of his life. Children who nurse for less than this tend to perform less well all through their school years. Weaning may be fairly easy at this age...but so is nursing! If you want to *avoid* weaning this early, be sure that you breastfeed willingly for comfort, not just for food.

If You Begin Weaning Your Baby at a Year...

you can avoid the expense and bother of formula. Your child's one-year-old body can probably handle most of the table foods your family enjoys. Many of the health outcomes this year of nursing has given your child will last her whole life. Without this year of nursing, she would have a less sturdy immune system, and would be much more likely to need orthodontia or speech therapy. The American Academy of Pediatrics recommends breastfeeding for *at least* a year, to help ensure solid nutrition and health for your baby.

If You Begin Weaning Your Baby at Eighteen Months...

you will have continued to provide the nutrition, comfort, and illness protection your baby expects, at a time when illness is common in formula-fed babies. He's had time to form a solid base for his growing independence. And he is old enough that you can work together on the weaning process at a pace he can handle. Antonia Novello, a former U.S. surgeon general, said, "It is the lucky baby, I feel, that nurses to age two."

If Your Child Weans When She Is Ready...

you can feel confident that you have met your baby's physical and emotional needs in a very normal, healthy way. In cultures where there is no pressure to wean, children tend to breastfeed for *at least* two years. The World Health Organization, UNICEF, and the Canadian Paediatric Society strongly encourage breastfeeding through toddlerhood. Your child's biology seems geared to weaning somewhere between two and a half and seven years; it makes sense to build his brain and bones from the milk that was designed for the job. Your milk provides antibodies and other protective substances as long as you continue nursing, and some of those benefits continue for a lifetime; you may find that neighbors who formula-fed have more frequent doctor visits and even more hospitalizations for their children for years to come. Research indicates that the longer a child breastfeeds, the higher his intelligence. The longer you breastfeed, the lower your breast cancer risk. And children who were nursed long-term tend to be very secure and independent, yet connected to their parents.

The end of breastfeeding is a big step for both of you. If you do wean before your child is ready, be sure to do it gradually if you can, and with love.

KATHY DETTWYLER'S OIL WELL

Anthropologist Kathy Dettwyler, PhD, compares breastfeeding to an oil well in your backyard. The income the first year is spectacular! Maybe it isn't as great the second year, but why would you cap the well and lose it? What if the income keeps dwindling? Will you cap the well? Maybe at some point the return isn't worth the noise and having the trucks go back and forth. But the well itself doesn't run out. You'll keep getting checks until you cap the well.

The importance of breastfeeding is greatest to a newborn. But that doesn't mean it isn't incredibly valuable at two years old. There's never a day when it stops being valuable, and no one but you can say when the trucks and the noise outweigh the size of the check. If you and your baby are enjoying breastfeeding, there's absolutely no reason you should stop at any particular time, and there are loads of reasons to continue. The "checks" will keep rolling in *for both of you* for as long as you both want to nurse.

How to Wean Faster than Nature Intended

Whatever the situation, weaning still works best for both of you if it's done as gradually as possible, to minimize the emotional effect on your baby and to allow your milk supply to decrease so you don't risk plugged ducts or mastitis. Weaning cold turkey can be upsetting to both your baby and your breasts. (See "Weaning Your Baby Abruptly," below, if you're stuck with that scenario.)

Make time for plenty of attention and cuddling. It's part of learning new ways to connect besides nursing. Try to be as flexible as you can. There might be days that he just needs more mommy time and you take a temporary step back. That's okay. He might be teething or coming down with a cold, or he might just need the reassurance that he's still your baby. Take it slow and cut back again when he seems ready.

The way you go about weaning will depend largely on how old your baby is. Here are some age-specific weaning strategies.

Weaning a Baby Under Six Months Old

Unless you have access to donor milk, weaning a baby under six months means transitioning to formula, so you'll need to talk to your doctor about what's appropriate. The first formula you try might not agree with your baby, so it may take some trial and error. It's a good idea to pump for any dropped feedings during the first week or so, while you make sure your baby can tolerate formula. More than one mother has discovered that continuing to breastfeed is easier than the eczema, irritability, or digestive problems that suddenly crop up. Some babies who can't tolerate formula at first can be eased into it over time, or can tolerate it better if it's tried again a few weeks later. In the meantime, keeping your supply up lets you swing right back into nursing if need be.

You can start by offering just one bottle for the first two or three days to give your baby (and your breasts) a chance to get used to the change. If your breasts feel uncomfortable from this missed feeding and you aren't pumping as insurance against possible formula problems, express just enough milk to feel comfortable, but not enough to drain your breasts. You're signaling them to slow down milk production.

Then add another bottle for a day or two, gradually increasing the number of bottle-feedings and decreasing the number of breastfeedings. The last nursings to go are usually first thing in the morning, naptime, and bedtime. As your supply keeps dropping, at some point your baby will probably indicate he wants a bottle instead of your breast even at the favorite feedings. The whole process could take two weeks or more. Since breastfeeding means more than just food, your baby may not bottle-feed as often as he breastfed. *It's important to make up for the comfort feedings by giving more cuddles, snuggles, and attention.*

Once you're down to his favorite times, you may find you don't have to do anything more. One or two or three feedings a day may be manageable for you. They take no more time than you'd be giving to the baby anyway, they give him your milk for a bit longer, and your supply will probably be low enough that your breasts are never uncomfortable.

Weaning a Baby Six Months to One Year Old

It may be helpful to refer to the information about how to wean a baby under six months, since you'll probably be using bottles and formula. For an older baby on solid foods, you may not need to feed quite as much formula.

The United States and United Kingdom recommend human milk or formula rather than cow milk for the entire first year. Canada's guidelines allow for cow milk from nine months on, provided the baby received human milk instead of formula *until* nine months. Their reasoning? Formula causes tiny intestinal bleeds in many children, which compromise their iron stores. But children need a good iron source throughout their first year. If they've lost iron through long-term formula-feeding, they need a better iron source than cow milk for those last three months.

Weaning a Baby One Year or Older

At this age, you can probably skip formula altogether, though you'll still need alternative ways to comfort, reassure, and connect. A time-honored way to encourage weaning is "don't offer, don't refuse." You stop offering the breast voluntarily, but you don't refuse if he asks for it. It helps to avoid the places where you usually sit down to nurse, spots that mean nursing time.

Distraction often works, too. When your child asks for a quick nursing, you can instead offer him a healthy snack like cut-up fruit instead. Some mothers have a spot in the refrigerator for the toddler's snacks so he can help himself. A cup of water or diluted juice might be especially helpful in very hot weather when "snack nursing" is mainly to quench thirst.

Naps and bedtime may be harder. Some mothers taper away sleepy-time nursings by saying they will nurse only as long as the length of a song they sing or play on a CD or iPod. Or you could count to a certain number (the count can go just as fast or slow as you need it to go). Tamara knew she was pushing too hard when her toddler pleaded, "Don't count!"

Try replacing the nap and bedtime feedings with other rituals that cue your child to begin feeling sleepy. Cuddles, rocking, backrubs, lullabies, and favorite books, poems, and stories are very soothing. You can make this a snuggly time by holding your child closely, maybe letting him lean his cheek on your breast. Introduce these strategies along with nursing at first. For example, sing a lullaby while you nurse. A few days later, just sing for a while and finish up with nursing. After a few more nights, the lullaby alone may work to put her back to sleep. Diana memorized the book *Goodnight Moon* and still recites it each night to her three school-age boys, who swear they can't go to sleep without it. It may also help to have your partner take over bedtime duties.

Talk with your child about what's going on and why you need him to wean. He may understand a lot more than you expect. There are some books about weaning that that you can read together, like *Maggie's Weaning* by Mary Joan Deutschbein, available through llli.org. Some mothers even plan a "weaning party" with their child to celebrate the finish line, letting him take the lead on the guest list, foods, and activities, and maybe having him pick out a toy that he can have once he's weaned. Many long-weaned children remember their weaning parties fondly. Consider *not* using a birthday as weaning day so the excitement doesn't spiral too high. And be prepared for your child to say at bedtime, "I changed my mind." You needn't follow through if that's how your child feels; another day can be weaning day. Parenting is full of false steps, half steps, advances, and retreats.

Weaning Your Baby Abruptly

Weaning abruptly is rarely necessary; it's worth a second opinion from someone who understands both your situation and breastfeeding. If you do have to wean suddenly, it's best to reduce your milk supply as slowly as you can to avoid a breast infection. When your breasts begin to feel uncomfortably full, remove just enough milk to feel comfortable again. This will help you stay comfortable while giving your breasts the signal to shut down production. It may take a week to ten days to feel like you don't have to remove any more milk, and you may be able to express drops of milk for a year or more, but eventually your breasts will stop making milk completely.

To speed the process of milk reduction, some mothers have found it helpful to use sage (think sage tea), parsley (think tabouli), or peppermint oil (as in many breath mints). One or two doses of over-the-counter pseudoephedrine (ask the pharmacist for brands) may also help things along. Caution: a supply drop from pseudoephedrine may be permanent, so be very sure of your need to wean before trying it. Breast binding has not been found to hurry the process, but you may find a supportive bra comforting.

Provide plenty of snuggles during this sad and confusing time. An older baby may understand that your "nummies" (breasts) are broken (especially if you put adhesive bandages on them), but he may do better if you wear a dress or tucked-in shirt that can't be opened or lifted by searching hands. A younger baby may need a lot of walking and singing; a still younger one may adjust quickly to a bottle but will be grateful for your warmth and bare skin during his meal and perhaps the real skin of your finger to suck on afterward.

If you are a co-sleeping family, it might help to have your partner sleep alone with the baby for a time, while a new pattern of no nursing is established. You're in an emergency situation, and emergencies often call for less-than-ideal arrangements.

Whatever his age, your baby is losing something important, just as you are, and you both have a right to mourn. If possible, change as little else right now as possible. While leaving your baby for a weekend in order to wean may feel less stressful to you, not having the center of his universe around for such a big change probably makes it extra hard on the baby.

Night Weaning

What if you just don't want to nurse at night anymore? Maybe you're hoping for uninterrupted sleep but want to keep nursing during the day. It's important to think this through, because early night weaning is a risk factor for early weaning.

Babies wake at night for different reasons. The child of a working mother, for instance, may use nighttime to reconnect after many hours of separation. Nighttime feedings may contribute significantly to some babies' nutrition right into toddlerhood. Night waking can be associated with teething, illness, or allergies. If you have a younger baby, you may need to pump at least once in the night to keep your supply strong, which partly defeats the purpose of the night weaning. But an older child may be able to learn to get back to sleep after a brief awakening. Replacing bedtime nursing with cuddles and lullabies, as described in the section "Weaning a Baby One Year or Older," might help, but of course this just substitutes one way of helping the baby get back to sleep with another. That's fine if your reason for night weaning is to increase your chances of getting pregnant, for example, or if you want someone else to settle the baby while you sleep. But in many cases, you end up with a baby or toddler who still wakes at night and you actually have to put more energy into getting him back to sleep than before!

Unfortunately, that's why some parents resort to letting the baby "cry it out." Their goal is for the baby to find her own way to get back to sleep without any help from the parents. But research has shown that this is very stressful for babies. And if your baby needs to breastfeed for nutrition during the night, her weight gain may falter. Eventually children do start sleeping for longer periods at night, although some night waking is still normal through the preschool years. Making sure that your child eats and drinks enough through the day and has plenty of exercise may help him sleep as much as he is physically and developmentally ready for.

If your child is old enough to understand basic concepts, you might be able to explain to him that you aren't going to be nursing at night anymore because the nummies have to go to bed at night, too. Some mothers tell their children that they have to wait for the sun to come up. Some mothers of toddlers assign one breast to daytime nursing and one to nighttime nursing, just to cut things down a little.

With any of these moves, you'll know soon enough whether the time is right. Many a mother who tried to night-wean and was met with hysterics tried a few weeks later and found her child fussed a little for a night or two and then slept soundly. If you're responsive to your child's changing needs, you can encourage longer night stretches without pushing her past her developmental limit. When Diana tried the "wait until day" approach with her son Ben, he started to wake her several times during the night to ask, "Is it Day yet?" So they waited a little longer to try again.

Night Weaning to Prevent Cavities

Historically, children who nursed all night had little or no decay until the advent of decay-inducing foods. Because today's kids eat so many of these foods, dentists often tell moms that they shouldn't nurse at night. But human milk itself rarely contributes to decay and actually has tooth-strengthening properties, so night weaning isn't likely to help. You'll find a full discussion in Chapter 12.

How Weaning Feels

Mothers whose children wean after several years of nursing often feel a mix of nostalgia, wistfulness, and relief, but the feelings tend to be muted because the process is slow and the weaned child is ready for more mature interaction. Those mild looking-back pangs have been felt by mothers for eons before us. If this is your last child, your sadness may be deeper because you know you won't be a nursing mother again. Consider some little celebration for yourself to put a different spin on it. This is, after all, quite a turning point!

If you weaned before two years or so, the strength of your feelings about it might surprise you. You may revel in your non-nursing status but also feel weepy or super-sensitive for a time. You may feel a sense of rejection if your child stopped too easily. Be gentle with yourself as you both find your new footing.

SOME GOOD WEANING BOOKS

Adventures in Tandem Nursing: Breastfeeding During Pregnancy and Beyond, by Hilary Flower
How Weaning Happens, by Diane Bengson
Maggie's Weaning, by Mary Joan Deutschbein
Mothering Your Nursing Toddler, by Norma Jane Bumgarner
The Nursing Mother's Guide to Weaning, by Kathleen Huggins

A Fond Farewell

Many women can tell you vividly about their breastfeeding experiences, even when they're elderly. Weaning is an important transition—really the end of a process that began at conception—and the end of a unique intimacy. Women who have both nursed and bottle-fed often recognize a difference in the relationship with their children. Indeed, having older weaned children ourselves, we can tell you that we see the effects of the close relationships that began with breastfeeding continuing in our children to this day. Maybe weaning never really happens completely. As one little nursling said, at a final nursing of his own choosing, "Mama, your milk will last me forever."

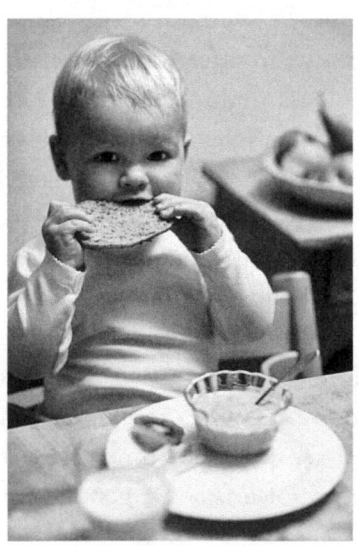

SEVENTEEN

Alternate Routes

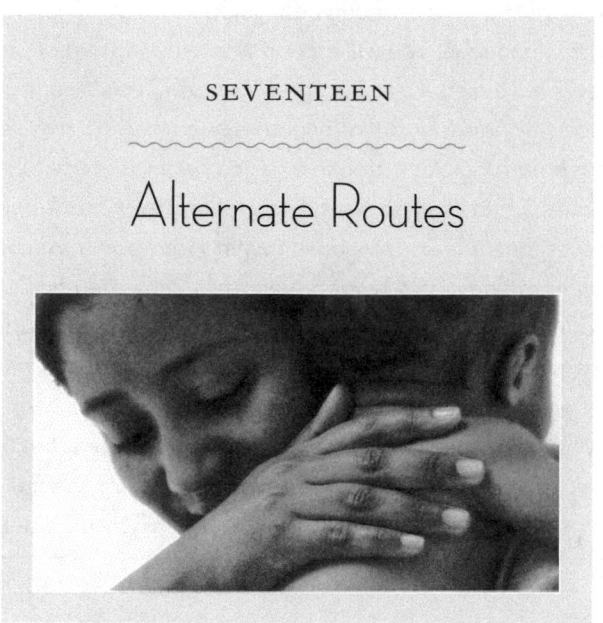

"*I am often asked to describe the experience of raising a child with a disability. It's like this...*

"*When you're going to have a baby, it's like planning a fabulous vacation trip to Italy. You buy a bunch of guidebooks and make your wonderful plans. The Coliseum. The Michelangelo David. The gondolas in Venice. You may learn some handy phrases in Italian. It's all very exciting.*

"*After months of eager anticipation, the day finally arrives. You pack your bags, board the plane, and off you go. Several hours later, the plane lands. The stewardess says, 'Welcome to Holland.'*

"*'Holland!?' you say. 'What do you mean, Holland?? I signed up for Italy! I'm supposed to be in Italy. All my life I've dreamed of going to Italy.'*

"*But there's been a change in the flight plan. You've landed in Holland, and there you must stay. The important thing is that they haven't*

taken you to a horrible, disgusting, filthy place, full of pestilence, fam-
ine, and disease. It's just a different place.

"So you must go out and buy new guidebooks. And you must learn
a whole new language. You will meet a whole new group of people you
would never have met. It's just a different place. It's slower-paced than
Italy, less flashy than Italy. But after you've been there for a while and you
catch your breath, you look around and you begin to notice that Holland
has windmills… and Holland has tulips. Holland even has Rembrandts.

"Yet everyone you know is busy coming and going from Italy, and
they're all bragging about what a wonderful time they had there. For
the rest of your life, you will say, 'Yes, that's where I was supposed to
go. That's what I had planned.' And the pain of that will never, ever,
ever, ever go away, because the loss of that dream is a very, very sig-
nificant loss. But if you spend your life mourning the fact that you didn't
get to Italy, you may never be free to enjoy the very special, the very
lovely things about Holland."   —Emily, remembering 1987

WHILE BREASTFEEDING IS usually fairly straightforward and uncomplicated,
some situations can be challenging. This chapter focuses on the more common of these situations to give you specialized help. Since these experiences can vary so much from one mother and baby to another, it may also
be very useful to contact a local La Leche League Leader or International
Board Certified Lactation Consultant (IBCLC) to give you personal guidance and support.

Exclusive Pumping

Most mothers who pump their milk do it either temporarily, until their
babies can breastfeed, or on a part-time basis while separated from their
infants. But some women pump exclusively. Maybe you wanted your baby to
have his normal food, but didn't feel comfortable breastfeeding. Or maybe
breastfeeding never went well and you or your baby eventually decided that
bottles were easier.

This happened to Diana West with her first baby, Alex. She didn't have enough milk because she had had a breast reduction, so she had to supplement. She started out using an at-breast supplementer, but over time she used bottles more and more. Eventually Alex refused to nurse, preferring the faster flow of the bottle. Diana pumped and fed Alex her milk (in addition to the supplement) for the next fourteen months. While she grieved the loss of their breastfeeding relationship, she felt wonderful knowing he was getting normal nutrition and anti-infectives from her milk.

As Diana knows from her personal experience, exclusive pumping is very different from breastfeeding even though both involve lactation. Breastfeeding is child-driven, happening when the baby is hungry or thirsty, or just wants to nurse for comfort. It rarely happens on a regular schedule or for the same length of time, but varies from day to day according to the child's growing needs. Since pumping is mother-driven, it's likely to happen on a more consistent schedule that revolves around her daily routines. Consistency is definitely good, but it lacks the many little top-offs that really help keep milk production strong. So most exclusively pumping mothers have to make extra efforts to keep their supplies up, and the regimen takes enormous dedication.

How Often Do You Need to Pump if Your Baby Doesn't Breastfeed?

This seems to vary greatly from mother to mother. There isn't a set standard minimum below which a supply will dry up. Most women will keep making some milk so long as some milk is being removed.

If you started out exclusively pumping from the beginning or the early weeks, it can be useful to pump more frequently at first. A newborn generally nurses *at least* eight to twelve times in twenty-four hours. One approach is to aim for ten expressions per day; not to fall below eight. The more you can do in the first few weeks, the better. Ideally, you'll need to pump an average of 25 to 33 ounces (750 to 1,000 ml) daily by the time your baby is two weeks old. This sets your milk supply high and may give you a freezer stockpile to help compensate for any low times later on. Pump whenever you think of it—even for short times—so that you're not just doing it on a set schedule. Once your supply is stable, at about six weeks, you can experiment a bit to see how many times you need to pump each day to get the amount your baby needs. Some women can get by on fewer pumping sessions than others need.

Keep in mind that milk is made most quickly when the breast is least full; the fuller your breasts are, the slower milk is being made. If you let them get too full for too long, milk production will slow down dramatically. After a while, you'll get a feel for when it's time to pump—follow your body's feedback rather than the clock and your supply should be fine. After those first six weeks, whether or not you pump at night depends on how long your breasts will let you go without becoming uncomfortably full and how much you can pump during the day to meet your baby's needs. It's a good idea to pump at least once at night during the first six weeks as part of establishing a solid supply.

What Kind of Pump Do You Need?

Most women are able to remove the most milk with rental-grade pumps. Renting this kind of pump can be costly but will still be far less than the expense of formula plus the increased health care expenses.

Supply Problems

Making enough milk is a common challenge for moms who are exclusively pumping. This often seems to happen around four to six months. Sometimes the issue is that the baby is getting too much by bottle—our tips in Chapter 18 for bottle-feeding in a breastfeeding-supportive way might come in handy to make sure your baby is being fed in a way that doesn't give him more than he needs. One way to know for sure if overfeeding is the problem is weight gain. So long as he is gaining appropriately, then all is well. But if you've ruled out overfeeding, then you may need to take some steps to increase your production. See "Low Milk Supply" in Chapter 18 for strategies.

How Often Should Your Baby Be Fed Your Pumped Milk?

Human milk is digested more quickly than formula, so an exclusively human-milk-fed baby is likely to need to be fed more frequently than a formula-fed baby. Just because he's being bottle-fed doesn't mean he can't be fed on demand. Any rooting signs (fists to mouth, turning his face strongly to one side, sticking out his tongue, or making sucking motions with his mouth) can be indications that he wants to feed. Since he isn't getting sucking opportunities at the breast and sucking is important for a baby's sense of soothing, a pacifier may be appreciated after bottle-feedings.

Staying "Pumped"

It can be really tough to keep pumping without the emotional satisfaction of breastfeeding. Other mothers who are in the same boat can make your experience much easier to cope with—and you can do the same for them. There's a very active forum just about exclusive pumping on the La Leche League website at llli.org. There is also an e-mail group just for exclusively pumping moms at pumpingmoms.org.

Premature Babies

When you have a premature baby, breastfeeding may be the last thing on your mind. Your first concern is whether your tiny, fragile-looking baby will survive and be healthy. Seeing your newborn with tubes and monitors attached can be frightening. And you probably feel helpless to do anything for your baby while the hospital staff bustles about, adjusting this dial and changing that setting.

Yet you are *hugely* important. Your baby knows your voice and your smell and will respond differently to your touch than she will to anyone else's. Even the most fragile baby will benefit from hearing you talk to her and from your gentle touch. Research has shown that premature babies cannot stabilize as quickly with standard medical technology as they do in simple skin contact with their mothers!

Hospital policies about skin-to-skin contact vary, and your baby's age and developmental stage are factors. We encourage you to spend as much time as you possibly can with your baby skin to skin on your chest. The transition from Isolette to you or you to Isolette can be difficult for premies; it's easier on your baby if your stays are at least a couple of hours long. Susan Ludington-Hoe's book *Kangaroo Care: The Best You Can Do to Help Your*

Preterm Infant gives a lot of information, with hints on making your baby's experience in the neonatal intensive care unit (NICU) better.

Kangaroo Care

When you hold your baby skin-to-skin for long stretches of time, research has shown:

- Your baby's oxygenation levels and breathing rates are more regular and stable, in harmony with his heart rate.
- His heart rate is slightly higher, showing a positive response to being close to you.
- You have the ability to warm and stabilize your baby's temperature better than an incubator, and will automatically adjust your own temperature to raise or lower your baby's to his optimal level.
- He is more likely to breastfeed more easily, and your milk production increases.
- He will have a better immune system, with less vulnerability to allergies and infections in his first year.
- You will feel closer to your baby—a help in healing the trauma of the premature birth.
- There are no downsides.

This all sounds lovely until you turn each of these items around: the premature baby who is *not* in Kangaroo Care with his mother

- Is not as well oxygenated and has less stable heart and breathing rates
- Has more trouble keeping a stable temperature
- Has more trouble with breastfeeding; his mother also has a poorer milk supply
- Has a depressed immune system, with more vulnerability to allergies and infections in his first year
- Has more bonding issues

Clearly, Kangaroo Care should be the standard of care. As the mother of a premature baby, your body is central to your baby's good health, whether he finishes developing inside your body or outside it. That's why Kangaroo *Mother* Care was devised, taking Kangaroo Care a step further.

KANGAROO MOTHER CARE: GOING KANGAROO CARE ONE BETTER

Most hospitals recognize the value of Kangaroo Care by now, but it's a form of care in which the hospital is the primary caregiver and the mother helps out when she can. Kangaroo *Mother* Care changes the arrangement. The mother acts as the primary caregiver, wearing the baby in a special wrap nearly twenty-four hours a day, and the hospital provides backup care and expertise as needed. The approach was refined in African hospitals that lacked the equipment of most Western facilities. When their babies were matched with babies receiving standard Western care, the babies receiving Western care didn't do as well!

Very few hospitals are even aware of Kangaroo Mother Care yet, but the idea is spreading. If you would like to learn more, check out kangaroomothercare.com or *Hold Your Prem* by Jill Bergman with Nils Bergman.

Your Milk Is Incredibly Important for Your Premature Baby

Your milk is different from the milk of a mother whose baby was born full-term, and contains more of the nutrients your preterm baby needs. Formulas, even special premature formulas, increase the risk of damage to your baby's sensitive and immature digestive system and make it more likely that she'll get infections and illnesses, especially *necrotizing enterocolitis* (NEC), a very serious condition that premature babies on formula are at high risk of developing. In some hospitals, the most premature babies (under 1,500 grams at birth) have milk fortifiers added to the milk their mothers pump for them. These fortifiers are intended to increase levels of protein and some other nutrients to help the baby gain weight more quickly during the early weeks. Attempts are under way to provide fortifiers that are human-milk-based rather than cow-milk-based, which would reduce the risk of allergies and illness. You can ask if they are available if you're told your baby needs a fortifier.

Building Your Milk Supply

A primary goal at this stage is to build your milk supply. For the first few days, when you are producing colostrum, hand expression will probably work better. You won't produce large amounts, but that's okay—your baby is tiny! When you notice your milk supply increasing, you can start using a breast pump. If your baby is being fed by *nasogastric tube* (a tube going from her nose down to her stomach) or bottle, it's ideal to pump or hand-express before each feeding so that your baby can have the fresh, just-pumped milk. Any extra can be refrigerated or frozen in case you have to be away for any future feedings.

Frequent pumping is important to build your milk supply. Your future milk production is based on the amount of milk removed in these early days. If you pump less now, there will be less milk six weeks down the road. For lots of information on pumping, see Chapter 15.

Seeing all the milk you're pumping that your baby can't begin to use yet may make you think it isn't important to pump so much. But your little baby who looks so tiny now is going to grow really fast, probably doubling her size in a few months, and before you know it she'll need every drop of a full milk supply. It's better to overproduce in the beginning so you'll have enough later, when your baby catches up. Remember to do a little hand expression after you pump during these early weeks; it could make a real difference for your overall supply. Breast compressions while you pump can help increase the amounts, too.

It's common for mothers of premies to see an occasional temporary dip in milk production. Being the mom of a premie is one of the most stressful experiences any mother can have. Maybe you got some bad news about how your baby is doing or you're finding it difficult to juggle demands at home with being with your baby in the hospital. Breast compressions while pumping can be especially helpful during these times.

If you are consistently having trouble making as much milk as your baby needs even though you're pumping at least eight times a day, you might find that an herb or medication (a *galactagogue*) increases your production (see Chapter 18). Check your planned approach with a breastfeeding-knowledgeable doctor. For more detailed information about milk production problems, see *The Breastfeeding Mother's Guide to Making More Milk* by Diana West and Lisa Marasco.

"I had to get help when I didn't have enough milk for my pre-term baby. I felt incredibly anxious. The first time I phoned a La Leche League Leader, there was no answer, and it took two weeks to get enough courage to phone again. I've thought about why I found it so difficult to ask for help. I finally realized that I was afraid that I would be told that there was nothing I could do to produce enough milk (which was what I was being told at the hospital). I had come to believe this and made that second call to ask about getting an at-breast supplementer because nurturing my baby at my breast was far more important than nourishing him with milk from my breast. When Anne, an LLL Leader, said to me, 'You don't need a supplementer, Jill, you are going to be able to breastfeed your baby,' I felt so happy. I believed her because she sounded so confident that I was going to do what I wanted to do. And I did."   —Jill

Breast or Bottle First?

At first your baby may be fed by nasogastric tube. After the tube is removed (or if it isn't used at all), some hospitals have a firm policy that the baby needs to be drinking from a bottle before she can try breastfeeding, or that the baby must take bottles before being discharged. The research doesn't support this. Bottle-feeding is *more* stressful for a premature baby than breastfeeding; a tiny baby has more trouble coordinating sucking and breathing with a bottle. If the baby doesn't seem to be ready to handle the flow of milk from the breast, he can "practice" by nursing on your breast right after you've pumped (he'll get a little milk in the process).

If you are doing Kangaroo Care, you may find that at some point your baby starts moving down your body and heading for your breast. He may even latch on without much help from you. This is an excellent sign that your baby is developmentally ready to breastfeed. Some babies will need more help than others, and sometimes a *nipple shield* can make it easier for the baby to latch on and nurse effectively (see Chapter 18). Because premies lack the fat pads in their cheeks that help fill the space in a full-term baby's mouth, they have to work harder to create enough suction. They have to pause often, and with every pause your nipple can slip away. With a nipple shield in place, your baby doesn't need to work as hard either drinking or pausing. It's certainly worth trying to breastfeed without a shield first, but keep it in mind if your baby seems to need some extra help.

Premature babies in hospitals are often kept to a fairly rigid schedule of feedings every three or even four hours, with the goal of not tiring the baby too much. But the baby who is in skin-to-skin contact with his mother will probably have the energy and interest to nurse more frequently.

If you don't feel up to debating this with the hospital staff, you may decide to go along with their instructions in order to get home more quickly. If that's what happens, don't be discouraged. Feel confident that if you keep your milk production going well, you'll be able to breastfeed.

> *"Mark was born nine weeks early. He needed a respirator at first and his weight dropped. That was a scary thing when he was already so tiny. But I knew the important thing was to get pumping right away so I'd have milk for him when he was ready to eat. I pumped every three hours around the clock and sometimes more. It was hard, but it helped to feel like I was doing something for him.*
>
> *"When he was breathing on his own, I started doing Kangaroo Care with him, but the hospital nurses were very resistant to the idea. I could stay overnight in the hospital's 'care by parent' room, but the nurses kept telling me it was too stressful for him.*
>
> *"Then they told me he needed to have a bottle before he started to breastfeed. I knew this wasn't true, but I was desperate to get him home, so I went along with them. Once he would take the bottle okay—filled with my milk, at least—the nurses said I could start breastfeeding him once a day. Then three times a day. If he didn't get enough, I had to top him up with a bottle.*
>
> *"Finally they let us go home, still partly bottle-feeding, partly breast-feeding. The nurse warned me not to breastfeed him too much because it would tire him out. I thought he was doing pretty well at the breast. But when we got home, I felt quite discouraged and anxious. How would I manage the pumping and bottle-feeding and breastfeeding?*
>
> *"I talked to my LLL Leader, who helped me put it all into perspec-tive. It was clear that I had plenty of milk—I was pumping more than he could eat in a single day. He was nursing well. So I tossed out the bottles and went to full-time breastfeeding, and we never looked back.*

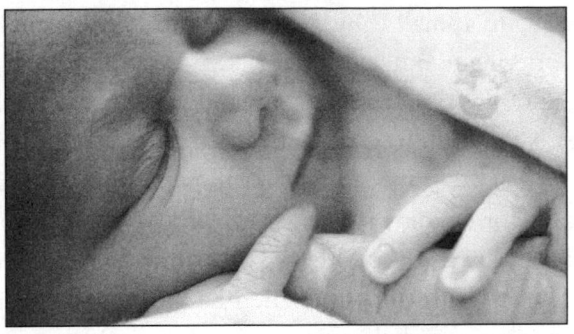

By the time he was three months old he was a big, plump baby. People who saw him couldn't believe he'd been born early."   —Julia

When Your Premie Breastfeeds

Expect to feel a bit anxious and nervous the first time your baby breast-feeds. He probably still seems impossibly tiny! Try a laid-back nursing position first. If you've been doing Kangaroo Care, you've likely been in this position many times: get comfortable semi-reclining, with some pillows to keep you comfortable, and relax with baby tummy down on your chest. He may move over to the breast all on his own, with a little help and support from you.

In the beginning, he may not nurse for very long. Some premature babies latch on, take a couple of sucks, then promptly fall asleep. No worries. He's just feeling very happy and contented. He can be fed some milk through a tube while he rests in your arms, and you can try again when he wakes up. (When he doesn't take much or enough from the breast, you'll need to pump after breastfeeding to remove the milk to keep your supply up.)

Providing a little extra support while he nurses may help. Sometimes the clutch hold position, where the baby is positioned on his back next to your side, with your hand supporting his neck and the base of his head as he feeds, works well for premature babies. You may also want to try breast compressions, squeezing your breast as the baby sucks to increase the flow of milk if the baby's suck isn't very strong. (Be cautious with this if you have a generous milk supply, though, since too much milk can be a bit overwhelming to a small baby. If you feel you might flood him, you can pump before offering to nurse.)

Expect some transition time at home. Your baby will be shifting from infrequent feeds to more frequent ones. You may need to initiate feedings at first. He may or may not need a little support from supplemental feeds at first. Your doctor or midwife will monitor his weight gain closely; wet and poopy diapers are not a reliable way of estimating whether or not your premature baby is getting enough. When he nurses, your baby will probably have more pauses and shorter sucking bursts than a full-term baby. Carrying him, in a wrap designed for Kangaroo Mother Care or in a sling, will help him grow faster, saving him calories by keeping him in his "natural habitat." Since premies are so tiny, check with someone knowledgeable about carriers and premature babies. Staying in touch with your LLL Leader or other breastfeeding helper can make any transition go more smoothly for both of you.

When should your baby-with-two-birthdates (the real one and the due date) start solids? That's up to him! See Chapter 13 for information on baby-led solids. It works for premies, too.

Near-Term Babies

A baby born between thirty-six and thirty-nine weeks may not be technically premature. But they often seem to have some immaturity and need extra help in the first several weeks to get the hang of breastfeeding. They also may go right from sound sleep to furious ("zero to sixty"); have trouble tuning out noise and distractions; have difficulty coordinating sucking, swallowing, and breathing while breastfeeding; have difficulty regulating their body temperature; have jerky and inconsistent rooting and sucking reflexes; have low muscle tone and not enough fat in their cheeks for stability and easy feeding; and they tire quickly during feedings.

Here are some ideas that may help your near-term baby breastfeed more easily:

- ☼ Minimize stimulation: lights down, TV off, voices quiet, less handling.
- ☼ Keep your baby skin to skin to keep him warm and secure.
- ☼ Until he reaches his due date, wake him for feedings if he sleeps longer than three hours.

- ☼ Consider the laid-back breastfeeding position to give your baby stability and support during feedings.
- ☼ If you sit up, try using your hand cupped under his chin while nursing to support his chin and cheeks.
- ☼ Use breast compression and massage during feeding to make nursing easier for him.

Multiples

The most common worries about breastfeeding twins, triplets, or more are having enough arms and having enough milk. We hope you'll have some help to give you a few extra arms to hold the babies, but you're the babies' best source for milk. Fortunately, you'll probably have plenty of milk, because the more placental tissue you have (and you have more with twins than with one baby, and still more with triplets), the more milk-making tissue your body creates.

Breastfeeding is particularly important for multiples that are also premature (as most are today). If they have to spend time in the NICU and are unable to breastfeed at first, pumping your milk for them with a rental-grade pump will be essential (see "Premature Babies").

Once your babies are home, you'll need to pay close attention to their diaper output and weights to make sure they are getting enough milk. Sometimes it's tough to keep the numbers straight for each baby, so it might help to have a separate color-coded clipboard or notebook for each of them. Don't be surprised if one nurses better than the other(s) at first. Just like all babies, some catch on faster and some have less developed neurological reflexes or even tongue restrictions that can prevent effective milk removal. Alternate the breast each baby gets to keep your milk supply evenly stimulated. Also be sure you're allowing each baby to nurse as long as he needs to.

Should You Nurse Two at the Same Time?

Nursing two babies at once can sure save time and the babies will stimulate milk releases for each other, but there's a huge learning curve in figuring out how to manage it, and it can feel overwhelming at first. So don't feel like it's something you *have* to do right away. What may work best for you is to

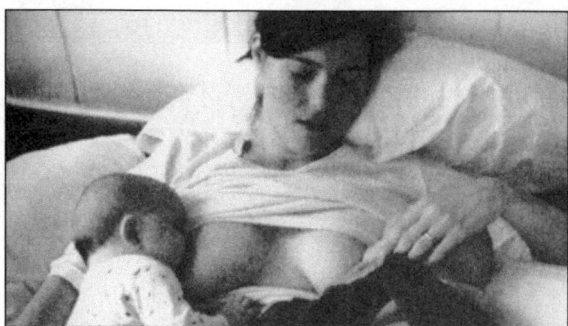

Laid-back breastfeeding for two!

take the time now to figure out how to nurse each baby effectively for his individual personality and needs. Later, when the babies are more mature and you're in your groove, you can try adding in a second baby after the first has latched on. You can nurse them both in the clutch position (so their heads are close together but their bottoms are tucked under your arms), or you can lay one across the other. Pillows can be your saving grace—some companies make nursing pillows just for nursing twins. Or try laid-back breastfeeding for two: sit fairly upright with a baby held along your body in each arm, their chests and tummies against you, as if you were carrying two tall sacks of flour that you're trying not to spill. Let each baby rest a cheek on a breast, and settle back comfortably. Now move your arm and body to drag or stroke a nipple across first one baby's cheek and then the other's, stimulating each to latch on in turn. Another mother's temporary solution, born of desperation, was to put both babies on the couch and kneel on the floor in front of them! Creativity and flexibility are your best friends now—there's no right and wrong so long as the babies are getting enough milk.

You may feel that you're glued to your couch when you're nursing twins or more. An enlightening moment for one mother of multiples came when she met a mother of grown twins, who told her, "Oh, I still remember fixing and feeding and washing all those bottles!" Breast or bottle, feeding twins or triplets is a demanding undertaking. But breastfeeding gets to be more and more fun. Washing bottles doesn't.

"The first try was hilarious. If you're holding a baby in each arm, what do you do when a newborn loses the nipple? Wish for a third hand,

that's what! I soon discovered pillows, and we've got the system down pat now. For a couple of frantic weeks, they refused to nurse at the same time. But with practice and the aid of pillows we finally discovered a lying-down position that is comfortable for all three of us. The nicest part is that now I can doze off while nursing, whereas before I sat upright until both were finished. That made for short nights! Looking back now, I realize I did little else but nurse the babies in those first couple of weeks. But now here we are at five months and things are going fairly smoothly—most of the time!" —Paula

Supply Problems

What if you're having trouble making enough milk? Some mothers of multiples do, often because the babies were conceived with fertility treatments for a hormonal problem that prevented conception and now is affecting milk production. This is a complex topic with many possible full or partial solutions. For in-depth information, consult *The Breastfeeding Mother's Guide to Making More Milk* by Diana West and Lisa Marasco or a Leader or Lactation Consultant.

Don't Forget to Take Care of Yourself

One of the most important factors to taking care of multiples is taking care of *you*. This is a time when the help of caring friends and family is not just helpful but absolutely necessary. Sure, you need more arms to hold the babies, but you need a lot of TLC (Tender Loving Care) right now, too, which includes plentiful, well-balanced meals and lots of hydrating fluids. (A foot rub or two wouldn't hurt, either!)

There are a lot of great stories from mothers of multiples on the llli .org website. Karen Gromada, mother of twins, IBCLC, and former LLL Leader, has written a wonderful comprehensive book about nursing multiples called *Mothering Multiples*.

"When time was a factor, I nursed the twins together, sitting in a rocker, with Jill on Judy's lap. Otherwise, I found it much easier to nurse the babies separately. I would awaken one about half an hour before the

other was due to get up so as to avoid nursing them together. Of course, I alternated so that one twin wouldn't always have 'first pickings.'

"If one was still hungry after nursing on one side, I would offer the other breast. Then the next one would begin on the side last nursed by the other. Usually the last to be nursed would be the first to wake up hungry. There were times when they would want to nurse again after only one and a half to two hours, and this served to increase my milk supply to meet their demands. Usually it would take two days of very frequent nursing and they would again be satisfied with a less demanding schedule.

"I always made sure the twins nursed at least every three hours and would awaken them if necessary. At night, all I had to do was scoop the hungry one into bed, doze and nurse until the other one awakened, and then switch. This was a marvelous system for me because it gave me the sleep I needed."   —Carolyn

Relactation

Relactation is about restarting milk production after it has been stopped for a while. You might have thought you didn't want to or couldn't breastfeed and then changed your mind. Or maybe your baby really needs your milk because he's having problems with formula. Whatever your reason, bringing back your milk supply for your baby is well worth the work.

How Tough Will It Be?

If you started out with a full milk supply originally, it will probably take about the same amount of time to get it back as it has been since you stopped breastfeeding (or pumping). If you never had a full milk supply or if it's been several months since you weaned, getting full production going might not be realistic, but it's almost always possible to get *some* milk production back.

Keep Baby Well Fed

As you work to bring back your supply, make sure that your baby is being fed adequately. You can gradually replace formula with your milk (ideally at the breast) as your supply increases, but your baby's intake should never be decreased during the transition. What you can do during this time is begin getting him used to feeding techniques that are more similar to breastfeeding, like those described in Chapter 18.

Restarting Milk Production

Is your baby willing to nurse fairly well even though there's no milk yet? If so, this alone can bring your milk back, although your baby will need to be supplemented during the process.

If your baby is reluctant to nurse or won't nurse very long, you can pump to begin stimulating your breasts to make milk again. Because you need the best stimulation possible, it's usually best to use either hand expression or a rental-grade pump, making sure the flanges fit well. Hand expression can be very effective when you are producing small amounts of milk. (Definitely read Chapter 15 for hints about expressing and pumping effectively.)

Pumping might not feel very comfortable at first (a thin coating of lanolin on your nipple tip can help), so feel free to work up to a full pumping as slowly as you need to. The first sign that milk production is starting up again will be a feeling of breast tenderness and possibly fullness. Then you should start to see some drops forming on your nipple when you express. They may be clear at first but soon will be white. Gradually the volume will increase. You'll probably begin to see good results in two to six weeks.

One option to speed things along is to use a galactagogue, an herb or medication that increases milk production. It is important to take these ONLY after you're nursing or pumping regularly to remove the milk that they will help create. When it comes to building a supply, galactagogues are the frosting on the milk removal cake. They never substitute for milk removal itself. Many mothers have been successful in increasing their milk by nursing and expressing alone, so it is worth trying this before you go to galactagogues. For information about them, see Chapter 18.

Enticing Your Baby Back to the Breast

If your baby is reluctant to nurse, remember that breastfeeding really is your baby's default setting. She has lots of instincts that can help guide her back to the breast. The most important thing as you go along is to be gentle and patient. You're *enticing* your baby to breastfeed—there's no way to *make* her do it.

In addition to feeding bottles in the breastfeeding-supportive ways described in Chapter 18, keeping your baby skin to skin for long periods during the day can go a long way toward helping her reacclimatize to your body and smells. Take baths together, lounge around in bed together, co-sleep. Keep your breasts a comforting place to be so she has positive associations with them. Laid-back nursing positions can also be really helpful while you encourage your baby to nurse.

If your baby is reluctant to take the breast, you can try using an eyedropper to drip milk onto the nipple as she latches, or have an at-breast supplementer set up so she gets milk right away. If she still won't latch, you could try when she's sleepy, when she first wakes up, with a little milk smeared on your areola, or any other way that you can think of. Sometimes it takes a lot of ingenuity and creativity. Some babies used to the feeling of bottle nipples will latch if the mother uses a nipple shield (see Chapter 18, which also has information on bringing baby back to the breast after nursing strikes). Do consult with your La Leche League Leader, International Board Certified Lactation Consultant, or other breastfeeding helper. They should have other ideas in their bag of tricks. It's all about "baby steps" in encouraging your baby back to the breast.

It will probably help to keep pacifiers away for the time being so that she is more motivated to satisfy her sucking needs at your breast.

Once your baby is nursing and gaining well and you are producing more milk, you can start reducing supplements gradually.

- Reduce supplements by very small amounts, maybe ½ ounce or less (5 to 15 ml) each feeding, every few days so your baby continues to get plenty of milk.
- At times of the day when you feel as though you have more milk (such as first thing in the morning), you may be able to reduce a supplement by ½ to 1 ounce (20 to 30 ml).

- Keep an eye on your baby's wet and poopy diapers so you know that he's taking plenty of milk.

Be prepared to take things more slowly if your baby becomes fussy or seems hungry. During the transition from bottle to breast, it's important to weigh your baby regularly on a reliable scale—maybe the one in your doctor's office—to make sure she is getting enough. If she isn't, you can give her more expressed milk (or formula if necessary), but don't cut down on the nursing or pumping.

Be sure to take care of your own needs during the journey. If you let yourself get run down, you may not be able to hang in there for the payoff. And don't try to do it all yourself. This is a time to reach out to all your breastfeeding-supportive friends, family, and online buddies. Gather a cheering team to celebrate your successes and console you when you feel frustrated, because there may be days when you feel discouraged. This experience can have a lot of ups and downs, and days of two steps forward, one step back. On the tough days, it can help to repeat a mantra like "Babies are born to breastfeed, and I am a breastfeeding mother."

"I had been looking forward to breastfeeding William, but as soon as he suckled for the first time I noticed it was very painful. I persevered, but after ten days we began using bottles and I stopped breastfeeding.

"Seven weeks of tears and depression followed. I finally telephoned Sally at my local breastfeeding clinic. She said if I felt that bad about my experience and was determined enough, why didn't I try to relactate? She referred me to Kerry, an LLL Leader, for more information. Kerry explained that it would take a lot of work and that I would need support from my family because of the time and effort involved. I felt that I needed to try.

"I started taking medications and expressing each breast for fifteen minutes with a pump, aiming for eight to twelve pumping sessions a day. With a young baby and two other children to care for, this was no small task.

"I got a lot of satisfaction from feeding William at least some of my milk from a bottle. We spent a lot of time having skin-to-skin contact, getting him to love the smell of my skin. I also used a nursing supplementer, a bag of milk I hung from my neck with two fine tubes running down to *my nipples. Will didn't like this. I tried using special nipple shields, but he would not latch on to them. I resigned myself to bottle-feeding my expressed milk.*

"One day when he was five and a half months old, he was licking my T-shirt. I offered him the breast, and he latched on and fed like a complete natural from that day forward. I was able to fully breastfeed him! He became a much more contented child and I felt a much closer bond with him, though it had been hard to imagine how the bond could have been closer.

"It was a hard and very emotional battle but worth every bit of effort. I look at him now and feel very proud of what we achieved."

—Kathy

Induced Lactation

Bringing in a milk supply without having been pregnant is becoming much more common as more mothers realize it's possible. You may have an adopted baby or your baby may have been born with the help of a surrogate or female partner. For many women who bring in a milk supply without pregnancy, the goal is less about the milk and more about connecting deeply to their new baby. But with new advances in the science of lactation, the chances of getting a good milk supply or even a full one are much better than in years past.

If you have infertility difficulties that have prevented pregnancy, one issue to consider is the possibility that underlying hormonal problems could affect lactation. This is especially likely in cases of polycystic ovary syndrome (PCOS), when breast tissue may be underdeveloped. Other hormonal issues, such as thyroid problems, may not affect fertility but can still affect lactation. So it's important to treat any known conditions (to the extent that you can) while you begin working to induce milk production.

Nursing Without a Milk Supply

If you're starting with a newborn or a baby who is willing to take the breast, you can begin nursing right away with an at-breast supplementer filled with donated milk or formula (see Chapter 18). Depending on your baby's cooperation, you also may be able to entice him to nurse for comfort in between feedings without the tube.

How to Induce a Milk Supply

Your approach depends a lot on whether or not your baby has been born, how old he is, and what you feel comfortable doing. You have many options.

Stimulating the Breasts

The most basic way of getting a milk supply started is simply to stimulate the breasts in a way that tells them to make milk. This can be done by frequent (eight to twelve times a day) nursing, hand expression, or pumping. The more stimulation, the better; starting each session with some breast massage often helps. For more thoughts on pumping, see Chapter 15.

You probably won't see milk for a while, and that doesn't matter. You're just trying to send the message to your breasts to *start* making milk.

If you're nursing with an at-breast supplementer, your breasts will eventually start making milk that your baby will get along with the milk from the tube. The first milk that comes won't be colostrum, but more like a birth mother's mature milk. After you feel like you have a fair amount of milk, try nursing the baby every now and then without the supplementer, or pinch the supplementer closed at the beginning of the feeding to help him drain your breast more fully.

As your milk increases, it can be hard to know how much is coming from you and how much from the tube. One way to get an idea is to weigh both baby and supplementer on a sensitive scale before and after the feeding. Any increase in weight came straight from you! Weighing him in this way every week or so can give you an idea of how much your milk supply is increasing. If you're already nursing with an at-breast supplementer, you can pump the other breast at the same time for even better stimulation. If you don't have the baby yet, hand expression or pumping will begin stimulating your milk supply. Hand expression can be great because it provides a lot of tactile stimulation, but most mothers use a high-quality rental-grade pump to get the best of both worlds. Be sure the flanges fit well (see Chapter 15 for pumping tips).

But there's no need to be so scientific unless you want to be. You may prefer, as many do, just to trust to the magic of it all. Successful breastfeeding isn't measured in units, any more than love is.

> "Breastfeeding is as much about a relationship and way of responding to your babies and children as it is about the food they receive. Nursing our two sons, who came to us through adoption seventeen months apart, allowed me to experience the same closeness that I enjoyed and loved with our biological daughter. I loved being able to nurse them at night and at times during the day without the need for a supplementer. I found that when each of our sons was a little bit over age one, he was taking enough table foods and drinking enough other fluids from a cup that I stopped using the supplementer completely, but continued to nurse them in a normal toddler pattern, until one was over four and the other three and a half years old." —Bonnie

Simulating Pregnancy Hormones

Many mothers who have induced milk supplies find that they can build a bigger supply faster by using hormones and galactagogues to simulate the process that builds the lactation infrastructure during pregnancy. The general idea is to simulate the hormones of pregnancy and then of birth and breastfeeding. The effect on your supply depends on how long before your baby comes you can start the process. But if you have to do it all quickly, you'll probably still make more milk than you would by just pumping or nursing alone.

You may or may not go through *all* the side effects of pregnancy (nausea, cravings, weight gain), but if all goes well, the infrastructure will develop and your breasts will begin feeling tender, just as in an actual pregnancy. Hormonal treatments to build a milk supply suppress lactation at first, so they are generally not appropriate for mothers who are already nursing another baby. Talk to your doctor, because certain hormones are not safe for some women.

Lenore Goldfarb, a lactation consultant in Canada, created a standardized hormonal protocol for induced lactation that's available on her website at asklenore.info/breastfeeding/induced_lactation/protocols_intro.html.

Colostrum from the Birth Mother

Since an induced milk supply does not provide colostrum, many mothers have asked the birth mother or surrogate to pump her milk for a limited amount of time for the baby. Some birth mothers and surrogates are pleased to be able to offer this healthy start in life. One birth mother shared that providing her milk helped her cope with the adoption process.

When Adoption Doesn't Happen

As adoptive parents know only too well, there is always the possibility that the birth mother may change her mind and keep the baby—a heartbreaking situation. When the adoptive mother has been preparing her body hormonally for many months, the loss can be even more devastating. Understandably, many mothers decide to discontinue their preparations for breastfeeding temporarily, knowing they always have the option to resume preparations when they're ready or when a new baby is on the horizon.

"As with anything in life, not everything is guaranteed. Adoptions can fall through. My husband and I experienced this with our first effort to adopt. I began nursing Anna within half an hour of her birth, using an at-breast supplementer for the first time. I was so happy that Anna was a good nurser, and her birth mother was happy I wanted to breastfeed her. At six days, the adoption agency called to tell us that the baby's birth father had revoked his consent for the adoption. We were stunned and worried, but the agency believed that the birth father would change his mind again.

"We continued caring for Anna. I was very excited to find I brought in a full milk supply by the time she was five weeks old. Unfortunately, the birth father did not change his mind, and our family was forced to part with Anna when she was eight weeks old. After losing Anna, I rented a pump for a while, but found that I needed to focus on healing my heart and caring for my seven-year-old daughter. I figured that if I could induce a milk supply once, I could do it again.

> *"A friend helped me very much by telling me, 'There's another little baby who needs you more.' I hung on to this thought, and within two months our adoption agency called us about another birth mother who wanted to meet us. We had a wonderful outcome this time.*
>
> *"With adoption, as with many things in life, we find we are more resilient than we might have thought. I have no regrets for having nursed Anna while she was with us. It meant a great deal to me to love and parent her the way I believe is best for babies and families."*
>
> —Bonnie

INDUCED LACTATION RESOURCES

Breastfeeding an Adopted Baby and Relactation, by Elizabeth Hormann, IBCLC

Adoptive Breastfeeding Resource Website—fourfriends.com/abrw

Adoption.com—breast-feeding.adoption.com

Ask Lenore—asklenore.info/breastfeeding/abindex.html#adoptive _breastfeeding

La Leche League International—llli.org/NB/NBadoptive.html

Maternal Challenges

Even with a challenging situation, breastfeeding often makes life easier. A mother whose daily life is already complicated by blindness, hearing impairment, a wheelchair, a chronic illness, or needing to recover from an acute illness or injury can breastfeed her baby without the added hassle of preparing, assembling, or cleaning bottles of formula. Since formula-fed babies generally have more health problems than breastfed babies, breastfeeding can also save many trips to the doctor. Emotionally, breastfeeding does wonders for our self-esteem, self-confidence, and sense of normalcy about mothering.

The hormonal shift that results from breastfeeding can also reduce the symptoms of chronic illnesses such as rheumatoid arthritis, multiple sclerosis, lupus, and diabetes. Some even go into temporary remission.

A mother who has diabetes and breastfeeds can reduce her child's chances of developing both type 1 and type 2 diabetes in adulthood. Pregnancy and lactation do change insulin requirements, and unless these are managed, milk production can be affected. Monitoring blood sugar and adjusting medication or insulin dosages accordingly is important. (It's perfectly safe to take insulin while breastfeeding.) It's also possible that your newborn's glucose levels will be monitored more closely at first, possibly even requiring time in the NICU. Keeping your own blood levels well controlled during pregnancy and keeping him in skin-to-skin contact after birth will help keep his blood sugar stable and minimize the need for interventions. Hand-expressing and storing colostrum during pregnancy will also help in case your milk is slow to transition to full volume, which is common with type 1 diabetes.

Most medications necessary for treating physical challenges are compatible with breastfeeding. See the section on medications in Chapter 18.

HIV

The recommendations on infant feeding when a mother is HIV-positive are still changing. Some evidence suggests that HIV can be passed on to the baby through breastfeeding, but there aren't any published studies confirming that the virus in human milk is actually infectious. And if it *is* infectious, we don't know if there is enough in human milk to infect the baby.

Research has clearly shown that the risk of an infant contracting HIV from an infected mother is much higher if the baby is both breastfed *and* receives formula supplementation than if he is exclusively breastfed or exclusively formula-fed. Yet a mother with HIV who lives in an industrialized country, such as the United States, Canada, or New Zealand, probably will be told by her doctor not to breastfeed.

The World Health Organization states that the most appropriate infant feeding option for an HIV-infected mother depends on her individual circumstances, including her health status and the local situation; she should consider the health services available and the counseling and support she is likely to receive. Exclusive breastfeeding is recommended for HIV-infected women for the first six months of life unless replacement feeding is acceptable, feasible, affordable, sustainable, and safe for them and their infants. When these conditions are met, avoidance of all breastfeeding by HIV-infected women is recommended. Given the lack of research proving that babies breastfed by HIV-positive mothers are more likely to get sick and die than babies who are formula-fed, there are some doctors in industrialized countries who occasionally and quietly support breastfeeding by an HIV-positive mother.

In 2001, AnotherLook, a nonprofit organization dedicated to gathering information, raising critical questions, and stimulating needed research about breastfeeding in the context of HIV/AIDS, was formed. In 2008, an AnotherLook position paper concluded, "For the overwhelming majority of HIV-exposed babies, the weight of current evidence favors exclusive breastfeeding for six months to prevent mother-to-child HIV transmission and to prolong the lives of already infected babies. Thereafter HIV-free survival for the majority of older babies is likely to be enhanced by promotion of continued breastfeeding with the addition of complementary foods for up to two years or beyond, in line with current guidelines outside the context of HIV."

For more information about breastfeeding with HIV, visit AnotherLook (anotherlook.org), WHO (who.int), and UNICEF (unicef.org). If you are HIV-positive and opt to nurse your baby, be sure to research all the issues very, very carefully. This is a complex issue, with very few solid facts.

Diagnostic Tests and Therapeutic Procedures on the Breast During Breastfeeding

If you find a *persistent* lump in your breast while you're breastfeeding, your doctor will probably want to have it examined and tested as soon as possible, without waiting until you've stopped breastfeeding. These tests could include imaging techniques, tissue sampling, or even removal of the entire suspicious area. Or if you have a lung or heart problem, you may need to have incisions through breast tissue to reach the affected organs. How much these tests affect breastfeeding and your ability to make milk depends on what's done and what stage of lactation you're in.

Imaging Procedures
There are many technologies for looking inside human tissue without actually cutting into it. The tests that are most likely to be used for examining breast,

heart, or lung tissue are ultrasound, mammogram, magnetic resonance imaging (MRI), positron emission tomography (PET) scan, 2-methoxy isobutyl isonitrile (MIBI) scan, electrical impedance tomography (EIT) scan, computed tomography or CT scan (also known as computerized axial tomography or CAT scan), thermography, diaphanography, or ductogram. None of these imaging procedures will affect your ability to make milk.

The ability of the procedure to harm the milk itself depends on which type is used. *X-rays, mammograms, MRI, and CT/CAT scans are completely safe.* The radiation doesn't collect in the milk. You may be told to wean before you can have the procedure because the results can be more difficult for the radiologist to interpret during lactation, when the breast is denser. But it isn't impossible, just more difficult. So there is no need to stop breastfeeding or to pump and dump for these types of procedures, although you will find the tests more comfortable on an empty breast. Occasionally a woman who is being tested for breast cancer is asked to wean in order to get a clearer image. Ironically, weaning increases the future risk of breast cancer both for the mother and for her baby girl! It may make more sense to find a more experienced radiologist.

Radiopaque and radiocontrast agents used in imaging procedures are not absorbed, so they are also absolutely safe for breastfeeding. Research has not found any problems in babies who have nursed after their mothers have had radiopaque and radiocontrast agents.

However, radioactive isotopes and particulate radiation *do* contain radiation that can be absorbed by the body and appear in the milk supply, so a mother can't breastfeed until her milk is clear of the radiation (which can be tested in most hospitals). In the meantime, she'll need to pump and dump to keep her supply up and clear the radiation from her milk, and she may need to avoid close contact with her baby. Typical times range from hours to one month, so it's important to check the agent being used, the typical time to clear, and the possibility of alternatives ahead of time. See Hale's *Medications and Mothers' Milk* for details, check out Google "LactMed," or go to toxnet.nlm.nih.gov/cgi-bin/sis/htmlgen?LACT for information and recommendations. Before any procedure that requires short-term suspension of breastfeeding, it helps to pump and build up a freezer stash of milk that can be given to the baby when breastfeeding isn't possible. If an agent requiring long-term suspension of breastfeeding is necessary, it is still possible to maintain a milk supply until the level of radioactivity is considered safe, then resume nursing. Yes, it's been done successfully!

Tissue Sampling Procedures

The procedures for removing tissue from a suspicious lump in your breast for closer examination range from needle aspiration to wide-angle biopsy. Needle aspiration isn't likely to have any impact at all on your supply or the milk itself, but you may have some bruising of the breast and some (harmless) blood in your milk right after the test. Because a biopsy removes more tissue, potentially damaging glands, ducts, and nerves, it is much more likely to affect milk production capability. Incisions near the areola, especially in the lower outer area, are more likely to damage the nerves that affect milk release. Incisions that run across the breast (like a section of a ring around the breast) are more likely to damage lactation tissue than incisions that run parallel to the ducts (like a spoke on a bicycle wheel). An incision that requires tunneling through the tissue to reach a mass deep in the breast is more likely to damage glands and ducts, as well as nerves, than an incision to reach a mass close to the skin. To make sure, you can request that your surgeon mark the proposed incision site. However, though it makes sense to ask your surgeon to place the incision vertically, away from the areola, and tunnel as little as possible to preserve your lactation capability, it may not always be possible.

Just as with imaging procedures, while it's more difficult to do a biopsy on a lactating breast, there's no research that shows that it's a problem. Milk won't slow healing and may actually keep the incision cleaner due to the immunological properties of human milk. And even though you may have stopped breastfeeding days, weeks, or even months prior to the procedure, your breast doesn't stop making milk overnight, so there's almost always going to be some milk still in the breast. But, as with imaging procedures, you and your surgeon may find the procedure easier if your breast has been drained as fully as possible beforehand.

Expect some leaking while you heal; try to think of all those wonderful anti-infectives washing the wound. You can hold a compress firmly over the incision while you nurse, to minimize additional leaking. If you've had a vacuum drain inserted, you'll continue to drain milk until it's removed.

Breastfeeding with Cancer

If you have cancer or have just had surgery to remove it, but you're still lactating and you'd like to continue breastfeeding, you may hear a lot of conflicting information. You may be told that it will be too tiring for you and that you need to wean to save your strength. That's your decision to make! You might even hear that your baby can get cancer by nursing on an affected breast. There's absolutely no research to indicate that this can happen. Experts believe that it's simply not possible. What *can* happen is that a breast that has had radiation treatments may no longer produce well, may be rejected by the baby because of changes in the breast or milk, or may be painful during nursing. But there's no evidence that breastfeeding can lead to recurrence. Your choice of whether or not to use that breast is entirely yours.

You also might hear that your baby will naturally refuse to nurse on a breast with cancer or that your first clue that something was wrong with your breast was that your baby refused to nurse on it. But there are also case studies of babies who did not reject the cancerous breast. And babies may also refuse to nurse from a breast when the taste of the milk or the volume changes, or because they have an earache. Reasons are many, and cancer is rare. So if your baby refuses to nurse from one breast, don't worry that it means you have cancer. If your baby begins to refuse one side *and* you have an unexplained change in your nipple or breast appearance, check with your doctor.

Unfortunately, breastfeeding during chemotherapy is not safe because the chemotherapy drugs are incredibly toxic and do transfer into your milk. Pumping to whatever extent you would like is an option, maintaining a toehold on a milk supply until your chemotherapy is completely over, and then relactating to whatever extent you choose. If you decide to wean for surgery or treatment, read Chapter 16 for ways to end breastfeeding that will minimize the impact on your child and your breasts.

Previous Breast and Nipple Surgeries

All previous breast and nipple surgeries, including breast reductions, breast augmentations, and nipple inversion release surgeries, can affect future milk production, especially surgeries that damage nerves and ducts. The extent of the damage depends on where the incisions are located, how much tissue is damaged, where any implants are placed, how the surgery healed, and how long it has been since the surgery. Incisions around the lower outer part of the areola are more likely to damage the nerves that affect milk release—you can tell if the nerves were affected or have healed by how much sensation you have in your nipples. Implants above the muscle are more likely to reduce milk production than implants below the muscle. In most cases, mothers have more milk when their surgeries were longer than five years ago because the ducts and nerves have had a chance to regenerate.

If you've had any incisions or surgery on your breasts or nipples, you'll need to monitor your baby's weight gain closely in the first couple of weeks. If supplementation is necessary, there are ways to do it that still support breastfeeding, and there are many methods that can effectively increase your milk production (see Chapter 18). For more information about breastfeeding after breast surgery, see *Defining Your Own Success: Breastfeeding After Breast Surgery* by Diana West, and her website, bfar.org.

Babies with Special Needs

The baby born with a disability or medical problem needs the stimulation, attention, and closeness that naturally happen with breastfeeding even more than a healthy baby does. For instance, the growth harmones in your milk go a long way toward intestinal healing. You benefit, too, since breastfeeding helps you to focus on your baby as a baby first and foremost. If your baby has a health problem that complicates nursing, remember that breastfeeding is nearly always possible and is important for both of you. If you know in advance that your baby may have extra difficulties, you might want to express some colostrum during your pregnancy and save it for when the baby arrives. Contact your local LLL Leader for information and support.

"I did not know anyone who had ever breastfed, but I was sure it would be natural and easy. When Stuart was born, he seemed perfectly healthy and robust. However, he was not interested in breastfeeding.

The nurses were not very supportive and kept suggesting bottles of water and formula, but he was not interested in the bottles, either. And he had never passed any meconium stools.

"Luckily, the staff pediatrician was alert and suspected Hirschsprung's megacolon disease. (A child with this disease does not have a functioning lower part of his large intestine. Therefore, he does not pass stools. Eating can make it worse.) When Stuart was three days old, he underwent a lengthy and relatively new surgery. He was given a series of biopsies of his colon and a colostomy.

"The staff told me to take pills to dry up my milk and to forget about breastfeeding. Somehow I found the courage to refuse the dry-up pills. An LLL Leader guided me through handling swollen breasts and milk expression, and she offered me much more—the belief that I would still be able to breastfeed my baby.

"Stuart was the biggest baby in the neonatal unit. The nurses there, unlike the ones I'd seen previously, were extremely supportive of breastfeeding. Stuart's surgeon was thrilled that I would be breastfeeding. He was an Israeli doctor and a pioneer in the new colon surgery Stuart had undergone. The surgeon believed that breastfeeding would increase the odds of success.

"During his first year, Stuart and I spent many days and nights in the pediatric surgical wing of the hospital. Each visit interrupted our ability to breastfeed because of the surgical procedures and IVs. During his final surgery, around his first birthday, the surgeon removed the lower two-thirds of his colon, connected the remaining section to his anus, and closed the colostomy. Stuart healed well. Breastfeeding helped both of us through a very tough year."   —Gloria

Down Syndrome

The immunological properties in your milk are very important if you have a baby with Down syndrome, because she is more susceptible to respiratory and ear infections and cardiac problems. But it can be harder to breastfeed her because she may be very sleepy in the first few weeks and have weak facial muscles, a high palate, and a large tongue that can make it hard for her to suck effectively. You may need to pump after feedings and supplement with your pumped milk to make sure your supply stays high and she gets enough milk. There are oral stimulation exercises that can help with her ability to maintain suction. A board certified lactation consultant can share these with you, and your LLL Leader can provide support as you breastfeed your baby with Down syndrome. Your baby will have her own timetable, and latching and nursing effectively may simply be farther down the road for her than for most babies. Patience and pumping have brought many, many babies with Down syndrome to full breastfeeding by four or five months. That may sound daunting at first. But it's definitely doable, and your persistence can have huge lifelong payoffs for your baby's health and development.

Cleft Lip or Palate

A baby with an opening in his palate has difficulty creating suction, which makes it difficult to remove milk effectively no matter how he is fed. With a cleft of the soft or hard palate, milk can flow into the nasal cavity, causing the baby to cough or sputter and often making any kind of feeding difficult. These clefts are traditionally repaired only in the second half of the first year, when the baby's mouth is bigger. However, repairing a cleft palate immediately after birth has several huge advantages. Weight gain and health are generally better because the baby can eat normally or nearly normally right from the start. And "normally" can include breastfeeding! In addition, fetal healing—the rapid, excellent healing that an unborn or new born baby is capable of—may improve the quality of the repair. If your surgeon is unwilling to perform a very early repair, you might want to ask for a second opinion and seek a surgeon with experience in these earlier surgeries.

One possible aid for an unrepaired hard palate is a palatal obturator, a device like an orthodontic retainer that covers the roof of the mouth and the cleft and is replaced frequently as the baby grows. It can be made with a smooth surface that's comfortable for your nipple. Be creative with positioning; holding your baby upright may reduce the sputtering and nose leaking that are common. Find a good helper, and remember that time at the breast can be wonderful for a baby, whether or not milk is involved.

If your baby has a cleft lip but his palate is fine, you may be able to breastfeed with few or no changes. A soft breast can "fill in" the cleft, or you can use a finger to seal it so your baby can nurse. Try different positions if the first one doesn't work well.

If your baby will be having corrective surgery, it might help to know that babies can receive human milk up to four (possibly two) hours before general anesthesia. Research has shown that it's both safe and comforting for them to nurse right after they wake up from the surgery. Surgeons are generally more familiar with bottle-feeding and may tell you that your baby can't nurse for several days post-surgery. You can point out that a breastfed baby's upper lip is relaxed, not pursed, and puts no stress on the stitches.

If your baby isn't able to remove milk effectively until a repair is done, you can keep your production up through regular and thorough pumping with a good-quality pump. Your milk, which is very important as your baby faces the immunological challenge of surgery, can be given to him with a special feeding device that does not rely on suction. A board certified lactation consultant can be very helpful in giving you techniques and support.

> "My husband and I showed Dr. Johnson the information about nursing. He enthusiastically agreed to allow me to breastfeed soon after the surgery. He assured me that if any stitches pulled out after nursing, it would not harm Peter in any way to have him quickly replace a stitch. He agreed it was important that Peter be comforted. After surgery, when Dr. Johnson appeared and saw that Peter was nursing happily, he commented that it was nice to see him calm and not crying so soon after surgery." —Tammy

Cystic Fibrosis and Other Metabolic Conditions

Breastfeeding your baby with *cystic fibrosis, celiac disease,* or other malabsorption problems can protect him from respiratory infections and help him gain weight more normally. In fact, it can do this so well that the initial symptoms may not show up until later than they otherwise might have.

A baby who has *phenylketonuria* (PKU), which is normally tested for at birth, cannot digest the amino acid phenylalanine but still needs small amounts to grow normally. Fortunately, human milk has less phenylalinine than cow milk formula, so it's usually okay for a baby with PKU to breastfeed at least part-time, while also receiving supplements of a special-ized formula. The problem is usually that the baby needs to get a certain ratio of milk to formula and it's hard to know just how much milk he got by breastfeeding unless the baby is weighed before and after feedings. For-tunately, there is another way to do it: the amount of human milk that is appropriate for PKU is determined and then subtracted from the estimated total amount that the baby should be getting in order to grow appropri-ately at his age and weight. The remaining amount is how much formula is needed. Since this is a guesstimate, it's necessary to check the baby's pheny-lalanine blood levels periodically.

Babies with *galactosemia* are unable to digest galactose, the sugar that lac-tose, the main carbohydrate in human milk, breaks into during digestion. Unfortunately, weaning to a specialized lactose-free formula is necessary. There is another type, called *Duarte galactosemia,* that does not usually require weaning. Your doctor will be able to tell you which form your baby has and whether you'll have to wean.

Lactation After a Baby's Death

Sadly, many families experience the death of a baby through miscarriage, stillbirth, or death shortly after birth or later through an illness or accident. Mothers who face this terrible loss are also in the difficult position of cop-ing with the milk that continues to be made.

If your baby was miscarried in the second or third trimester of preg-nancy or died at birth or shortly after, you'll usually be discharged from the hospital fairly soon. When your milk comes in, engorgement is likely, but ice packs, anti-inflammatory medication, and other remedies recom-mended in Chapter 18 will help relieve the discomfort.

Milk releases can happen spontaneously by thinking about the baby, hearing another baby cry, or hugging someone. Absorbent nursing pads may be helpful until your milk production decreases.

Sometimes women are worried that removing milk to ease their dis-comfort will only encourage more milk to be made, but it's actually the best thing to do to stay comfortable and prevent a breast infection. The point is to remove just enough to be comfortable, but not enough to drain your breasts well. Taking a hot shower or using warm wet compresses on the breast just before pumping or hand-expressing may help the milk flow more easily. At first you may need to do this several times a day, but over a week or two, the milk will gradually subside until the day comes when you no longer feel discomfort and don't need to remove any more milk. Some herbs (sage, peppermint, parsley) can slow milk production. Pain medication may also help.

While these approaches can minimize the physical pain, the emotional pain can be more intense. Some mothers feel that continuing to lactate so the milk can be donated to a milk bank helps them feel they are doing something positive to help other babies. They may see the milk as their body's tears, or as their baby's gift to another. There are many milk banks that are pleased to receive donated milk. To find one in North America, visit hmbana.org., in Europe, europeanmilkbanking.com and in Australia, mothersmilkbanking.com.au.

Taking Care of Yourself

Your baby's needs may feel overwhelming at times, and you may feel that there is just no time or energy left over for you. Because you are so essential to your baby, it's important that you get the nurturing, good nutrition, support, and care that you need. Don't hesitate to ask for help or call on your network. That's why we're here!

EIGHTEEN

Tech Support

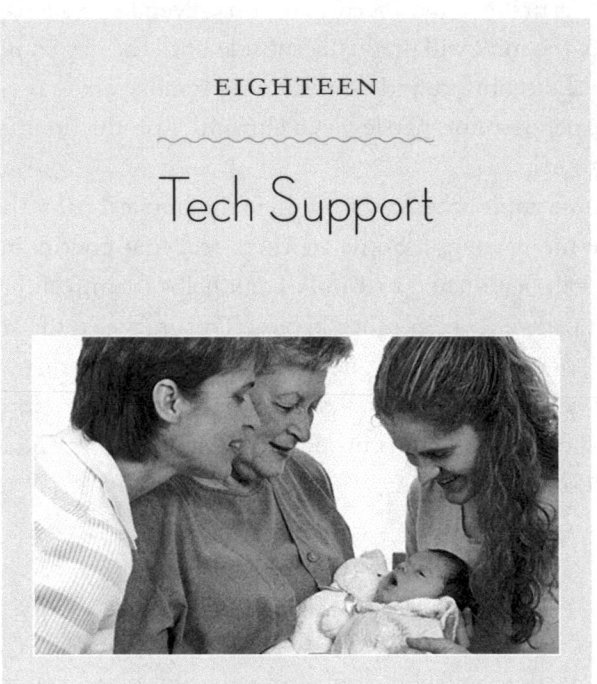

LIFE ISN'T PERFECT. If you've used a computer, you've probably run into a problem or two. What then? Well, you don't toss the whole thing out the window. You might mess around a little to see if there's a quick fix. Maybe you check the manual or look online. But in the end you often have to call tech support—the real person who can listen to your problem and talk you through the solution.

Sometimes breastfeeding needs a little tech support, too. Consider this chapter the first step. It isn't a real person; it's just a book. So if the answer you're looking for isn't here, find an LLL Leader, International Board Certified Lactation Consultant, or other helper trained in the more technical aspects of breastfeeding. And do it soon! Breastfeeding DOES work, even though there are challenges sometimes. Most likely all you need is someone to talk you through some solutions, a breastfeeding tech support person.

What if you went to the relevant section of this chapter, followed the ideas, fixed the problem, and things still aren't right? Well, having one issue doesn't mean you don't have another. Tongue-tie can cause nipple damage that leads to mastitis, and treating the mastitis doesn't make the tongue-tie disappear. Oversupply can cause a nursing strike. Engorgement and jaundice often go together. Nipple pain can cause you to delay nursings, which can drop your supply. And so on.

You may have to peel away a few layers of problems to find the happy mother and baby buried under them. The fastest way to accomplish that? Find that tech support person and keep working through the layers. You'll get there.

WHY HELP CAN HELP

There is no book that will give you all the answers. There is no strength of character that will get you through every problem. There is knowledge that you can get only in person from an experienced helper.

We've been where you are right now. We understand the feelings of disappointment and, yes, embarrassment or shame that can go along with being blindsided by a problem when you thought you had prepared so well. We understand that you want to get it right on your own. But if things aren't right, a Real Person can help you move from a too-short, gritting-your-teeth breastfeeding experience to a long and lovely one. It may take just a moment's help, it may take a few phone calls or visits, you may need to find more than one helper. The difference it makes can be dramatic. But first you need to reach out.

Alcohol During Breastfeeding

Mothers have enjoyed alcohol while breastfeeding since time began. It's generally safe in moderation.

The Back Story

Alcohol is present in your milk at the same level as in your blood, and rises and falls along with it. If you know your blood alcohol level, you know your milk alcohol level. However, babies don't metabolize alcohol nearly as well as adults do, and when there's alcohol in the milk they seem to take less milk than they would otherwise. Combine that with the slowed milk release that can result from alcohol, and your supply and your baby's growth can be compromised if you drink substantial amounts regularly. A beer or glass of wine a couple of times a week is unlikely to matter, and the effects decrease as your baby gets older.

What You Can Do

If you want to minimize the alcohol your baby gets, try nursing right before you have a drink—your milk will be alcohol-free again within two or three hours.

Bariatric (Gastric Bypass) Surgery

You can definitely breastfeed after bariatric surgery, but you'll need to pay close attention to your own nutrition.

The Back Story

Doctors commonly recommend not getting pregnant until at least two years after the surgery because of the calorie restrictions that limit nutritional absorption, particularly of vitamin B_{12}, calcium, folate, iron, and protein.

What You Can Do

Vitamin and mineral supplements may be necessary to ensure that your milk is fully nutritious. And you may need periodic blood tests to confirm that you're retaining enough of the nutrients from your supplements. Try to consume at least 90 grams of protein each day. It's also important to investigate and treat any underlying causes of obesity, such as polycystic ovary syndrome (PCOS), insulin resistance, or thyroid problems, any of which can decrease milk production.

Blebs

Now *there's* a new word for your vocabulary! A *bleb* is a little white spot on the tip of a nipple that looks as if there's milk stuck in a nipple pore. Maybe there's a bit of skin over the surface of it, maybe not. Maybe there's a plugged duct in your breast behind it, maybe not. But it can *hurt* when your baby nurses, like squeezing a pimple. Ow! When you get rid of a bleb, the contents may come out as little granules that you can feel between your fingers, or as a tiny ribbon like toothpaste. Or it may just disappear during a nursing (going *harmlessly* into the baby). Once it's gone, any backed-up milk generally clears quickly.

The Back Story

Maybe a bit of skin grew over the nipple pore and held milk in. Maybe a plug moved down from within the breast and couldn't make it through the nipple opening. Maybe a plug formed right there within the nipple. However it happened, a bleb seems to be a plugged duct with the plug right at the nipple opening. If milk has been stuck there for a while, it thickens where you can see it and feel it, and creates a stress that isn't supposed to be there, like having a grain of sand in your nipple.

What You Can Do

Because we aren't sure how they form, there are lots of possibilities for treatment. If it isn't causing any pain or problem, you can ignore it. It might last for weeks or months, and then you discover that it's gone. Or you can try one of the following. In each case, it's also helpful to wash the area with soap and water once a day, and use a small amount of antibiotic ointment for a few days after the bleb clears, to help ensure that it doesn't come back.

Make the plug smaller. Soak a cotton ball in vinegar and wear it over your nipple inside a bra. Milk has a lot of calcium in it, and vinegar dissolves calcium deposits.

Make the nipple pore softer. Soak in the tub or shower, then soak a cotton ball in water, olive oil, or canola oil (corn or peanut oil could encourage allergies) and wear it in your bra over your nipple. Putting some gentle heat over the cotton ball—a sock filled with rice and heated in the microwave, for instance—may help. Or soak your nipple in a cup of warm water to which you've added 2 teaspoons (10 g) of Epsom salts. Then see if nursing, gentle manipulation, or pressure from behind will squeeze the thickened milk out.

Open the skin over the pore. You can ask your health care provider to open it gently with a sterile needle, or do it yourself with a well-sterilized (in a candle flame, for instance) needle. Pick carefully at it from the side; that top layer of skin should have no feeling in it, but the skin underneath may be sensitive. You can use sterile tweezers to peel back any tiny flaps of skin that cover the opening. Manipulate your nipple or have your baby nurse to remove the bleb.

Treat the plug higher up. Check out "Plugged Ducts," below, for ideas.

Blood in Your Milk

Your baby spits up a little and you notice that the milk is streaked with red. You express a little milk from the side where he last nursed—and there's blood in your milk!

The Back Story

Blood in your milk can come from more than one place, *and it's rarely a concern.*

The blood may not be in your milk at all. Sometimes a crack in a damaged nipple opens up and bleeds as the baby sucks; taking care of the nipple will stop the bleeding.

Imagine an old, seldom-used faucet that gushes orange-colored water from its rusty pipes when you first turn it on. That's the image that led to the name *rusty pipe syndrome,* seen most often in first-time mothers whose breasts and milk ducts have been growing rapidly during pregnancy. As the ducts fill with milk, the expansion can cause some oozing of blood that is harmless and stops within a few days.

Bruising, a baby who bites or clamps, a too-strong pump, or other minor breast damage can cause temporary bleeding. Teresa was getting a heavy box down from a shelf in a closet when it slipped in her hands and the corner hit her breast. Later that day her three-year-old commented on a funny taste in the milk, and sure enough, when she hand-expressed, she could see a little blood. This minor bleeding in the ducts can last for several days.

Small, harmless growths in the ducts called *papillomas* can sometimes bleed into the milk. You may have one larger papilloma and may be able to feel it as a tiny lump, or you may have a group of small ones that can't be felt. These are more common in women thirty-five and older.

What You Can Do

In most cases, nothing is needed. The milk is fine. The baby isn't likely to be bothered by the blood in your milk (although in large quantities it can cause some harmless tummy upset), and it should disappear on its own. *Very* rarely, a bloody discharge from your nipples could be a sign of a more serious problem. While this is unlikely, if you are not able to identify other causes and bleeding persists for a week or more or keeps recurring, check with your doctor. You don't have to wean while tests are done to determine the cause of the blood.

Breast Abscess

A gradually discoloring bulge on your breast, probably surrounded by redness, could be an abscess. It's more clearly defined than a plugged duct, and probably extremely tender to the touch. Basically, an abscess is a pocket filled with pus that has no place to go. You may or may not have a fever as well.

The Back Story

Abscesses are not common. They can follow poorly managed mastitis—stopping nursing during mastitis, for instance, instead of continuing to nurse, or not taking antibiotics when mastitis is clearly getting worse and worse. Or they can happen as a result of poorly managed nursing—following a schedule instead of your breasts and baby. Very rarely they can also happen for no clear reason.

What You Can Do

An abscess requires prompt medical care. Drained by a medical professional using a needle or a small incision, it should feel immediately better. As with any breast surgery, a radial incision, like the spoke on a wheel, will probably cause less internal damage than one that cuts across the spokes. You'll probably be put on antibiotics to clear up any lingering bacteria. If there was an incision, you may have a drain put in—like a small section of rubber band resting in the incision—to ensure that the surface doesn't heal before the inside does. You can nurse through the whole interesting adventure. Hold a piece of gauze over the incision when you nurse, to reduce milk flow through the incision and to keep any drainage away from the baby. There's no need to wean for the surgery, and you can expect slow, steady, healing. See Chapter 17 for more information about breastfeeding and breast surgeries.

Breast Lumps

As a nursing mother, you can expect lumpy breasts, and you'll get to know your breasts better than you ever did before.

The Back Story

The lumps will shift location and change, getting larger and smaller as your breast empties and fills. Lumps that come and go are not a cause for any concern. If there's a particular lump that is persistently there, it may require some investigation.

An uncommon type of breast lump is a *galactocele* (ga-LAC-toe-seel), which is a section of duct that has formed a pocket of pooled milk. It usually feels like a smooth, round, movable sac within the breast. The milk inside gradually develops the consistency of butter or oil. And there it stays.

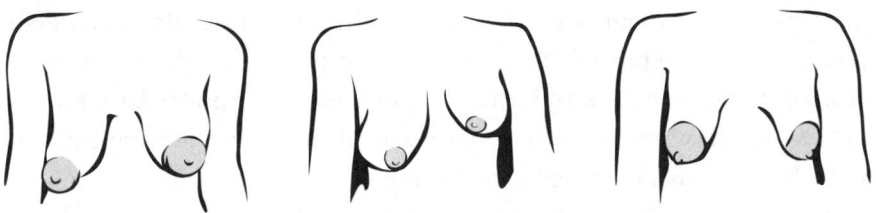

These breasts may or may not make enough milk.

What You Can Do

A galactocele can be suctioned out with a needle while you're lactating, but it will probably return because the emptied sac is still there, happy to refill. If you want to, you can have it surgically removed when you've finished nursing.

A mammogram or sonogram can investigate a persistent lump. Weaning is not necessary. Nurse or express milk as thoroughly as you can ahead of time, both for your own comfort and to provide as un-milky a picture as possible. Mammograms and other X-rays of the mother pose no risk at all to the nursing baby. The same is true of a needle or incisional biopsy—weaning is not necessary.

With any breast surgery, an incision that radiates from your nipple like the spoke on a wheel will cause the least damage. There's no need to wean to have the surgery. See Chapter 17 for more information about breast procedures during breastfeeding.

Breast Tissue Insufficiency

Insufficient glandular tissue, or *breast hypoplasia* (hypo=less, plasia= growth), can be an exception to the all-breasts-work rule, because these types of breasts have less milk-making tissue.

The Back Story

Hypoplastic breasts are different from small breasts. They're tube-shaped rather than melon-shaped, or have very little tissue on the underside, or are separated by a hand's width or more. They may differ dramatically in size, and one or both of the areolae may be puffy. *But appearances can be deceiving!* Some women with breasts that fit these descriptions have nursed babies—even twins—with no problems at all. And since nursing tends to build breast tissue, the simple act of nursing tends to increase the amount of milk we can make, for this baby and future babies.

What You Can Do

If you sense that something isn't right, or if your breasts match what we've described and didn't make enough milk with a previous baby, talk to your tech support person and look over the sections on low supply and supplementing. We know a lot more than we knew even a few years ago. Certain galactagogues might be helpful. *The Breastfeeding Mother's Guide to Making More Milk* by Diana West and Lisa Marasco is a great resource for further information.

Colds and Other Illnesses

Sometimes you get sick. Sometimes your baby does. Does it matter?

The Back Story

You and your baby have been a unit ever since she was conceived. More and more health facilities talk about "the breastfeeding couple" as almost a single person. And no wonder! Your baby not only lives on your milk, she shares your immune system. By the time you know you're sick, you've started passing not only the illness but your immunities on to your baby. To stop nursing now would be to deprive her of the best of your immune system when she needs it most. The reverse is truly remarkable. If your baby picks up an illness that *you* haven't been exposed to, she passes those germs to you through nursing, and *within the breast itself* you begin making antibodies and passing them back.

What You Can Do

There are very few illnesses that require any kind of mother/baby or baby/milk separation. The Centers for Disease Control and Prevention (cdc.gov) and the World Health Organization (who.int/eng) both have information on breastfeeding during specific maternal diseases and vaccinations. Bottom line: with very few exceptions, keep nursing!

Illness in babies can come quickly, hit hard, and leave just as quickly. Nursing provides fluids and nutrition when other foods and drink are refused, and serves as excellent pain relief.

If you are vomiting and/or have diarrhea, you might see a small dip in your milk production. Drink enough to stay hydrated, and know that your milk will increase as you recover. Most medications that you might need are compatible with breastfeeding. You can double-check with anyone who has a copy of Hale's *Breastfeeding and Mothers' Milk*. Take care of your own health to help prevent or reduce the severity of illness in either one of you. Adequate rest (if possible) and a diet rich in vitamin D, antioxidants, zinc, and omega-3 fats can help keep your immune system in good shape. And that helps keep your baby's in good shape, too.

Colic

Colic is the catchall description when a baby cries hard at least three hours a day, usually late in the day, for unknown reasons. It tends to start in the early weeks and is usually gone by about four months.

The Back Story

Some colic is probably caused by oversupply, which has its own section in this chapter. Some is probably caused by reflux, which also has its own section. Both oversupply and reflux are much more likely to be a problem when meals are large and widely spaced, and reflux is worse when the baby lies down. Babies who are carried most of the day not only have the reassurance of their mothers but also tend to have small, frequent meals and stay upright much of the time, all of which help with reflux and oversupply, and may make colic better. But some colic is caused by factors you just can't uncover and may be related to personality or temperament.

What You Can Do

If your baby is colicky, first make sure that he isn't just clamoring to eat again and you're holding him off because of sore nipples or watching the clock. Next, try carrying him. Many fussy babies settle down when they're allowed free access to their mother's body and breasts. But many others are still unhappy. Some ideas:

- Remember the phrase "contact, carry, walk, and talk." Research indicates that these steps, used in sequence as needed, can significantly reduce crying in many babies. Most of the suggestions that follow are variations on that theme; it seems that mothers agree with the research!
- Respond right away. Research shows that responding before the baby gets worked up allows you to calm him more easily.
- Use a soft carrier as much as possible, so that your baby is close to your body, upright, and easily fed.
- Use the Magic Baby Hold from Chapter 6.
- Get into the tub together.
- Use the "I Love U" massage from William Sears and Martha Sears's *The Fussy Baby Book.*
- Save errands for the baby's fussy time, to entertain him.
- Dance with him.
- Put the baby in a sling or blanket "hammock" and swing him either head-to-toe or ear to ear, whichever works.
- Check out the sections in this chapter on oversupply, reflux, and food sensitivities.

Your baby isn't doing this to drive you crazy, and his crying doesn't mean you're doing something wrong. This time is even more unhappy for him than it is for you. He needs you now more than ever. Having a baby with colic is tough, but it *does* end. In the meantime, find a circle of friends that you can complain to! (Hint: LLL meetings!) They may have suggestions and they'll surely have lots of empathy. Two good books on fussy babies are *The Fussy Baby Book* by William Sears and Martha Sears and *Colic Solved* by Bryan Vartabedian.

Eating Disorders

If you have a history of anorexia, bulimia, or other eating disorders, you can still breastfeed. You may need help (from a physician, counselor, or nutritionist) in managing your symptoms, though.

The Back Story

If you've had an eating disorder in the past but your weight is stabilized and you're eating normally, you shouldn't have any trouble making enough milk, and the quality will be just as good as anyone else's. If you're still struggling with an eating disorder, though, the quality and quantity of your milk may be affected. Even if there are nutritional deficits in your milk, formula is still inferior.

What You Can Do

It will be important to follow your baby's weight gain carefully, and you may find it helpful to talk to a counselor or nutritionist about ways to maximize your nutrition. Supplementation (see the section on it, below) may be needed if your milk supply is low.

Engorgement

Engorgement is too much fluid in a breast. In the first week after birth, it's a combination of milk and increased circulation. Engorged breasts feel heavy, full, tender or painful, hot. Over-fullness can make latching difficult. Without a well-nursing baby or some other means of frequent, effective milk removal, that heaviness and warmth can expand into tight, shiny breasts that are too congested for milk to leave, the way a cold can make you too stuffy to blow your nose.

The Back Story

In the first three to five days after birth, milk production blossoms. Blood circulation to your breasts increases to get the "milk factory" up and running. And lymph flow increases to remove waste products. As one mother said, "After the birth, all that fluid that was in your ankles rushes up to your breasts to see what's going on." If you've had IV fluids during labor, some of the fluid the tubing pumped into your body will also go to your breasts.

The baby's role is to keep things moving by nursing frequently. As long as milk is taken out well and often, you're unlikely to feel anything more than some heaviness and warmth, although the occasional mother finds herself engorged even with an effectively nursing baby.

Do you have lumps under your arms? That's milk-making tissue that you never knew you had! Sometimes it connects to the rest of the breast and will drain along with it, and sometimes there's no outlet. Even if it doesn't drain, it'll slowly subside and not return.

Engorgement can also result if your baby suddenly sleeps through the night or spends several days boosting your supply for her growth spurt and then spends a day happily napping while you cope with your no-longer-needed bounty—or whenever you go an unexpectedly long time between nursings. But in those cases, it's just milk, and easy to relieve with nursing.

It's important to resolve engorgement as quickly as possible to avoid compounding the problem as more milk is made. Like a stuffy nose, the fuller the breast, the more difficult it is to move the milk. *Extreme* engorgement can damage a milk supply.

What You Can Do

During labor avoid IV fluids, which can significantly increase engorgement. After birth (and at any time during breastfeeding), removing milk from the breasts is critical to helping the other fluids drain as well. It won't make the engorgement worse or result in too much milk. Once the breasts are completely softened, engorgement doesn't usually return. If you find engorgement becoming a problem after your baby is born, some of these ideas may help:

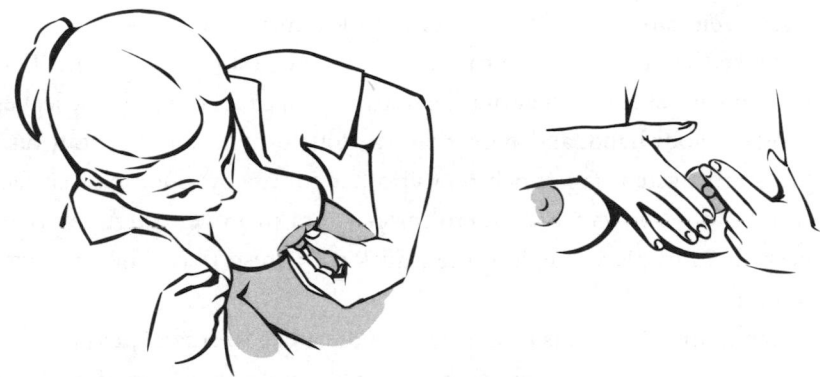

Reverse Pressure Softening—Use fingertips or finger lengths to press fluid back.

- 💡 Keep your baby with you, and nurse as long and as often as he's willing, beginning as soon after birth as possible.
- 💡 If your breast is too firm for your baby to latch onto, you can use "Reverse Pressure Softening" to push fluids back away from where your baby's mouth needs to be, and soften a "landing platform" for him so that he can attach deeply and remove milk effectively. Press steadily with the length of your index fingers on either side of your nipple's base, where your baby's upper and lower gums will be. It may work best to put your first joint opposite your nipple, and you can use more than one finger if you like, especially on the lower-jaw side. Press for the length of a lullaby, then immediately offer to nurse. Or press all the short-nailed fingertips of one hand around the base of your nipple to make five little dents. Try this at least every hour or so.
- 💡 If your baby can't breastfeed even with Reverse Pressure Softening, gentle hand expression or pumping on a low setting might help (too high and it pulls more fluid into the areola, compounding the problem).
- 💡 Moving your breasts gently may help drain lymph fluids. Massage them gently, lift them, move them around in ways that don't hurt.
- 💡 Lie flat on your back when you rest. Gravity will help drain fluids away from your breasts.
- 💡 Part of engorgement is inflammation. Ask your doctor for an anti-inflammatory medicine that's compatible with breastfeeding (most over-the-counter brands are).

- ☼ Use green cabbage (red can stain), which may help reduce swelling. Remove the outer leaves in case there are any pesticides on them. Tear off some inner leaves, tear out the hard central stem, crumple the leaves gently in your hand, and apply them to your breast (not over your nipple, so the taste isn't left behind to bother your baby). Doesn't that feel wonderful? You can wear them inside a bra or under a tight shirt to keep them in place. Replace the leaves with fresh ones whenever you want to.

- ☼ Inflammation responds best to cold. Wrap a bag of frozen peas (or carrots) in a small towel and use it as a cold compress, alternating about twenty minutes on and twenty minutes off, as much as you like. Refreeze as needed. If you feel like a hot shower, let the water play over your back, not your chest. Same for a heating pad.

- ☼ If engorgement returns, try expressing as much as you can from both sides, getting right down to the "bottom of the barrel."

Fertility Treatments During Breastfeeding

If you are beginning fertility treatments while still breastfeeding, you may be told by your reproductive specialist to wean.

The Back Story

Weaning is often recommended by reproductive specialists because breastfeeding hormones can suppress fertility. There's usually no need to wean solely to be able to take fertility medications, because most are safe for breastfeeding.

What You Can Do

Whether or not you wean is a personal decision, weighing your and your baby's need for breastfeeding and your desire to have another baby now. Some mothers choose to ignore the advice, accepting that the fertility treatments may be less effective.

Food Allergies and Food Sensitivities

After the first month, when many cultures encourage a mild diet for mothers, most babies don't care what their mothers eat. Spicy foods, garlicky pasta, cabbage, and beans all suit the average baby just fine.

But you may have noticed that your baby seems especially distressed at times. She might spit up much more than normal, have green stools on occasion, have a lot of gas that may smell more than usual, and may have a rash on her cheeks or bottom. She may develop eczema as well. And you may start to notice a link between things you eat and these changes in your baby.

The Back Story

What you're seeing might be a food sensitivity or a true food allergy. When your baby is small, her intestines allow particles into her system more readily, and in some babies certain foods passed on through the milk can cause some of the reactions you see. That's a food sensitivity; babies usually grow out of these as their digestive system matures. Other babies are truly allergic to certain foods and react to the traces of those foods in your milk.

What You Can Do

Allergy testing doesn't work on young babies; the only way to figure out if a food is bothering your little one is to eliminate it from your diet and see if the symptoms improve. Most mothers start by trying to eliminate some of the foods most likely to cause a reaction. These seem to be:

- *Cow milk* (and products made with cow milk such as cheese, butter, ice cream, etc.). This can be especially tricky since cow milk is hidden in many prepared foods, and highly sensitive babies are bothered by even a small amount. Some also react to beef or veal.
- *Soy products,* including tofu, soybeans, soy milk, soy ice cream, etc. Some babies who are sensitive to cow products may also react to soy products.

- *Eggs.* Some babies will also react if their mother eats chicken.
- *Citrus* fruits and juices.
- *Wheat* and wheat flours.
- *Corn.* Another tricky one, because it can appear in many forms, including corn syrup (found in many prepared foods) and corn chips.
- *Caffeine* in foods such as coffee, tea, and cola drinks.
- *Chocolate* bothers some babies. (If that's the case for you, please send any you are given directly to the authors.)

You can try eliminating just one food at a time, waiting at least a week or two to give it a fair trial. No change? Add back the food you eliminated and try something else.

Or try a *rotation diet*. If you eat a particular food (say, cheese) on Monday, you don't eat anything with dairy in it on Tuesday, Wednesday, or Thursday. Then you can have dairy again on Friday. Perhaps on Tuesday you ate tofu, so you wouldn't have any soy products again until Saturday. Each food is eliminated for a cycle of four days. As you follow this diet, track your baby's symptoms, trying new combinations and noting when she seems most fussy.

Some feel a rotation diet may not give enough time for certain foods to be eliminated completely from your milk or from the baby's system. But it can help identify the offending food fairly quickly without disrupting your own diet too much, and then you can try eliminating it for a longer period of time.

The occasional mother starts from the other direction, eating a limited diet of, say, lamb, pears, rice, and squash—all low-allergen—and adding other foods one at a time.

At some point your doctor may suggest a *food challenge*—reintroducing a suspect food to see if the baby reacts. It's a way of confirming that, yes, that food is what your baby is sensitive to. If your baby's symptoms were mild and you've been longing for cheese, you may want to try it. If the baby doesn't react, you can start to reintroduce dairy, but take it slowly. Some babies can tolerate a small amount of a food they are sensitive to, but react once it reaches a certain level.

If your baby's earlier symptoms were fairly intense, you might opt not to do a food challenge. After all, your baby is doing well now, and you've figured out how to get by without dairy in your life. Many mothers decide to wait until the baby is a year old, when most sensitivities and some allergies are outgrown, before trying a food challenge.

Hospitalization or Surgery—Your Child's

When your little one needs surgery or hospitalization, your presence and your breasts can be immensely consoling.

The Back Story

Hospitals used to keep parents away, and they saw how badly it worked for their little patients. Now they usually welcome mothers everywhere but in the operating room. The biggest challenge can be getting permission to nurse before and after surgery.

What You Can Do

Many hospitals can arrange a bed next to your child's or provide a bed you can share. You may be able to put rails up for co-sleeping. If you can't be with your child, leave behind an article of your clothing with your familiar smell. Or you may be able to take shifts with your partner or other family, staying awake to hold a sleeping child. Mothers have crawled into oxygen tents and draped themselves over bizarre frameworks to nurse in odd positions. Remember the pain-relieving power of breastfeeding, and nurse through any procedures that you and your child want to. Bring a notebook and keep a record of procedures, vital signs, doctors, whatever. One notebook veteran said the staff quickly began consulting *her,* because she was obviously keeping close track of her child's care.

A fasting period before surgery will almost certainly be required—but keep in mind that human milk digests more quickly than formula and so a shorter fasting period is appropriate. Nursing should be acceptable until four hours, perhaps as little as two hours, before surgery. Letting the baby nurse for comfort from a pre-pumped breast might satisfy everyone. You should be able to nurse again as soon as your baby wakes from the procedure. It is not necessary for him to eat or drink other fluids to "prove" that he can nurse. Hospitals are often amazed at the calm and uneventful recovery of breastfeeding children; your nursing relationship and its outcome may make it easier for the next mother and baby to travel your path.

Hospitalization or Surgery—Yours

You may need to be in the hospital while you are breastfeeding. Does that mean you'll have to wean?

The Back Story

Many hospitals now have a policy of keeping mothers and nurslings together, usually requiring that someone help you care for the baby. If your hospital doesn't have such a policy, maybe you can help create it! Be prepared to go higher up in the chain of command if necessary.

What You Can Do

Hospital policies rarely take breastfeeding mothers and babies into account. That works to your disadvantage...and to your advantage. If you state your case assuming they'll cooperate, they often will because no protocol says they shouldn't. The American Academy of Pediatrics says, "Should hospitalization of the breastfeeding mother or infant be necessary, every effort should be made to maintain breastfeeding, preferably directly, or by pumping the breasts and feeding expressed breast milk, if necessary." Most hospitals with maternity facilities have a breastfeeding specialist on staff who can be your ally.

Rather than asking if it's okay, you can explain that you'll need to have your baby with you much of the time to avoid compounding your health problem with mastitis. They may require that you meet your baby in the lounge or waiting room on your unit. When you're mobile, that can be a reasonable compromise. As the staff gets to know you, it's surprising how many rules relax.

If possible, talk with the anesthesiologist about the drugs that will be used. In almost all cases, breastfeeding is fine as soon as you're alert enough to hold your baby. An occasional mother experiences a drop in supply after surgery, as if her body is mustering its resources to take care of her first. Frequent nursing will almost always bring it back up. If you're concerned, try to have some milk tucked away in the freezer at home ahead of time.

You may be able to use one of the hospital's pumps, but you may be required to purchase the parts that connect to it. It will help to arrange for a pump ahead of time. If you nurse thoroughly or express milk before surgery, that will give you the longest comfortable stretch possible. Consider showing a family member or nurse how to use the pump; more than one mother has had someone relieve her full breasts when she was still too muddled to do anything about it herself!

Mothers with arms in casts, legs in traction, and heads in metal "halos" have come up with all sorts of creative ways to position their babies for nursing. Ask the nursing staff for any help you need. In general, expecting the best from others is the best way to get it.

Hypoglycemia

The baby with hypoglycemia has low blood sugar (*hypo*=less, *glycemia*= sugar).

The Back Story

A baby kept away from his mother burns more calories and can become jittery and distressed if his blood sugar level gets too low. A baby whose mother is diabetic can be born on a "sugar high" and can come crashing down after birth. Fortunately, just being skin to skin with his mother can raise a baby's blood sugar, *whether or not he eats while he's there.* Unfortunately, some hospitals want to check the blood sugars of all babies, especially those designated as "large," whether they show symptoms or not, and have thresholds below which they'll want to supplement, whether or not there are symptoms.

What You Can Do

The Academy of Breastfeeding Medicine has a thorough, research-based protocol at bfmed.org that you can share with your doctors if needed. Some of its main points:

- Breastfeeding within the first hour after birth is important.
- Babies with no risk factors or symptoms should not be tested.
- At-risk babies should be screened until their blood sugar normalizes.
- There is *no* evidence that hypoglycemic infants *who show no symptoms* should be treated.

If supplements are needed, the preferred order is the mother's own milk, donor human milk, elemental formulas, and partially hydrolyzed formulas. Standard formula is the *least* desirable option.

Hypothermia

A baby with hypothermia is a baby who's gotten cold (*hypo*=less, *thermia*=heat).

The Back Story

Hypothermia wasn't a problem in the days when mothers held their babies against their own bodies from birth. Nothing has been found to warm a baby better than his mother. Nothing. Babies in warmers, Isolettes, and incubators all take longer to warm up and don't warm as thoroughly or hold their temperature as well as babies who simply stay with their mothers.

What You Can Do

Keeping your baby with you, his skin against your skin, with a blanket over you both, is the best prevention for hypothermia. Being snuggled toasty warm in bed with you is also a good way to prevent...

Jaundice or Hyperbilirubinemia
(*too much bilirubin*)

Babies can develop yellowed skin and eyes in the days following birth. A little jaundice is normal and good. The bilirubin that causes it is an antioxidant common to all mammals. However, too much bilirubin, a condition called *hyperbilirubinemia,* or jaundice makes a baby sleepy and less interested in eating, and can be downright unhealthy.

The Back Story

Before birth, a baby needs more red blood cells because he's in a low-oxygen environment. After birth, he breaks down the excess cells. The bilirubin they contained is excreted in poop, not pee, so milk (not water) is the most important way to prevent excessive jaundice.

Whether jaundice deserves treatment depends in part on when it occurs and to whom. Babies don't build up bilirubin from breaking down blood cells until they're two or three days old, so the baby who has high bilirubin on his first day is more likely to have something else going on. Premature or ill babies are more at risk from building up too much bilirubin than healthy, full-term babies are. The jaundice that can occur from not having enough bowel movements tends to be fading by about five days of age, as milk becomes more plentiful, so jaundice that persists beyond then may be a case of so-called breastmilk jaundice.

Don't worry about breastmilk jaundice. Healthy, thriving babies (maybe *especially* healthy, thriving babies) may have a harmless "suntan" for weeks or even a couple of months. But what about the not-enough-bowel-movement jaundice, sometimes called not-enough-breastmilk jaundice?

What You Can Do

Bringing bilirubin down to normal levels involves food and light.

1. *Food*—Formula brings the bilirubin number down faster than human milk does, *but at a lifelong price,* since formula increases the risk of so many short- and long-term problems. With human milk, the bilirubin

number comes down a bit more slowly, at no risk and enormous benefit to your baby. So do your best to provide your own milk, or donor milk, and get help if your baby isn't nursing well.

2. *Light*—Hospital "bililights" produce wavelengths that are absorbed by the bilirubin in the baby's skin and blood, making the bilirubin change into a form that is excreted faster. You can ask to have the lights over both of you so your baby is unstressed and has ample access to nursing. Babies need to have their eyes covered when they are under the bililights. Bililights may also be available as a blanket or wrap that you can use at home. With the blanket type of lights, the eyes do not have to be covered. Be prepared for some poop the color of creamed spinach in your baby's diapers as the bilirubin is eliminated.

3. *Food, one more time*—Keep your baby with you so you can keep the breastfeeding going strong. It's your first and best ally against jaundice.

Low Milk Supply

Sometimes a baby *is* growing too slowly. The good news: there are ways to help both the baby and the milk supply.

The Back Story

If your baby really isn't getting enough milk, it's important to figure out if he's not *taking* enough milk because you're not *making* enough, or if you're not *making* enough because he's not *taking* enough, or if he's taking plenty but not using it well. These are three completely different issues that your tech support person can sort out with you.

Among the reasons babies can have trouble taking enough milk are the way the baby is held at the breast, the frequency and length of feedings, prematurity, tongue-tie and other mouth issues, and muscle and neurological issues. Probably least commonly, babies with an underlying illness such as a bladder infection or heart defect may not eat well because they don't feel good, or may eat plenty but burn through it too quickly. Most of the time, your supply would have been good at the start, gradually declining.

Among the hormonal reasons mothers can have trouble making enough milk are thyroid problems (which can cause problems with milk release), polycystic ovary syndrome, and other fertility issues. Most of the time these would result in a low milk supply from the start.

Structural possibilities include breast hypoplasia and previous nipple or breast surgeries. Here, too, you'd likely have had a low supply from the start. And of course there may be more than one thing going on.

What You Can Do

First of all, your baby needs to be well fed. If the problem was spotted early enough, you may be able to increase your supply quickly enough to meet his needs. If necessary, donor milk or formula can fill in the gaps.

By far the most common causes of poor weight gain are babies who are not nursing often enough or not nursing well enough. Weight gain can begin to spiral down as a result, and a little tweaking turns everything around. So your first step might be offering the breast more often and rereading Chapter 4. But figuring out what's going on isn't always that easy. Having a skilled helper to work with usually makes all the difference here.

Once you have an idea of what the problem might be, you can develop a plan for fixing it. Increasing milk removal through some added pumpings, combined with hand expression and breast compressions, is a standard approach. Chapter 15 has detailed information about hand expression and pumping. A galactagogue—any substance that increases milk production, including herbs, foods, and prescription medications—may add to the boost that good milk removal provides.

Some of the more common herbal galactagogues used with success by women in Western cultures are goat's rue (often used for insufficient glandular tissue and breast surgery situations), shatavari (often used for hormonal support), fennel (often used for milk release problems), alfalfa, and fenugreek. Foods such as barley, brown rice, and oatmeal may also help. Prescription galactagogues are domperidone (Motilium), often used to increase prolactin; metoclopramide (Reglan, Maxeran), often used to increase prolactin; and metformin (Glucophage), often used to stabilize blood sugar. A knowledgeable tech support person can help you find the right galactagogue and dosage for your situation. If you choose to use a galactagogue, it's important to tell your doctor, even if she or he disagrees with your use of it, because there is always the possibility that it can interfere with other medications or cause reactions. Avoid herbs that can decrease your supply, such as parsley, sage, and peppermint (in large quantities), and medications such as pseudoephedrine, hormonal birth control (especially when introduced before four months postpartum), bromocriptine, ergotamine, and Methergine.

There's much, much more to know! *The Breastfeeding Mother's Guide to Making More Milk* by Diana West and Lisa Marasco can lead you step-by-step through the entire process of discovering what's going on and finding a treatment that can help you get the best result.

Almost every plan for improving low weight gain needs frequent adjustment as you go, so keep an eye on your progress and stay in touch with your helper. If your helper is out of ideas and things still aren't working, ask her to refer you to another resource. There's almost always something more that can be done, and it's *never* too late to increase your supply!

Mastitis

Maybe you discover a warm, red, sensitive area on one breast (almost never both unless both haven't had milk removed in a while). Maybe you're running a slight fever, or you're beginning to feel flu-like aches and chills. These are all signs of mastitis. About a third of nursing mothers experience mastitis at some point, usually in the first few months. It can come and go like a whirlwind, sometimes lasting only a few hours. Other times it can hang on for the better part of a week.

The Back Story

Mastitis isn't necessarily an infection. The suffix *-itis* just means "inflammation," the process in which protective substances in your body rush to wherever infection is threatening, trying to head it off before it starts or end it before it gets too bad. That physiological process can cause pain, redness, fever, and chills. If there is no infection, an antibiotic won't fix it. Sometimes, however, there *is* an infection. Infection-based mastitis that doesn't clear with some straightforward breast care (described below) tends to clear within a day of starting the right antibiotic, which is usually begun a day or two after symptoms begin. Non-infection-based mastitis usually clears on its own in two to four days. Do the math, and you can see that a lot of mastitis gets "cured" by antibiotics that didn't do anything. But there's no easy way to tell which type you have.

Typical causes of mastitis are nipple damage that lets bacteria in, milk that isn't removed regularly and well, and a body that's just generally run-down. That usually translates to nipple trauma from a baby who isn't latching well, infrequent or inefficient breast emptying, something that routinely presses on certain milk ducts (such as a poorly fitting or underwire bra, or a backpack), or trying to do too much on too little sleep with too little food ("holiday mastitis" is common).

What You Can Do

If you're feeling ill, your doctor may want to see you, or may phone in a pre-scription for an antibiotic. Since you may not have an infection, and taking antibiotics when there's no infection serves no purpose, you can wait to fill the prescription, using it only if you decide you need it.

The basics for mastitis treatment are simple: Empty Breast, Lots of Rest. Empty Breast means plenty of nursing or milk expression. Try to keep that side nice and soft without neglecting the other side. Since this is inflam-mation, cold may be helpful. If it feels good, you can use the same cold treatments listed under "Engorgement," above. Gentle heat may also be helpful; do what feels best to you. An over-the-counter anti-inflammatory drug can help make you more comfortable; check with your doctor (the common anti-inflammatories are considered safe for breastfeeding).

Lots of rest means don't stand if you can sit, don't sit if you can lie down, don't try to stay awake if you can sleep. Feet up as much as possible. Favorite books, magazines, music, TV, or movies. A pitcher of juice or water nearby. A stack of diapers, a plateful of easy snacks (that you didn't fix, if possible), a comfy pillow. You're sick. You'll get better much faster if you *behave* that way!

Diane DiSandro, a La Leche League Leader and IBCLC, suggests a "bag of marbles" massage. Hold your breast in your hands with interlaced fingers. Pretend it's a bag of marbles and with a gentle kneading motion shift the marbles all around inside the bag. Do this several times a day. Her reasoning: breasts have abandant lymph vessels that carry away the body's waste. Lymph flows best when our bodies move around, but we tend to hold breasts rigid inside a bra for most of a day. Give your breasts a chance to move and your lymph system just might perform better!

If you're not getting worse, you can keep up the standard treatment of Empty Breast and Lots of Rest for twenty-four hours. If you're still holding your own, see what happens over the next twenty-four hours. If you're not improving, consider the antibiotic. If you do start on an antibiotic, remember to take it *all,* even if you feel better immediately. Partially completed courses of antibiotics can cause mastitis to come back again stronger because it never really left.

If mastitis happens more than once, talk to an LLL Leader or other tech support person to see if you can figure out what's going on. For more suggestions, see the Academy of Breastfeeding Medicine's mastitis protocol at bfmed.org/Resources/Protocols.aspx.

Medications and Breastfeeding

We know to be careful about medications during pregnancy, but what happens *after* your baby is born?

The Back Story

The mother who takes a medication or drug *before* her baby is born "mainlines" it straight to her fetus. Then her own liver and kidneys go to work metabolizing and excreting the drug for both of them, and their shared blood levels drop together. A key difference between mother and baby, of course, is that the mother is fully developed, while the baby is growing limbs, organs, head, and brain.

After the baby is born, any medication goes from her digestive tract to her bloodstream to her milk to the baby's digestive tract to his bloodstream. It's a long, contorted path that means he gets a very, very diluted form of the drug, at a time when he is much more completely developed. But he also has to rely on his own organs to metabolize and excrete the drug, and his liver is still pretty immature, especially during his first month or so.

Some drugs do tend to concentrate in milk, while others appear in even lower amounts than in the mother's blood, and others may be blocked from entering milk at all. In general, the amount is very small.

Other points to consider:

- Some drugs aren't very well absorbed when swallowed, or have to be injected because they don't work orally. These are unlikely to be a problem, because your baby won't absorb them orally (from your milk), either. Some drugs don't leave your digestive tract and so never enter your milk.
- Some drugs are commonly given directly to babies in doses far, far larger than your baby would get through your milk.
- The older the baby, the better he deals with any medications.
- The baby who has started solid food automatically gets a smaller dose of your medication because he's no longer totally dependent on your milk.
- Older medications have longer track records with nursing mothers, but pharmaceutical companies often offer incentives for prescribing newer medications. If little is known about the drug that's recommended, ask if there's an older equivalent about which more is known.
- Your breasts are not sealed containers; the level of a medication in your milk rises and falls along with the level in your blood. "Pumping and dumping" is mainly to keep your supply high while you wait for your milk to clear. Fortunately, since most medications don't require missing even one feeding, pumping and dumping is rarely necessary.

What You Can Do

Check with a tech support person or pharmacist who has a current edition of Dr. Thomas Hale's *Medications and Mothers' Milk*. It's the most complete source of information, giving studies relating to each drug during breast-feeding, explaining how the drug's properties affect its transfer into milk and into the baby, and discussing how it might interact with other drugs, whether there are other drugs that might be a better choice, and whether the drug can affect the mother's milk supply. In contrast, the *Physician's*

Desk Reference or other literature produced by the manufacturers themselves often simply recommend weaning.

If you still have concerns, there's always wiggle room:

- You can nurse first, then take the medication.
- The baby's blood level can be tested.
- After five "half-lives"—the time it takes for half of a drug to have disappeared from your body—a drug is considered to have been used up. Hale's *Medications and Mothers' Milk* gives the half-life for many of the medications listed.
- You can nurse part-time.

For more information, you and your tech support person can consult the following resources:

- LactMed, the U.S. National Institutes of Health's Drugs and Lactation Database (toxnet.nlm.nih.gov/cgi-bin/sis/htmlgen?LACT)
- Dr. Hale's website (neonatal.ttuhsc.edu/lact)
- U.K. National Health Service *Quick Reference Guide for Drugs in Breast Milk* (ukmicentral.nhs.uk/drugpreg/qrg_p1.htm)
- The MotherRisk Program at the Hospital for Sick Children, Toronto, Canada (http://www.motherisk.org/women/breastfeeding.jsp)
- American Academy of Pediatrics policy statement *Transfer of Drugs and Other Chemicals into Human Milk* (aappolicy.aappublications.org/cgi/content/full/pediatrics%3b108/3/776)
- World Health Organization publication *Drugs in Pregnancy and Lactation* (whqlibdoc.who.int/hq/2002/55732.pdf)

If your choices are exposing your baby to a medication in your milk or exposing your baby to formula, you are generally choosing between a small or theoretical risk and a known risk with wide-ranging consequences. Formula *always* has side effects; the only unknown is how great they will be for you and your baby. The vast majority of the time, playing it safe means continuing to breastfeed, not switching to formula, even if medications are involved.

Nipple Diversity

We're all built differently, and most of us don't look like the women in the breastfeeding videos. Your baby will love your shape, whatever it is. But babies who are separated from their mothers, recovering from a medicated birth, or exposed to artificial nipples can have a difficult time. Here are some thoughts on common variations.

The Back Story

Most babies can give you a hickey by just sucking on your neck; they don't need an ideal nipple in order to latch, just a little matching of parts. Breast size says nothing at all about our ability to make milk, but there may need to be some matching of parts there, too.

What You Can Do

Flat nipples are really just "short-stemmed." Your baby will find them by their texture, taste, and smell and by seeking the point on your breast's natural contour where a nipple is usually found. You can rub or fiddle with short nipples to make them more prominent, or use your index finger to

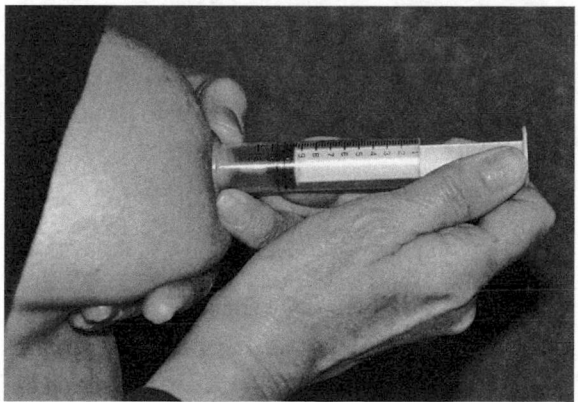

Drawing out an inverted nipple.

push up into the breast from underneath and help push your nipple out farther (this is called a "nipple nudge").

While you and your baby are learning, it's important to avoid bottles if at all possible because the longer artificial nipple isn't built like you at all and your baby can come to prefer the nipple that's easier to grasp. If nothing else works, a nipple shield may help, but make sure you're working closely with someone who's experienced with them, to help you use it effectively (see "Nipple Shields," below).

Some nipples aren't short; they just seem that way if you're really engorged. If this happens, try using the Reverse Pressure Softening technique described in the "Engorgement" section.

Inverted nipples tuck in instead of sticking out. You can try nursing after first working your nipple out by hand. Some self-correct during pregnancy, and there are commercial devices that help pull out (evert) the nipple, before or after your baby is born. Or you can make your own device. Ask your health care provider for a needleless syringe that's somewhat bigger in diameter than your nipple. Take the plunger out. Using a serrated knife, cut the needle end off and put the plunger in the "wrong" end. Now you have a little suction device with a smooth end that you can put over your nipple. Pull out on the plunger far enough to draw your nipple out, but not so far that it's uncomfortable, and keep the suction up for about a minute

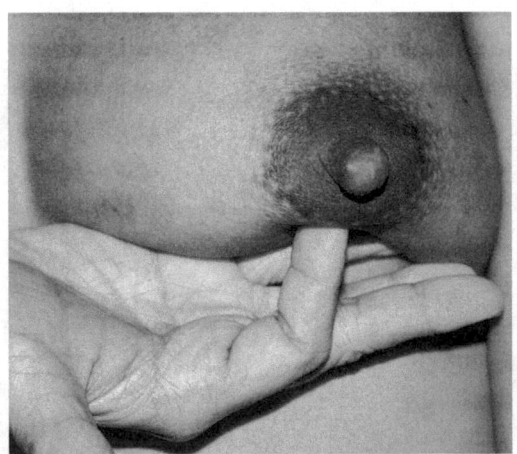

"Nipple nudge" to help baby latch on.

(two times through a leisurely rendition of "Rock-a-bye Baby"). If it fills with milk while you're waiting, pull back farther on the plunger to keep the suction up. To remove it, depress the plunger enough to stop the suction. Now quickly offer your breast to your baby.

Pumping briefly before nursing may also help. Or see the section above on nipple nudges and the section below on nipple shields. If your nipple won't evert at all, breastfeeding may be more difficult. Remember, though, it takes only one nipple to breastfeed.

Other nipple shapes are common. If your nipple tip is oval instead of round, try having your baby take the longer dimension from corner to corner in his mouth. If his mouth is just too small for your nipples at first, he'll grow into them. Until then, he may not be able to get much milk because he can't reach the milk ducts in your breasts, so trying to grow him just through nursing may not work. Time is on your side, though. Pump or hand-express to keep your milk supply up, keep him well fed, and nipples and mouth will soon match.

Babies can begin nursing—and nurse just fine—*months* after they're born. As one LLL Leader pointed out, "Right now, we need to keep your milk supply up and keep your baby fed. We can sort out the utensils later." See Chapter 15 for thoughts on keeping your milk supply high. See also "Low Milk Supply" and "Supplementing" in this chapter. He'll get there!

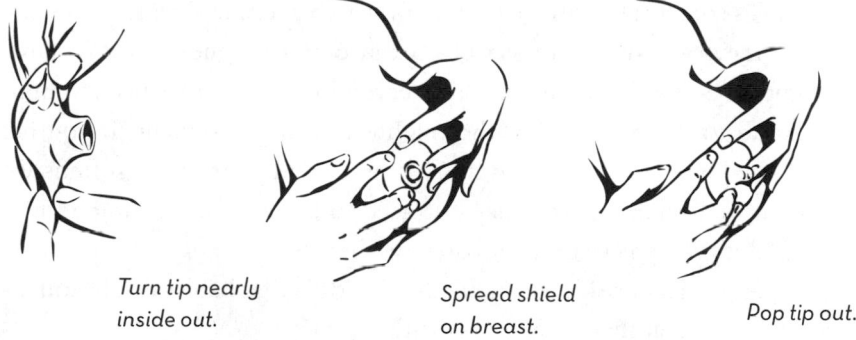

Turn tip nearly inside out.

Spread shield on breast.

Pop tip out.

Applying a nipple shield.

Nipple Shields

A nipple shield looks something like a hat made of silicone. It doesn't move or recede when a baby tries to latch, the way a nipple can, and can sometimes help a persistently non-latching baby, especially one who has gotten used to bottle nipples. It can also sometimes help a baby latch onto an inverted nipple. A nipple shield also makes it easier for premies who don't have a lot of energy or fat and muscle in their cheeks; it stays put when they pause, so less energy goes into holding everything in place. A nipple shield is often suggested as a solution for nipple pain but isn't usually helpful.

The Back Story

Experiment to see what size works best (premies may do best with the smallest size that's comfortable for you). It may help to turn the shield almost inside out, so that the stiff nipple section is folded back on itself. Now, when you put it in place, your own nipple is closer to the shield's tip. Then you can spread the rim into place (maybe moistened underneath to help it stick) and wiggle the nipple section to pop it out. It will draw a bit of your own nipple out at the same time, which means a better fit. If you compress your breast a few times, you may be able to add a few drops to the space in the tip—instant reward when your baby starts to suck. If your baby latches on deeply enough, his gums will land on the soft rim, not the stiff nipple.

Babies sometimes remove milk poorly with a nipple shield for the same reason they can't use a breast well (because of a tongue-tie, for instance) or simply because it's an unnatural intervention, so you may need to pump afterward to drain the breast thoroughly and to supplement. If you hear good swallowing (as described in Chapter 5) and your breast softens well in response to nursing, you may not need to pump after nursing with the shield. But keep an eye on your baby's weight.

One significant risk to using nipple shields is that babies can become so used to them that they won't nurse without them.

What You Can Do to Get Away from Nipple Shields

Your baby is built for your breast, but he doesn't know yet that he can make it work. He'll catch on. Here are some strategies that might help.

- 💡 Try removing the shield after the baby is fed, dozing, and still contentedly sucking. Many babies open their mouths and search for the nipple without opening their eyes, which can provide an opportunity to get the breast in there. He may then take it next time right from the start, while awake, or it may take a few times making the change in the middle of a nursing session.
- 💡 Try removing the shield in the middle of a nursing session. Pick a calm time to try. If he starts to get upset, give him what he wants and try again later. With an older baby you may need to wait a day or two between tries. Try rinsing your nipple and areola. A baby who is used to the bland taste of the silicone shield may be bothered by the taste of your skin at first.
- 💡 Coat your nipple and areola with your milk to make them more enticing.
- 💡 Wait for a time when your baby "just looks different." Sometimes something just changes.

Do not cut away the tip of the nipple shield a little at a time. That leaves a sharp edge with a silicone shield.

Nursing Strike

Sometimes a baby who has been nursing happily for months suddenly stops nursing altogether, refusing the breast when it's offered. This is different from baby-led weaning because it happens so abruptly. Often the baby is clearly unhappy but still unwilling to breastfeed. It's called a *nursing strike*.

The Back Story

The cause can be physical—a stuffy nose or earache, for instance—or emotional. Maybe there's been a move or new job; maybe you startled him when he bit you; maybe a loud noise startled him while he was nursing. A change in lotion, perfume, deodorant, or detergent; a low supply or change in milk taste; contact or negotiated nursings; or too many bottles or pacifiers may contribute to a strike. Babies who deal with oversupply problems may be especially prone to a nursing strike. The result is a baby who has lost his biggest comfort, his main food source, and his easiest way of falling asleep. And yet he turns away whenever you offer! Many babies on strike will continue to nurse, reluctantly or the same as always, at night. It keeps them fairly well fed and keeps your own hopes higher. Some babies won't nurse at all. It's a tough time for you both, and sometimes you never figure out the original cause. And even if the original problem is resolved, your baby still may not want to nurse. It's as though he doesn't realize that it was his stuffy nose that made breastfeeding uncomfortable—he thinks that breastfeeding itself caused the difficulties and he's reluctant to try it again.

What You Can Do

Don't be too quick to give the baby lots of other drinks and foods to make up for the milk he's missing. He's probably a sturdy little guy by now and may just need a little time. Do pump or hand-express your milk during this time, both to maintain your milk supply and to prevent plugged ducts or mastitis. If the strike continues for more than a day, you could offer your expressed milk in a cup—but avoid giving bottles if you can so that his sucking urge will encourage him toward breastfeeding.

Some time-honored approaches:

- 💡 Nurse the baby in his sleep. This is probably the most commonly helpful suggestion.
- 💡 Sing or rock your baby with your shirt open and see if he'll relax enough to latch.
- 💡 Nurse somewhere different—while walking around, while sitting in the car, at a friend's house, outside, or in a warm bath together.
- 💡 Offer in a whole new position—have him sitting facing you, for instance, or put him up against your shoulder and slide him down into a vertical position.
- 💡 Do a dance or baby bounce—starting small but getting bouncier and

bouncier—while holding him in a nursing position. (Stop if he doesn't like it.)

- 💡 Don't offer for a day or so, to let the tensions (whatever they are) cool. Then, for a day, keep your shirt up and your breast available but don't push the issue.

- 💡 And here's a wild one that worked for one mother: sit in an office chair holding the baby in your lap near but not at your breast, have someone spin the chair (not too fast) until you're a little dizzy, and then offer your breast. Sometimes being a little disoriented lets our instincts rise to the surface.

Whatever works may need to be repeated once or for a few days before everything smooths out. Almost all nursing strikes end happily, but they don't all end quickly; your Leader can be extremely helpful.

Oversupply

It often starts with a sigh of relief. Yes! You have milk! You can hear your baby glugging. You may hear milk hit the bottom of her stomach, or she pulls off, spluttering, and milk hits her in the face. Soon she's a fussy eater. Maybe she eats only when she's really hungry. She may bob on and off your breast, or twist her body, seldom nursing to sleep. Maybe she nurses eagerly until your milk releases, then she arches away as if she's angry. She may spit up frequently or need a lot of burping. Maybe she screams if you switch sides. She may gain splendidly but develop a rash. Her diapers may start out yellow, then turn green, maybe frothy or really mucousy. Nursing may become a struggle. You might wonder if you have milk after all, and her splendid gain may falter. She may fall on bottles of pumped milk like a starving child, or fuss over bottles as well as breast. And then comes the day, perhaps, when you see a streak of blood in her stools! What's gone wrong????

Relax! You've been blessed and cursed—like many of us—with an overabundant milk supply, also called *oversupply* or *overactive letdown,* and it's fixable.

The Back Story

Part of the problem with oversupply is just plain physical. Your baby is trying to drink from a fire hose, and it takes concentration and commitment to do that at every meal. Then there's the digestion part—fat and lactose (milk sugar).

The amount of fat in your milk can vary. Here's how: As the milk is made inside your breasts, much of the fat stays near the cells that make milk, while the rest of the milk flows down toward your nipple with the baby's sucking. If the baby hasn't nursed for a couple of hours and the milk has had time to collect in the ducts, he'll drink the lower-fat milk first, then the fat level will rise as the baby's continued sucking helps to bring down more of the fat. When he stops nursing, the fat gradually drifts back up away from the nipple, to be pulled down again next time the baby nurses (along with the new milk that's been made). If you have an overly generous milk supply, your baby has to drink quite a lot of milk before much of that fat starts getting pulled down.

The amount of lactose stays the same, but lactose is digested by an enzyme called *lactase,* produced in your baby's small intestines, on tiny finger-like projections. The lactase breaks down the lactose in your milk, your baby digests it, and she feels great…unless there's so much milk that the lactose overwhelms the lactase, or if something temporarily damages those tiny "fingers." Then the milk sugar starts to ferment, causing gas and maybe frothy green stools that can cause diaper rashes. Sometimes the damage is enough to cause small amounts of bleeding that show up in her diaper. (Don't worry! Intestines are sensitive but they're tough, just like your skin. Small injuries to an intestine are no more serious than a scratch on any other part of you.)

If you can drop your milk supply somewhat, your baby won't get full before she gets all the fat she wants. That will slow her digestion and give her lactase time to work. And if we can remove anything that's become an irritation to her while her intestines are riled up, they'll heal faster and regrow those tiny fingers faster so they can produce more lactase.

Some women with very small storage capacity may end up with a lot of force behind even a modest milk supply. These babies are more likely to be bothered by the fire hose than by truly irritated intestines. Nursing frequently so that there isn't that backlog of milk should help.

What You Can Do

If your baby isn't having any rashes or intestinal bleeding, you probably just have to quiet your supply down a little. Some possibilities to consider:

Nurse on just one side each time, nursing briefly on the other side *only* if you're uncomfortable and only enough to relieve the pressure. If your baby wants to nurse for comfort or conversation before the next full feeding, stay on the first breast. This lets your baby tap in to the higher-fat-content milk that lingers after a nursing, and slows milk production on the side he didn't nurse from.

Nurse on one side as many times in a row as you need to in order to soften it thoroughly before using the other side. Called "block nursing," this could mean you nurse on the same side twice, or all morning, or for six hours or even more at a time. If the other side is clamoring to be used, you can nurse on that side enough to keep from being uncomfortable. This is much more a matter of reading your breasts and your baby than your clock. The idea is to keep up some full-breast pressure on the side you're not using, but not keep it so full that you risk mastitis or pain.

Shift your position. Try the laid-back position in Chapter 4. Leaning back turns your fire hose into a fountain, which may be enough. Or try sitting up but hugging your baby's back and shoulders more closely, which tips her head back a bit farther and gives milk a straighter shot down her throat. The same fast flow that choked her before may be just fine now. Or try nursing lying down, which some babies prefer when there's oversupply.

If your baby has a rash or blood in her stool, it can indicate a really irritated intestine. In addition to managing for oversupply, it may help to remove other irritants temporarily. Consider removing the following one step at a time from both your and your baby's diet, not moving to the next step unless the first step doesn't appear to be enough:

1. Dairy and soy products
2. Artificial colors and preservatives
3. Anything that you might have binged on during pregnancy

Some mothers have had success by adding the herb sage to their diets. Certain medications can also help. Talk to your tech support person about other possibilities.

Or ignore all the above, and go back to nursing your baby however you choose. Sometimes we get too caught up in trying to limit our milk supplies. Sharing baths, co-sleeping, and nursing just for the pleasure of it can all be part of getting the happy times back.

If your baby's growth and behavior are fine but your baby's diapers are still green or frothy, or there's occasional blood, most doctors say you can ignore minor bleeding, which can take a long time to disappear. Formula-fed babies *often* have blood in their stool, whether it's visible or not, so switching to formula isn't a solution.

We tend to have more milk with each baby, so oversupply tends to be more likely with each baby. But nursing for any old reason at any old time and not bothering to use a second side unless one of you wants to can help prevent or solve most oversupply issues.

If your oversupply is severe, you might want to start your block nursing by expressing both sides thoroughly, so that you start with two breasts that are as softened as you can make them. You may need to repeat this several times before your supply begins to settle down.

Piercings

Body modification has been practiced since the beginning of time, and many more mothers today are getting piercings. The only types that could be problematic for nursing are those through the nipple or areola, but even these don't usually cause a problem.

The Back Story

Most nipples are pierced horizontally, which seems to work best for breastfeeding. Nipple piercings don't usually affect milk production, although they can add outlets in the nipples that can increase leaking.

Areolar piercings can damage the nerves that affect milk ejection. Both nipple and areola piercings can cause problems for milk ejection if scarring blocks the milk flow.

Jewelry left in place during nursing is a choking hazard. It can also affect latching or harm the soft tissues in the baby's mouth.

That's the bad news. The good news is that most of the time, if the jewelry is removed, nursing works just fine. Avoid getting a piercing while you are pregnant or breastfeeding, because the jewelry can't be removed until healing is complete, which can take up to a year.

What You Can Do

Remove nipple and areola rings or bars during feedings. Some mothers use insertion tapers or polytetrafluoroethylene (PTFE or Teflon) barbells between feedings to keep the holes open. If scarring has decreased your nerve response, you can use breast massage and compressions (Chapter 6) in addition to other milk release techniques (Chapter 15).

If the piercings close and you want to have them re-pierced, it's best to wait about three months after weaning to let the old holes heal completely.

Plugged Ducts

If you brush your hand over your breast and suddenly notice a firm, tender spot, you may have found a plugged duct. It may be the size of a marble or the size of your hand, depending on whether the plug is fairly far "upstream" (causing a small blockage) or "downstream" (backing up milk from a broader area).

The Back Story

Plugs can result from milk not being taken out—maybe because your baby suddenly sleeps through the night or you miss a feeding. They can also result from pressure on the ducts from a bra that's too snug or even a baby carrier worn for a long period of time that presses on your breast. Sometimes you never learn the cause. Plugs probably represent thickened milk. Our ducts are very small, and a bit of milk that thickens from not moving can presumably stop things up. A plugged duct can result in mastitis, go along with mastitis, or be nothing more than an isolated plug. Some women may be more prone to them because of the particular blend of fats in their milk.

What You Can Do

As with mastitis and blebs, the goal is to get the milk moving again. You can help keep that breast as soft as possible by nursing or expressing milk as often as you can. You can also try the following:

- Lay your baby on his back on the floor or bed, perhaps on a folded blanket so that the back of his head can drop off the edge and his chin doesn't tuck. Loom over him on your elbows so that your breast dangles, and nurse in that position so that gravity can help out.
- Nurse your baby with his chin pointed in the direction of the plug.
- Avoid wearing a bra, especially underwires.
- Wear a different style of bra.
- Use the "bag of marbles" technique described in the "Mastitis" section of this chapter.
- Use an electric toothbrush or massager against the plug, or see a physiotherapist for a painless ultrasound treatment to break up the plug.
- Take 2 tablespoons of lecithin (available in a health food store or pharmacy) daily, or one 1,200 mg capsule three to four times a day. Lecithin helps to break up fat particles and keep them from clumping. (Egg yolk contains lecithin, which is why it helps to smooth out mayonnaise.) After a few weeks of daily lecithin, some mothers who suffer chronic plugged ducts find that the plugs stop happening. (It may be necessary to continue taking the lecithin to keep plugs from returning.)
- Applying heat—with a warm washcloth or heating pad—right before nursing or expressing milk may help.
- And the old refrain—take care of yourself, eat well, get enough rest. (But you knew that. It's *doing* it that's hard.)

Postpartum Depression

Depression that hits after the birth of your baby, known as *postpartum depression,* lasts longer than the common and very short-term "baby blues." Here are the most common symptoms:

- A persistent sad, anxious, or "empty" mood
- Sleeping too much or too little
- Reduced appetite and weight loss, or increased appetite and weight gain
- Loss of interest or pleasure in activities you once enjoyed (including sex)
- Restlessness, irritability, or excessive crying
- Persistent physical symptoms such as headaches, digestive problems, or chronic pain
- Difficulty concentrating, remembering, or making decisions
- Feeling guilty, hopeless, worthless, helpless, or pessimistic
- Fatigue or loss of energy

If you are thinking about death, suicide, or harming your baby, don't wait. Get medical help right away. These thoughts are not typical of postpartum depression.

The Back Story

Postpartum depression can hit anytime within the first year, though it tends to start by about ten weeks postpartum. It usually lasts at least a couple of weeks and may strike as many as 25 percent of women in Western cultures. It's more common in women who have suffered depression in the past, and may be more likely following a traumatic birth, with mother-baby separation or breastfeeding problems, and in societies in which new mothers have little family and cultural support.

What You Can Do About It

Continued breastfeeding is not only one of the best things you can do to reduce or avoid depression, it's also the best thing you can do for your baby if you do become depressed. Babies of depressed mothers who bottle-feed are more likely to have developmental challenges due to her depression than babies of depressed mothers who breastfeed.

In mild cases, support, friendship, and help with breastfeeding may resolve the problem. If you still feel sad, talk to your physician, who may suggest medication. Most antidepressants are compatible with breastfeeding. Have your caregiver check Hale's *Medications and Mothers' Milk* for more information. Another great resource you can share with your doctor is *Non-Pharmacologic Treatments for Depression in New Mothers* by Kathleen Kendall-Tackett. Like other forms of depression, postpartum depression is helped more by both having someone to talk to about it and taking medication than by either one alone.

If you sense that your periodic unhappiness is something other than true depression, keep reading.

D-MER–Dysphoric Milk Ejection Reflex

D-MER is a little-recognized "glitch" that most affected women never talk about because they don't want to be treated for a depression that they suspect they don't have.

Alia Macrina Heise finally had her dream birth with her third baby—at home, unmedicated, peaceful, joyful. A wonderful beginning! By two weeks, though, she noticed that every time she nursed her baby, she felt worthless, hopeless, useless, and worse. She couldn't concentrate. Food looked disgusting, and there was a bad feeling in the pit of her stomach. But she had these feelings *only* when her milk released. And then, within a minute or so, it was as if the feeling had never happened. All the rest of the time she was a happy, confident, in-love-with-her-baby new mother.

She established a website, d-mer.org, and several *hundred* women responded: "I thought I was the only one." "Now that I know I'm not alone, I think I can handle it." "I had this more than twenty years ago."

We don't know much yet. Alia found several treatments that worked for her, described on the website, and went on to nurse her baby well into toddlerhood. If you suspect you have D-MER, you're not alone, and we hope there will be more answers soon.

Reflux

Gastroesophageal reflux occurs when the valve between the stomach and esophagus opens or does not close completely and stomach contents and acids rise up into the esophagus. All humans have reflux many times a day, babies more often than adults. Not all reflux is noticeable and not all reflux makes us uncomfortable. But when it's severe, the acids rising from the stomach into the esophagus can be painful.

The Back Story

Some of the symptoms of reflux in a baby include frequent swallowing between feedings; arching when nursing; pulling on and off the breast as if he wants to nurse but it causes pain; fussing in a car seat, when he's bent in the middle, or when lying flat; and salivating or having near-constant congestion or rumbly breathing. The opening from the stomach to the esophagus is usually on the right side, so anything that puts the right side higher than the left side may keep stomach contents down better.

What You Can Do

First, read the "Oversupply" section. Resolving oversupply can often cure reflux. Nurse often, so that his meals are smaller and your milk flows with less force. One of the reasons the Magic Baby Hold (Chapter 6) is helpful is that your baby's right side is higher if you use your left arm, which can be soothing. Minimize time spent in a car seat—the position puts pressure on your baby's stomach. Sleep so that your baby lies on his left side. Consider a wedge under the mattress to keep his head higher than his feet.

If your baby's symptoms persist or he seems particularly bothered, you can ask your doctor to evaluate your baby for reflux and refer her to a gastroenterologist. *Research does not support thickened feeds or simethicone drops,* but there are medications that can help. A good resource for further information about reflux is *Colic Solved* by Dr. Bryan Vartabedian.

Sore Nipples

You've probably heard a few stories about nipple pain. Some women will tell you that breastfeeding always hurts in the beginning and that you have to wait for your nipples to "toughen up." Not true!

The Back Story

The most common cause of sore nipples in the early days is a baby taking the breast poorly. Maybe he's tensing from not being allowed to do the job himself, maybe he's held in a position that doesn't allow him the mouthful he wants, or maybe birth medications have caused temporary problems.

Engorgement can lead to sore nipples when the breast becomes too full for him to get a good mouthful, and if he can latch at all, it may be very shallow (see "Engorgement"). If the problem is the way the baby is attached to your breast, you'll probably see a distinct change in the shape of your nipple when it leaves his mouth—it may look creased, have a white stripe, or have one side flattened.

Blebs, mastitis, tongue-tie, and thrush can all cause sore nipples and have their own sections in this chapter. Sore nipples can also be an early sign of pregnancy. (If that's the case for you, you may want to check out the section in Chapter 16 about breastfeeding while pregnant.) Less common causes for sore nipples include skin conditions such as eczema. Unlike baby-latching issues, these unhappy-skin issues can cause nipple pain even though your nipple isn't distorted or flattened when it leaves your baby's mouth.

What You Can Do

If your nipple is distorted, you can try letting the baby fix the problem by using the laid-back nursing position described in Chapter 4. One of the more mother-controlled latches described in Chapter 4 may also help. Maybe you can spend a day or half a day in bed, letting your baby work on getting a good latch in a relaxed setting. If your nipple is still distorted, take a look at the tongue-tie section below. If the pain relates to skin problems, one of the tools below may be helpful.

Nipple or breast pain is a message that something needs fixing; it's not meant to be a constant companion. The following tools may help, but only if you also address what caused the pain in the first place.

Your milk can help. Try hand-expressing a little milk after the feeding and let it dry on your nipples. The anti-inflammatory and anti-bacterial properties of your milk can heal not only nipple wounds but other skin and even eye infections—a reason to learn hand expression!

Purified lanolin is for nipples what lip balm is for lips. It helps keep the cells' own moisture intact. A healthy nipple doesn't need ointment, but if your nipple is chapped or slightly damaged, a light coating of purified (to reduce the risk of allergies) lanolin keeps newly formed cells from drying out and allows them to slide easily across the damaged area to bridge the gap more quickly. This "moist wound healing" can be very effective, but only if you address what caused the damage in the first place.

Soap and water, banned from nipples for years, is back! A nipple wound is like any other skin wound. It's a potential opening for bacteria and needs to be kept clean. There's no need at all to wash healthy nipples, but washing an injured nipple with a mild soap and water several times a day makes sense.

Hydrogels designed for nipples (sold with other breastfeeding supplies) feel cool and comfortable on your skin, don't stick to wounds, and protect your nipple's moisture balance while they protect from bumps and baby kicks. They're fairly expensive and can be used for only a few days before they become waterlogged with milk and must be replaced. Some mothers find them extremely helpful; others don't.

Over-the-counter antibiotic ointments stay in place much better than creams and may be less likely to cause irritation while they protect against infection. If you use a vanishingly small amount two or three times a day after nursing, it will be gone by the time your baby nurses again, so there's no need to wash it off. One way to hold it in place and create a moist wound healing effect is to put plastic wrap over your nipple after putting the ointment on. (Be sure to take the plastic off before nursing again, though!)

Breast shells are hard plastic domes originally designed to help flat or inverted nipples stand out, although the newer suction devices probably work better. If your nipples are very sore, the shells can act as armor, but they also tend to hold external (not the cells' own) moisture in, which can slow healing. If you like the idea of the shells, don't wear them at night because they can slide away from their intended location and cause further damage. Wash and dry them frequently to make sure they don't collect bacteria. You can use one when you're nursing to keep your baby from kicking your sore nipple, but leave them off as much as possible to speed healing.

Supplementation

Supplementing can be both emotional and confusing. Does your baby really need it? If so, what should you give and how much? And is there a way to give it that doesn't undermine breastfeeding? As with causes of low milk supply, we know a lot more than we used to.

The Back Story

Before you give your baby any supplementation, be sure he really, truly needs it. Giving unnecessary supplements—extra milk besides nursing—is a surefire recipe for decreasing your milk production because your baby will fill up on the supplement and take less of your milk. But if your baby truly isn't getting enough milk, and if the reason can't be eliminated quickly, he'll need that extra milk to grow the way he should.

While it's important to avoid unnecessary supplements, remember that a hungry baby *can't* try harder. Babies breastfeed better when they're calm and not frantically hungry. So while you're trying to fix any breastfeeding problem, it's important to make sure that your baby is getting enough milk, even if it means he has to have a supplement for a while.

What You Can Do

Before you begin supplementing, you may find it helpful to check with your LLL Leader or another tech support person. That person may be able to help you avoid it, or help you use it in a way that supports rather than undermines breastfeeding.

The best option for a supplement, of course, is your own milk that you've pumped or hand-expressed. If you don't have any expressed milk, then donated pasteurized human milk is the next best option.

One possibility for donated human milk is from one of the many milk banks in North America (hmbana.org) and throughout the world. Milk donors are screened for illnesses that can pass into the milk, which is then pasteurized and frozen. Milk from a human milk bank may be available through your hospital or from the milk bank directly with a prescription.

Not all requests can be filled because supplies are limited, so most donated milk goes to premature babies and those who cannot tolerate formula. The cost for human milk is fairly high, but it's covered by some medical insurance policies and government programs.

If you don't have enough of your own milk and donor human milk isn't available, then your baby's doctor can advise you about what to use for a supplement.

How much should you supplement? Only your baby knows the answer. Let's look at three different babies. The first baby has begun to complain about his intake since you've been packing for a move or preparing for the holidays. What supplement does he need? Probably just some extra nursing because things are basically going well and you've hit a small dip. The second baby has begun to grow more slowly. The supplement he needs may just be the extra that you pump while you get a minor nursing problem sorted out. He'll soon start refusing some of what you've pumped, and you can start phasing out the extra. Often you never find out exactly what the problem was, but a little pumping takes care of it for good.

The third baby's weight gain is faltering, and your supply isn't up to helping him gain at first. He'll need more in terms of supplementation. You'll probably be pumping to build your supply, but also giving your baby supplements in addition to what you've pumped. If your baby has been on "short rations" for a while and begins to be offered unlimited supplements, he may not take much extra at first, but then he may start to "pig out." His stomach had become accustomed to smaller amounts and takes a few days to be able to hold more. Paced bottle-feeding (see page 425) allows him to stop when he's full. After a week or so, you'll have a sense for what he needs at various times of day, and can offer the supplement before nursing. That allows him to finish at the breast, and probably also encourages better nursing.

Your baby may need to gain weight extra fast to catch up, because a baby is supposed to be gaining weight from birth on. If he falls behind and *then* starts growing at his normal rate, he'll stay as far behind as he was. He needs to grow *faster* than normal for a while in order to catch up, and that takes more food than normal. Once he catches up, his intake will settle down to normal, but until then, expect a steeper-than-average line on his growth chart. There's no other way he can get up to where he would have been.

How do you feed the extra milk? The best device for you is the one you feel most comfortable with.

Supplemental Feeding Devices

One possibility is a tubing device at the breast, sometimes called an at-breast supplementer. It's a simple concept that can be a bit tricky to learn. The idea is that soft tubing runs from a container of milk to your nipple, like a long, flexible straw. When the baby nurses, he takes both tubing and nipple into his mouth, and gets the extra milk as he sucks.

There are several commercial brands. Here's a homemade version: Use a regular baby bottle with a regular bottle nipple, and ask your health care provider for a #5 french feeding tube. (You can also use the tubing from a commercial supplementer device.) Cut a slightly larger hole in the bottle nipple tip, put your supplement in the bottle, and install the bottle nipple either right side up or projecting into the bottle. Either way works; it's just there to keep the milk from spilling and the tubing from wiggling, not to seal the bottle. Keep one end of the tubing below the milk in the bottle, and use a finger-length of medical or hair setting tape to hold the other end at your nipple. Run the tape along the tubing instead of across it, to keep the tubing secure on your breast. Many women find it easiest to run

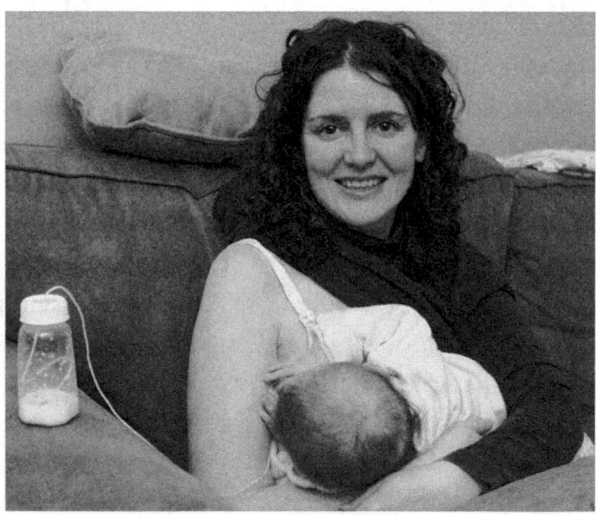

Homemade at-breast supplementer.

the tubing along their breast where the baby's tongue will be, but any position that gets the tubing inside the "sucking tunnel" of baby's upper lip and cupped tongue will work. Experiment until you find an arrangement that lets milk zip quickly from bottle to baby when he starts sucking. If you're having trouble, it helps to talk with someone who has experience with supplementers.

Devices for Supplementing a Breastfed Baby

Supplementing method	Advantages	Disadvantages	Comments
Spoon	Easy and quick for small amounts	Tedious and messy for large amounts	Especially useful with colostrum.
Eyedropper, syringe, or periodontal syringe (this last is harder to obtain, but with its curved, narrow tip can be used to supplement at breast)	Easy and quick for small amounts	Tedious for larger amounts	Try having baby suck on a finger at the same time, while he lies on your raised thighs (feet propped on coffee table, for instance). Make sure the tip doesn't poke the baby.
Small cup	Simple way to supplement small amounts for a few days	Can spill, wasting "liquid gold" and making intake harder to judge	To learn how, cup-feed an adult, and have that adult cup-feed you. Have the one being fed close his/her eyes.
Finger-feeder	Easy to learn	May not prevent nipple confusion	Use manufactured device, or use at-breast supplementer on finger.
At-breast supplementer	Baby is nursing!	Fiddly at first	Get help from someone familiar with their use.
Bottle	Easy to use	Can undermine breastfeeding	Paced bottle-feeding and finishing at the breast help a lot.

You've probably heard both good and bad things about bottles. They're the easiest way to supplement large amounts and don't have much of a learning curve. But a baby who is fed well with a bottle and not a breast can quickly come to prefer the bottle. And it can be discouraging to see your baby relax and fill up happily with the bottle when he didn't at your breast. Is it nipple confusion? Nipple preference? Flow preference? A baby simply going where he can get food most easily? Whatever it is, it's a real and common problem. Fortunately, new understandings about how babies feed from the breast and how bottles work have shown us ways to use bottles that work better with breastfeeding. See below for ways to bottle-feed that support breastfeeding.

One way to make breastfeeding more appealing to your baby so that he prefers it is to give the supplement *before* breastfeeding. This works for any type of supplementation device that's used away from the breast, especially bottles. You'll see your baby relax and fall asleep "milk drunk" at your breast, which is a great feeling. He'll most likely feed longer and better at the breast, and breastfeed more patiently even when the flow is slow. His increased interest may boost your supply faster.

There is a risk that the baby can fill up on the supplement and not breastfeed well, so don't give him *quite* as much supplement as you normally would, and see if he's satisfied with that lovely at-breast last course. If he doesn't seem to drain your breast after having the supplement, give him a bit less supplement next time. If he's still hungry after breastfeeding from one side, switch to the other. If he's still hungry, feel free to give him more supplement, but then bring him back to the breast again to finish the feeding.

Although it doesn't work for every baby or in every situation, this method of supplementing can often encourage a baby to breastfeed better. There is also a tear sheet in the back of the book with more ideas for feeding bottles in a way that supports breastfeeding.

When you've increased your milk supply and your baby's weight has caught up, you might find that he starts refusing to take as much supplement. This is your cue that the supplements won't be needed much longer. If he's still taking some though your supply has increased, try decreasing the amount slowly over several days and see if his weight stays up. If it doesn't, slow down and give it more time. For various reasons, occasion-

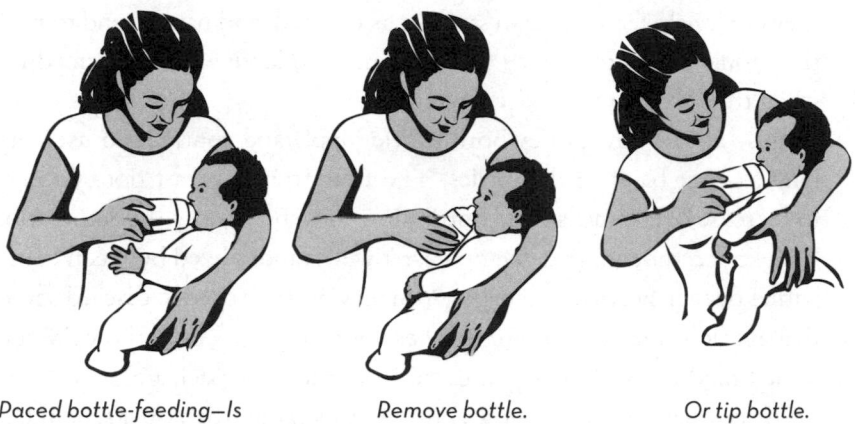

Paced bottle-feeding—Is baby stressed?   *Remove bottle.*   *Or tip bottle.*

ally mothers aren't able to get a full supply, so sometimes supplements are needed until the baby is eating a more varied diet.

Paced Bottle-Feeding

You can help your baby gain control over the feeding and avoid overfeeding by pausing the feeding periodically. If you see his forehead and eyes crinkle, his fingers splay and tense, his eyes widen, or his swallows turn to gulps, lean him forward slightly until the milk in the nipple runs back into the bottle. No need to unlatch him, and you can tip the bottle back again as soon as he likes. If you do take the bottle out, rest it in a "shhh" position against his lips so he knows it hasn't gone away. Then offer it again—and if he's not interested, let the feeding end.

Bottle-Feeding Techniques That Support Breastfeeding

There's a lot you can do to put your baby in control, just as he is when the two of you breastfeed. Consider these suggestions:

🔆 Choose a bottle nipple that is similar to your own nipples. If you have short nipples, for example, look for short bottle nipples. This will help minimize competition between the bottle and your nipple. (It's interesting to do this, isn't it? There's probably nothing out there that looks even remotely like you!) Avoid "orthodontic" nipples. Research shows that their shape isn't what your nipple looks like in the baby's mouth, they don't help teeth grow in straight as claimed, and babies tend to pull their tongues back in a way that's counterproductive for breastfeeding when they use them.

- ☀ Choose a slow-flow or newborn bottle nipple and continue to use it as long as your baby needs bottles. The flow from a breast doesn't tend to increase over time, so the bottle flow rate should stay the same, too. Remember, though, that the flow isn't well standardized between companies or even between packages. You may find you need to discard some that are slower or faster than the ones your baby likes, even if they're the same brand you always buy or came from the same package.
- ☀ Feed your baby when he shows hunger cues rather than on a schedule.
- ☀ Give the bottle in a way that's similar to how he takes the breast. Stroke the upright bottle nipple down the center of his lips to trigger him to open his mouth widely. When he does, lay the *base* of the nipple on his lower lip so he latches on to both base and narrower nipple section with a relaxed jaw.
- ☀ Reduce the flow by holding the baby sitting mostly upright so the bottle is mostly horizontal. (Don't worry about keeping the nipple full of milk so the baby doesn't swallow air. Any air just comes out his nose. It's rapid gulping, not smooth feeding, that results in swallowed air…and swallowed air just results in burps, not distress.) A more upright position also helps limit bottle-feeding-related dental caries and ear infections because milk isn't pooling in the mouth and throat. And it allows the baby to stop and start sucking when he wants to.
- ☀ Switch sides at least once a feeding to help prevent a side preference when breastfeeding. This also helps stimulate equal eye and facial muscle development.
- ☀ Allow the baby to decide when the feeding is ended. This isn't always when the milk is gone.
- ☀ See the page on bottle-feeding on the Tear-Sheet Toolkit.

Tattoos

Body modification in the form of tattoos has been practiced since the beginning of time, and many more mothers today are getting them to celebrate special events and transitions.

The Back Story

Tattoo ink molecules are too large to pass into your milk, so existing tattoos are completely safe for your baby. One risk of tattooing during breastfeeding is infection, which is less likely if the wound is kept clean and treated appropriately. Human milk banks will not accept donations from mothers who have had a tattoo done in the past twelve months because of the risk of hepatitis C, tetanus, and HIV from contaminated needles. Tattoo removal is usually done with a laser; the only risk of that is an infection from inadequate wound care.

What You Can Do

It makes sense to wait to get a tattoo at least until your child's first birthday, to give your body a chance to recover completely from childbirth. If you're planning to get a tattoo after that point, screen the tattooist carefully, choosing one who follows "universal precautions," including sterilization of the tattoo machine using an autoclave; single-use inks, ink cups, gloves, and needles; bagging of equipment to avoid cross contamination; and thorough hand washing with disinfectant soap. Don't be surprised if the tattooist wants to wait until after you've weaned; most won't knowingly tattoo a pregnant or breastfeeding mother.

Tobacco During Breastfeeding

Tobacco isn't good for anyone, but for the mother who smokes, breastfeeding is still a safer choice than formula.

The Back Story

A nursing baby is exposed to the nicotine and cotinine in her mother's system. Nicotine can lower your prolactin level, which can reduce not only your interest in breastfeeding but also your supply and the fat content of your milk.

What You Can Do

If you smoke, you can limit your child's exposure by smoking as little as possible, always going outside to smoke, wearing a "smoking jacket" that you take off before picking up your baby again, never smoking in the car with your child, and nursing before you have a cigarette rather than after. If you use a nicotine patch, be sure to take it off at night. If you decide to stop smoking, check smokefree.gov.

Tongue-tie

If your baby isn't latching on deeply or well despite all your efforts, or if your nipple comes out of his mouth flattened, it's possible that your baby has a *tongue-tie*—a tongue that can't move freely enough.

The Back Story

A baby can maintain a deep latch only if he can move his tongue without restriction. A membrane under the tongue, called a *frenum* (FREE-num) or *frenulum* (FREN-yew-lum), can be so tight that it prevents that free movement. The tongue can't lift or extend well enough to remove milk well, and it can abrade the tip of the nipple or compress it tightly, causing blisters or wounds or flattening one side of the nipple and shaping it like a new lipstick.

Many doctors and nurses recognize tongue-ties with the frenulum attached to the tip of the tongue, especially if it pulls the center of the tongue into a notch or heart shape. But not all understand that a frenulum can also attach just behind the tip of the tongue, in the middle, or at the base. And, unfortunately, frenula that are attached to the base of the tongue are the hardest to see and sometimes cause the worst problems.

Other signs of tongue-tie include a high and narrow palate (because the tongue can't lift to spread it), a tongue that rolls under or has a flat front edge when it's extended, a tongue that doesn't lift when the baby cries, or one with a crease down the middle. You might see a dip in the center of his tongue when he lifts it or when he cries—that's the frenulum pulling the

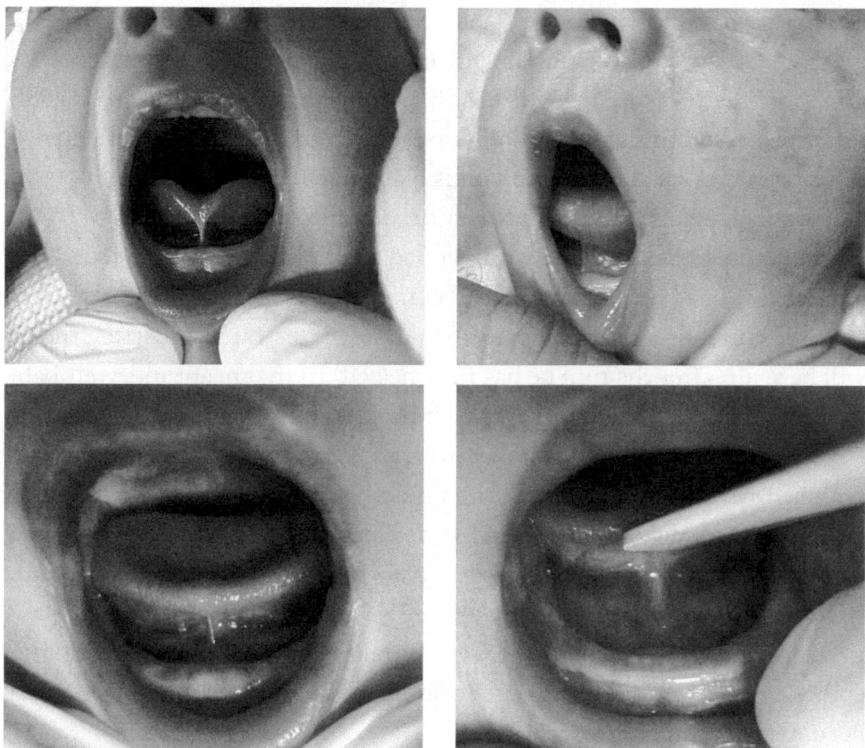

Tongue-tie: several types of restricted movement.

center of the tongue down. You might hear clicking when he nurses—that's caused by breaks in suction. A too-tight tongue may tire easily and quiver. Feedings might take a long time or he might tire out right away.

Some surgeons or dentists recommend waiting to see if the frenulum breaks on its own, but this rarely happens during the first year—a long time to wait! Babies with tongue-tie sometimes have difficulty using bottles, too. Untreated tongue-tie can cause later difficulty with speech, cleaning the teeth with the tongue, swallowing pills, licking ice cream cones, and kissing.

What You Can Do

If you suspect your baby is tongue-tied, you'll need to see a doctor to actually diagnose the problem and to treat it. Usually all that's required is a quick snip or two—called a *frenotomy*—by a dentist or doctor with a small pair of blunt-end scissors or laser in his office. Only local anesthesia is needed, or none at all. A cry from being held still, a drop or two of blood, and usually the baby latches immediately and nurses much more easily and effectively. Your Leader or lactation consultant is likely to have names of local doctors who do this, or check lowmilksupply.org/frenotomy.shtml.

Sometimes the frenulum isn't snipped deeply enough and a second trip is needed. But if your baby doesn't latch painlessly in the week or so after the procedure, don't worry. If the first nursing afterward was better, then it will be again after the tongue has fully healed. In the meantime, your baby is just holding his tongue back while it heals.

It can also take a baby a while to learn how to move his tongue better when he nurses, especially if he's older when it's snipped. (A lactation consultant can suggest exercises that may help.) That's one reason to have tongue-tie treated as soon as possible. Another is that the younger the baby is, the less blood and nerve supply there is in the frenulum, so the less it is likely to bleed or hurt. If your baby's frenulum is tight enough to limit his ability to remove milk but you decide not to have a frenotomy, you may need to pump for him as well.

Vasospasm

A nipple *vasospasm* happens when the muscles inside the tip of the nipple spasm so tightly that all blood is forced out of the nipple, turning the tip white, like a clenched knuckle, and then bright red when the spasm relaxes and the blood flows back in. You may feel stinging or burning following a feeding; some women feel a pain that shoots deep into the breast. You might feel it in one nipple but not the other. It can last several minutes and can occur even in between feedings. It's often misdiagnosed as a yeast infection.

The Back Story

Vasospasms usually occur as a result of nipple trauma—a nipple's way of saying, "Ow!" It's also fairly common in women who have had breast or nipple surgery, possibly due to nerve or tissue damage. Some drugs, including nicotine and caffeine, can contribute to vasospasm.

What You Can Do

You'll probably find that vasospasms resolve once the main reason for your nipple pain is addressed. In the meantime, to *stop* a spasm, you can try to squeeze blood back into the nipple by squeezing your nipple at the base (it will probably stop the pain immediately).

To *prevent* vasospasms, it may help to stay warm. Wearing a vest may help or holding the baby against that side after nursing or turning up the thermostat. Some mothers apply a warm washcloth to the nipple as soon as the baby lets go. Others use a blow dryer set on warm. Just cupping the nipple with your warm hand may help. Or use a buckwheat or cherry pit pillow, or a sock filled with rice and sewn or tied shut; microwaved on high for about a minute, they'll hold a gentle heat for quite a while. Keeping warmth *nearly continuously* over a nursing pad for seven to ten days may end vasospasms for good. Or talk to your tech support person about vitamin B_6, calcium, magnesium, or a short-term prescription medication.

Weight Gain Worries

Weight gain is one way that your doctor or midwife monitors how things are going with your baby's feeding and overall health.

The Back Story

Healthy babies can gain at very different rates. Scales can differ. Growth charts conflict. Sometimes everyone forgets to look at the baby as well as the numbers. And sometimes there really is a problem, and the scale can alert you and let you know when things turn around.

What You Can Do

If your doctor says your baby's weight gain is too low, a good first step may be simply to confirm the numbers. Since all scales are calibrated differently, it's very important to have your baby weighed on the same scale each time, wearing the same or similar clothes. Avoid weighing a fully fed baby one time and a hungry baby the next.

If the numbers are accurate, the problem might be that your fully breast-fed baby is being evaluated on a weight chart based on data that include formula-fed babies. Unlike formula-fed babies, breastfed babies tend to grow rapidly in the early months and slow down around four months. So your baby's "slow growth" at five months might be normal after all. The charts commonly used in the United States are provided by the Centers for Disease Control and are *not* based on exclusively breastfed babies. The best weight gain charts based on breastfed babies alone are available at the World Health Organization's website, who.int/childgrowth/en.

Once you've gotten accurate weight information, take a close look at your baby. Is she plump and rounded in appearance? Of course, if she was premature or born "small for dates," it may take a few weeks to get that chubby baby look, but slow-gaining babies who are doing well usually have rounded cheeks, plump thighs, and creases around their wrists and ankles. That plump look is a good sign; loose "puppy skin" on legs and arms should disappear with a week or so of good feeding.

How is she behaving and developing? Does she relax after feedings (hands open, arms limp) and stay content for at least a few minutes? Is she hitting developmental milestones for smiling, reaching for objects, etc.? Is she energetic? These are all good signs.

Are you seeing enough poopy diapers (in the first six weeks, at least three a day larger than the "okay" finger sign)? Another good sign.

If your baby is feeding as often as she wants, including plenty of con-versational nursings, seems plump, healthy, active, cheerful, and develop-mentally on target, but still is gaining slowly, what should you do? Maybe nothing. With everything else looking good, this may simply be your baby's normal growth pattern. Research has shown that babies in the lowest per-centiles during the first year do just as well in terms of later intellectual and physical development as babies in the higher percentiles.

Maybe your concerns are about the other side of the coin. If your exclusively breastfed baby has tripled his birth weight by three or four months and is already causing you an aching back, people may suggest supplements or solid foods because he's so big, or may warn you that your "chunky monkey" is on the way to a lifetime of obesity. No worries. Unlike formula-fed babies, exclusively breastfed babies who gain rapidly are not at increased risk of obesity. Most of these babies start to slow their growth by six months or so, and once they become mobile they tend to slim down quickly. They don't need solid foods sooner than their smaller peers. (If you haven't checked out slings, wraps, or other kinds of soft carriers for your baby yet, we'd encourage you to try a few—the right carrier will make all the difference when you're lugging around one of these "blue ribbon babies.")

Yeast Infections

When you have a yeast (*Candida*) infection on your breast, breastfeeding usually hurts. Your nipples are pink and shiny-looking, sometimes with flaking skin. You may feel a burning, itching, shooting, or stabbing pain during or in between feedings.

The Back Story

A yeast infection is caused by the same fungal organisms that cause vaginal yeast infections. You have these little yeasty beasties on your body all the time, but they cause pain only when there's an overgrowth. You may be at increased risk of an overgrowth after taking antibiotics (which you may have been given in labor) or if your iron levels are low. You're also at risk if your baby has a yeast infection (thrush) in his mouth, which usually appears as whitish areas on the inside of his cheeks and gums that leave a raw area if you try to wipe them away. You and your baby can pass a yeast infection back and forth, and either of you can have it without it being visible.

What You Can Do

If you suspect a yeast infection on your nipples or if your baby has thrush, consult with your doctor or breastfeeding support person. Gentian violet, an over-the-counter treatment used once a day for three or four days, is often helpful (although very staining), but sometimes a prescription anti-fungal medication is needed.

If you've been told you have a yeast infection but the problem persists after treatment, it's possible that it is really a bacterial (usually staph) infection requiring antibiotics, since the symptoms can be identical. Your tech support person may be able to help you find the most current research to share with your doctor.

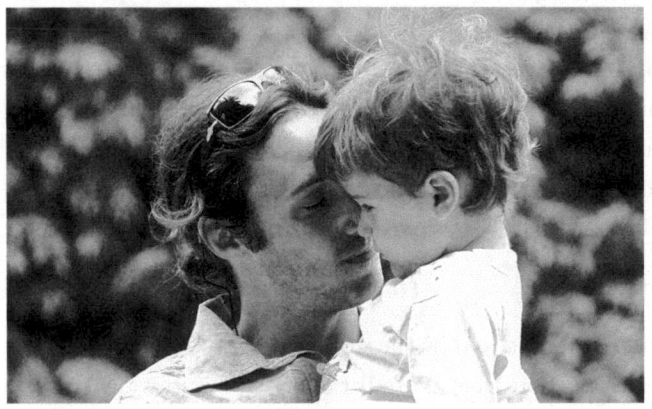

PART IV

La Leche League Resources

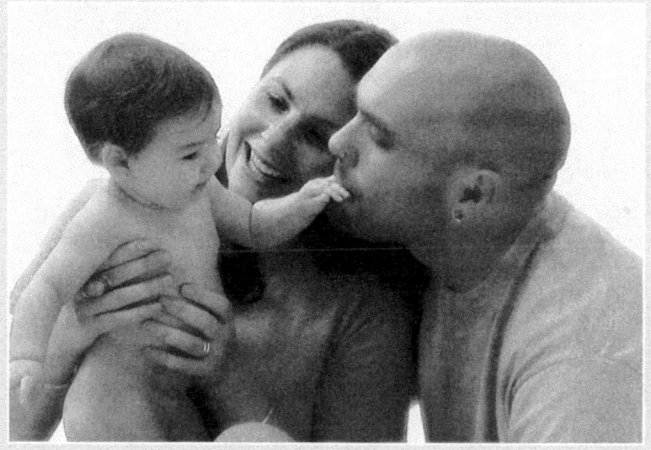

NINETEEN

About La Leche League

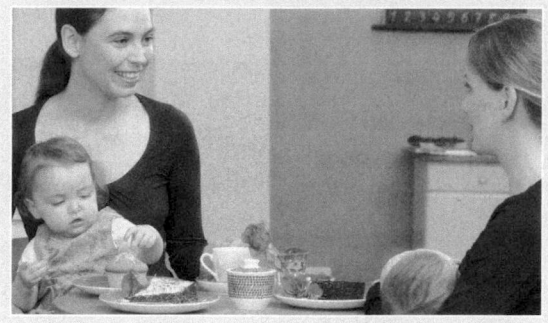

"*I* *went to my first La Leche League meeting to learn* *how to breastfeed my son Matthew sitting up, because in the hospital* *they'd only taught me how to do it lying down. My baby (who I thought* *was the most wonderful baby ever born) was completely bald except for* *a dusting of almost transparent blond hair. When I arrived at the meet-* *ing, the Leader said to me, "Oh, your baby has such a beautifully shaped* *head! He's gorgeous." I knew I had to come back because the Leader was* *obviously very intelligent and perceptive. Also, I did learn how to breast-* *feed sitting up, and I met a whole group of other women who understood* *how I felt about my baby and being a mother. I was hooked and have* *now been going to those meetings and getting to know more amazing* *women every month for thirty-one years.*"   —Teresa Pitman

"I found La Leche League when my first son, Alex, was about six months old. I was supplementing heavily because I had had a breast reduction, and I was worried about having to give him a bottle during the meeting. But the Leaders and moms welcomed me warmly, telling me I was a heroine for working so hard to give my milk to my baby. I left the meeting walking on air, feeling included in the Wonderful World of Breastfeeding Mothers. Over time, I became more and more involved with LLL, falling deeply in love with its sisterhood and philosophy of gentle, intuitive mothering."   —Diana West

---

"I almost walked out of my first meeting. All those mothers, all those babies! 'There is more to me than this,' I thought. But I came back once or twice (ho hum), and then I came with a toddler as a thank-you for their help with a nursing strike…and I 'got it.' This wasn't just about the mechanics of breastfeeding. This was about connecting with my child in fundamental ways, and being with other mothers who were making those same connections. Without La Leche League, I might have been a very different kind of mother. Our boys are adults now, with their own children. I watch them and their wonderful wives and how they're raising our grandchildren, and I think how fortunate I was; what if I hadn't gone back?"   —Diane Wiessinger

---

THE SEVEN MOTHERS who started La Leche League didn't have it easy. Most had difficulties themselves before finding information and support, and they wanted to offer that information and support to others. Millions of mothers today—this edition's authors among them—owe their breast-feeding success, directly or indirectly, to the organization that those seven women began.

The LLLove Story and *The Revolutionaries Wore Pearls* by Kaye Lowman and *Seven Voices, One Dream* by Mary Ann Cahill are excellent resources for more information about the history of La Leche League and the lives and perspectives of its founders.

How It All Started

At a church picnic near Chicago in the summer of 1956, two friends, Mary White and Marian Tompson, spent the afternoon breastfeeding and tending their babies while one woman after another approached them to say how impressed they were by how easy it seemed for them to care for their babies, with no bottles to warm or clean. These women all told a similar story. "I wanted to nurse my baby but..." "My doctor told me I didn't have enough milk." "My mother-in-law said the baby must not be getting enough because he wanted to nurse so often." "My baby lost interest after I started supplementing with formula." Over and over, Mary and Marian heard, "I tried to breastfeed, but I just couldn't."

Both Mary and Marian had experienced some of the same problems with their earlier babies. Ultimately, both of them learned what helped ensure success—and what was guaranteed to produce failure. They decided to try to help their friends and neighbors enjoy the same experience that meant so much to them.

First they made some phone calls to enlist the help of other successfully nursing mothers. Mary talked to her sister-in-law, Mary Ann Kerwin, and to Mary Ann Cahill, who casually mentioned the idea to Betty Wagner. Marian contacted Edwina Froehlich, who called her good friend Viola Lennon. Each had nursed one or more babies. Then these seven women invited their pregnant friends to a meeting at Mary White's home. What they offered mothers then—and what the more than forty-three thousand LLL Leaders who have followed them offer today—was simple: information, encouragement, and support, from one breastfeeding mother to another.

The meetings quickly outgrew Mary's living room, and the seven women found themselves with an organization in the making. Those were exhilarating times. Their phone lines (land lines back then) buzzed with local and long-distance callers. Unmedicated birth, breastfeeding basics, and mothering were their core topics. Mothers who had successfully breastfed and who were eager to help other mothers became La Leche League Leaders and started support groups in their own neighborhoods. Word spread around the country and eventually around the world that LLL had breastfeeding information that worked and that there were breastfeeding mothers available to help. In 1964 this rapid expansion led them to incorporate and officially become La Leche League International (LLLI).

The founders agreed from the very beginning that their families were their first priority. That understanding freed them to set aside LLL work when their families needed them. The seven founders wrote the first edition of *The Womanly Art of Breastfeeding* in 1958 between other chores, while babies and toddlers napped or played nearby. More often than not, the desk was the family dining table, with manuscript pages gathered up at mealtime. As their children grew and circumstances changed, some of them took on salaried jobs at the LLL office.

In the years since, in addition to raising their families, each of the founding women has contributed her particular talents to the growth of the organization. The recent deaths of Edwina Froelich, Betty Wagner Spandikow, and Viola Lennon still leave four active, passionate women participating in LLL projects.

OUR MISSION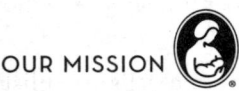

To help mothers worldwide to breastfeed through mother-to-mother support, encouragement, information, and education, and to promote a better understanding of breastfeeding as an important element in the healthy development of the baby and mother.

The La Leche League Influence

Many of the changes that have occurred in infant-care practices over the past fifty years can be traced to the influence of LLL. In 1956, the average American woman no longer participated in her own baby's birth. Many women feared birth, or didn't believe themselves capable of unmedicated birth. LLL encouraged women to trust their bodies; its founders were among the first women to promote the presence of husbands in the delivery room and a return to home birth for those who want it.

When La Leche League began, babies were routinely separated from their mothers following birth for as long as twenty-four hours. LLL spoke out: babies need their mothers, and mothers benefit, too, from early nursing and uninterrupted bonding. Today women are encouraged to hold and nurse their newborn babies immediately after birth. What was unheard of fifty years ago is common practice now, and well supported by research.

In 1956, babies were routinely introduced to solids between one and three months of age. But based on medical research and their own successes in keeping up their milk supply by watching for solids readiness the founders of LLL recommended postponing the introduction of solids to about six months. Today, the World Health Organization and many health organizations agree.

The mother of the 1950s was led to believe that she should rear her child according to the advice of "experts." Lynn Weiner, a historian and lecturer with the Department of History at Roosevelt University, believes that La Leche League's empowerment of women as mothers was the start of modern self-help groups and women's renewed control over family health care issues.

The women of the 1950s came to LLL with very basic questions: "How do I know if I have enough milk? How do I know when the baby is hungry? When will my child sleep through the night?" Women today still come to LLL in search of answers, encouragement, and the mother-to-mother support that we have become known for. And now research finds not only that this kind of support increases breastfeeding success but also that mothers sharing with others is a fundamentally female approach to problem-solving.

LLL has been contacted by mothers, fathers, doctors, nurses, lactation consultants, and other professionals throughout the world for its expertise on breastfeeding. LLL serves as a Non-Governmental Organization Consultant to the United Nations Children's Fund (UNICEF), the United Nations (UN), and the World Health Organization (WHO); acts as a registered Private Voluntary Organization for the U.S. Agency for International Development (USAID); is a member of the U.S. National Breastfeeding Coalition; is a member of the Child Survival Collaborations and Resources Group (CORE); and is a founding member and Core Partner of the World Alliance for Breastfeeding Action (WABA), a global network of organizations and individuals that is dedicated to protecting, promoting, and supporting breastfeeding. From its small beginning, LLL has matured into an experienced, well-seasoned, vital women's group that has helped change our world.

How La Leche League Can Help You

Today's La Leche League is a non-profit, non-sectarian organization with over three thousand Groups in sixty-eight countries around the world. Accredited Leaders are available to help mothers in person, through e-mail, and on the phone. LLL has helped millions of mothers breastfeed their babies, all through one mother helping a mother and that mother helping another.

La Leche League Meetings

La Leche League meetings are the heart of the organization. They are free, informal discussion groups, held in the homes of members or at easily accessible public locations, that cover the practical, physical, and psychological aspects of breastfeeding. An even less structured type of meeting is now also held in cafés and restaurants on a drop-in basis, where moms can share ideas and help, with Leaders on hand as a resource. LLL gatherings are a wonderful place for information and encouragement, and a ready source of new friendships among mothers who automatically have a lot in common. Your questions on any topic are welcome; they never need to wait! There are usually several mothers who can offer insights or suggestions from their own experience—or at least who have the same questions, which is reassuring, too.

Because breastfeeding is a relationship, it's bound to have its ups and downs. La Leche League gives you a safe place to complain, as well as to ask or celebrate. This is a place where you'll find understanding. You can come late, leave early, walk a fussy baby, change a diaper, and compare notes with other mothers who quickly come to feel like old friends. If you can attend at least one LLL gathering while you're still pregnant, you'll be much better prepared for breastfeeding because seeing other mothers breastfeed in person makes your own breastfeeding easier. Just seeing the face of the woman who'll be on the other end of the phone if you call can help! It's both fun and reassuring to watch the other babies thrive and grow month by month—a preview of your own baby's behavior a few weeks or months from now. You'll see how unique each baby is, and see the varied, comfortable ways in which different breastfeeding mothers and babies relate to each other. Naturally, babies and toddlers are always welcome at La Leche League.

Publications

LLL is one of the world's largest resources for breastfeeding information. We publish books, pamphlets, and informational sheets on topics such as breastfeeding, parenting, and nutrition; many are available in multiple languages. *The Womanly Art of Breastfeeding,* first published from a kitchen table in 1958, is in its eighth edition and has sold more than three million copies.

The website, llli.org, offers opportunities to learn more, as well as breastfeeding books and products. You can shop, read articles and LLL publications, browse the "Frequently Asked Questions (FAQ)" section, submit a breastfeeding question through an online help form, or talk to other mothers on the online forums. You can also find information in several languages, and find LLL contacts throughout the world.

Conferences

LLL conferences are held all over the world for parents and professionals. Speakers include doctors, nurses, lactation professionals, educators, researchers, authors, and parents who are experts in breastfeeding, parenting, childbirth, nutrition, child care, and related topics. And because the conferences always make a point of being completely family-friendly, they're not only horizon-expanding, they're always great fun.

Professional Support

LLL has a Professional Advisory Board with a Health Advisory Council, composed of doctors and health professionals from all over the world, that it consults about medical situations, about evaluation of new research, and for review of most LLL publications that include medical information. Complementing the Health Advisory Council are doctors throughout the world serving as LLL Medical Associates. A Legal Advisory Council and a Management Advisory Council complete the LLL Professional Advisory Board.

How to Find La Leche League

With more than three thousand LLL Groups meeting around the world, you probably have a Group nearby. The easiest way to find a Group in your area is to go to the LLLI website at llli.org/webindex.html. The webpage has listings for every country with a La Leche League presence, leading you to Groups in your area.

How You Can Help La Leche League

As a mother who has been helped by LLL, you pass along that gift each time you share birthing, breastfeeding, and mothering information and support with another woman. In turn, that woman will help another. This never-ending ripple continues in your community, improving it in ways that extend far beyond breastfeeding. LLL provides an infrastructure for reaching and improving the lives of women, babies, and families in the far reaches of our planet. Here are a few ways you can extend your help to other mothers by helping LLL in our important work.

Become a Member

Your annual membership helps LLL provide information and support to nursing mothers everywhere through:

- Publication and translations of our print, video, and online media providing scientific and mothering information to the global community
- Education of Leaders and Peer Counselors, particularly in under-privileged areas

- Information and resources for health care professionals
- A supportive, global presence for breastfeeding through work with private voluntary organizations and regional and international agencies and organizations
- Statistics, facts, and interview contacts for media around the world

Become a Donor

Your donation to LLL furthers our work in all the ways listed above. It can take many forms:

- Unrestricted and restricted gifts to LLL
- Corporate matching gifts, often available through your employer
- Recurring gifts—maximizing your donation to LLL through regular, monthly, or quarterly donations
- Planned gifts through your estate
- Gifts in memory of or in honor of a group or individual
- Donation of stocks and bonds
- The Combined Federal Campaign, in which U.S. government workers and military personnel around the world give to the organization of their choice via payroll deductions
- Participation in affinity programs

For more information, see "Creative Ways to Give" at llli.org/donate .html.

Become a Leader

By assisting mothers with the mechanics of breastfeeding and answering the many questions specific to breastfed babies, La Leche League Leaders help babies stay healthy and help mothers develop a relationship with their children that lasts a lifetime.

As a breastfeeding mother, you may notice that other mothers already value your breastfeeding expertise and ask you questions. If this is something you enjoy, consider becoming an LLL Leader. If you're already involved with an LLL Group, ask the Group Leaders for information about becoming a Leader. If there is no LLL Group in your area, visit our webpage at llli.org/LAD/TaLLL/TaLLL.html, e-mail us through our website at llli.org/contact/contact_us, or write to us at La Leche League International, c/o Leader Accreditation Department, PO Box 4079, Schaumburg, IL 60168-4079. LLL needs mothers like you who have enjoyed breastfeeding their children and who want to continue the ripples of breastfeeding support.

A Final Word from the Founders

In closing, we wish to acknowledge and express heartfelt thanks to those who have made important contributions to the development of La Leche League. First we would like to recognize two physicians, Dr. Herbert Ratner and Dr. Gregory White. As fathers of breastfed children and supporters of natural childbirth, these two doctors were a rarity in 1956. Without their unfailing support and guidance, it is almost certain that we who began LLL would have found it extremely difficult to face the criticism and sometimes hostility of the medical community toward two basic womanly functions—natural childbirth and breastfeeding. Our own enthusiasm for and appreciation of these two functions survived because of the solid backing of those two physicians. We are eternally grateful to them, and we thank them also on behalf of the breastfeeding mothers to whom we have passed on what we learned. Over time, many other courageous physicians, including Drs. E. Robbins Kimball, Robert Mendelsohn, Lawrence Gartner, and many others, have also openly supported our efforts and generously shared their knowledge with us, and we are grateful for their help. We also wish to recognize and gratefully acknowledge our volunteer LLL Leaders. It is the daily efforts of these thousands of generous volunteers that have built LLL. Without their continuing efforts over the years, we would not be the organization we are today.

TWENTY

Tear-Sheet Toolkit

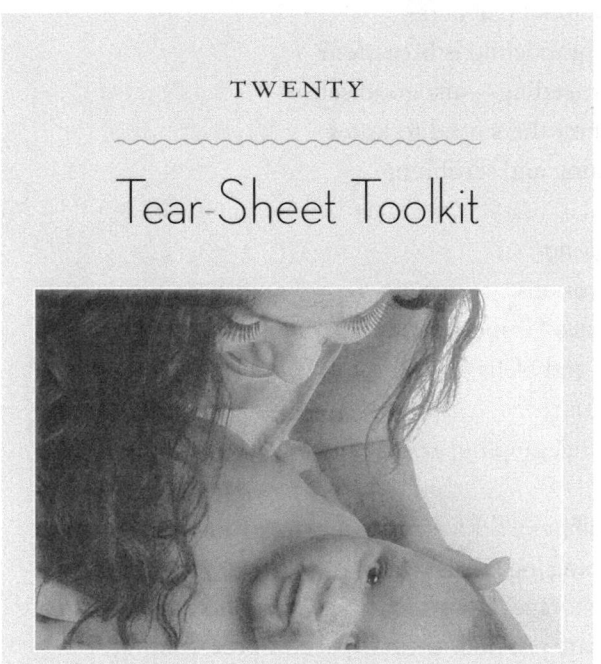

SOMETIMES YOU DON'T want a whole book. And sometimes you want to be able to tear something *from* a book! Here's your chance. Each page in this section is complete on its own two sides, ready to be removed. You can put these sheets on your refrigerator or by your computer, or hand them to your family or day care provider—whatever you need. Online copies are available at llli.org.

Early Breastfeeding

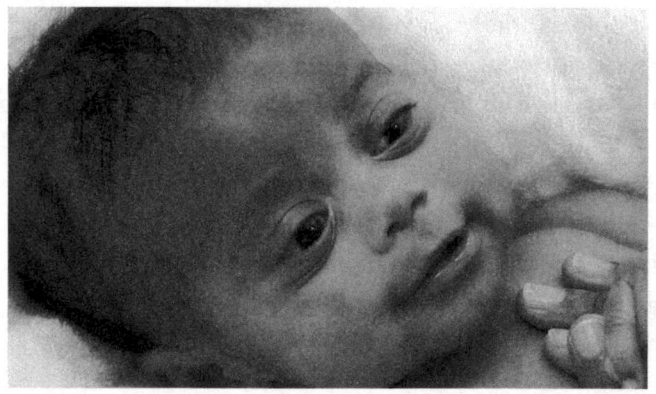

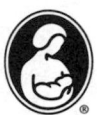

Laid-back Breastfeeding

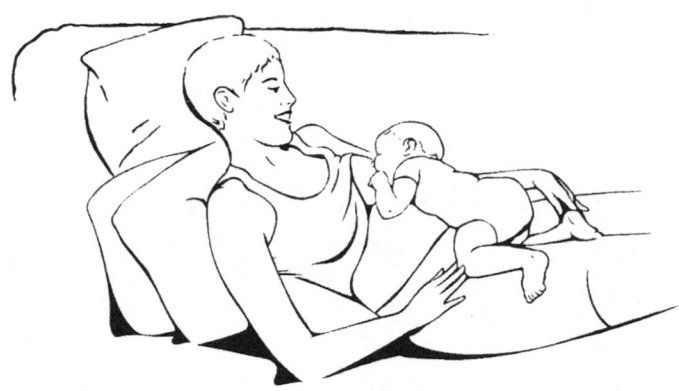

LAID-BACK BREASTFEEDING, or Biological Nurturing, means getting comfortable with your baby and encouraging your own and your baby's natural breastfeeding instincts. See biologicalnurturing.com for further information.

- Dress yourself and your baby as you choose.
- Find a bed or couch where you can lean back and be well supported—not flat, but comfortably leaning back so that when you put your baby on your chest, gravity will keep him in position with his body molded to yours.
- Have your head and shoulders well supported. Let your baby's whole front touch your whole front.
- Since you're leaning back, you don't have a lap, so your baby can rest on you in any position you like. Just make sure her whole front is against you.
- Let your baby's cheek rest somewhere near your bare breast.
- Help her as much as you like; help her do what she's trying to do. You're a team.
- Hold your breast or not, as you like.
- Relax and enjoy each other.

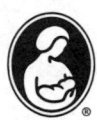

Early Days Diaper Log: The Bottom Line

(If it comes out, it must have gone in!)

COUNT ONLY POOPY diapers that have contents at least as big as the "okay" circle you make with thumb and forefinger. No need to count wet diapers. Poopy diapers tell more about how a baby is doing.

Circle the X when your baby has an "okay" poopy diaper.

If your baby is...	Expect *at least* this many "okay" diapers	
0–1 day old (first 24 hours)		
Black sticky poopy diaper	X	1
1–2 days old (second 24 hours)		
Brown sticky poopy diapers	X X	2
2–3 days old (third 24 hours)		
Greenish poopy diapers	X X X	3
3–4 days old (fourth 24 hours)		
Green to yellow poopy diapers	X X X	3
4–5 days old (fifth 24 hours)		
Yellow poopy diapers	X X X	3

My breastfeeding helpers:

Baby's health care provider _____

My health care provider _____

Local La Leche League Leader _____

International Board Certified Lactation Consultant _____

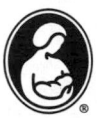

Waking a Sleepy Newborn

If your newborn sleeps longer than three hours at a stretch, but

- You had no birth medications
- Your baby stays in physical contact with you
- He feeds well when he feeds
- His diapers are on track (see the Early Days Diaper Log)

that's probably just who he is. Keep an eye on his poopy diapers and his weight.

If he's not gaining well and he sleeps more than three hours at a stretch, aim for at least ten nursings each day until he wakes on his own and has at least four good poopy diapers each day.

It will be easier to wake him to feed if you see some of the feeding cues listed on the next tear sheet. If he's sleeping and you try to lift his arm and it drops like a rock when you let it go, he'll be hard to wake. Try again in twenty minutes. Things to try:

- Dim the lights, pull the drapes. It's easier if he doesn't have to squint.
- Undress him partially or completely. Put him on your chest.
- Stroke him and call his name. Rub his feet.
- Lay him down and roll him gently from all the way on one side to all the way on his other side.
- Hold him along your forearms, head in your hands, feet at your elbows, and lift him from nearly horizontal to nearly vertical and back, as you talk to him.
- Wipe his face with a damp cloth.
- Put a little colostrum or milk in his mouth—just a bit, waiting for him to swallow before adding more.

He might latch and nurse in his sleep in a laid-back breastfeeding position, or he might take sips from a spoon. Feed him in whatever way works for you.

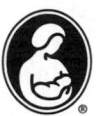

Feeding Cues

- A baby starts with subtle nursing cues—eyes moving beneath eyelids, eyelids fluttering before they even open, hands coming toward face, mouth movements.

- Then she adds more obvious ones—rooting toward your chest, whimpering or squeaking.

- If you offer to nurse now, she'll probably take your breast gently and easily.

- As her hunger builds, her body and mouth tense. She breathes fast or starts to cry.

- Once she's crying, she'll have a harder time latching. Crying is a *late* sign of hunger. Calm her down before trying to feed her.

- Breastfeeding is easier if you answer her requests instead of waiting for her demands.

- Don't wait for your breasts to feel full. A full breast has already started to slow down production.

- Offer even if she's not asking, anytime you like.

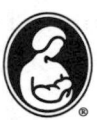

Feeding the Non-Latching Baby:
One Possible Approach

Birth to 6 hours—skin contact
- Keep the baby skin-to-skin and gently encourage him to breastfeed.
- If birth was medicated—hand-express colostrum by end of first two hours.

By about 6 hours—begin regular hand expression
- Continue keeping the baby in skin-to-skin contact with you.
- Express drops of milk on your nipple to encourage him to latch on.
- Hand express colostrum into a spoon, spoon-feed baby every 2–3 hours and when either of you wakes at night.
- Removing milk from your breasts is as important as feeding the baby.

As milk volume increases—hand-express or pump, use nipple shield, finger-feed or bottle
- Continue as much skin-to-skin contact, laid-back, and holding as possible.
- Pump at least 8–10 times in 24 hours (including at least once at night) finishing with hand expression. Massage before and/or during pumping, hand express afterward.
- Consider a nipple shield to help the baby latch.
- With increased milk volume, finger-feeding or a bottle may work.

By the end of the first week—help, patience, confidence
- Continue skin-to-skin/holding as much as possible.
- Express at least 8–10 times per 24 hours, tapering off as baby begins to nurse.

- You may want to express extra and store in the fridge to be a feeding or two ahead. Adding a couple of extra pumping sessions for a day or two will help.
- Stay in touch with your Leader or other breastfeeding support.

Babies sometimes take weeks to breastfeed well. Keep your supply going. If we can teach a tiger to jump through a flaming hoop, we can help a baby do what he is designed to do!

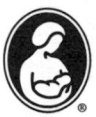

Hand Expression

- Wake your breasts up—shake, massage, move them
- Fingers on opposite sides of your areola
- Press back toward chest
- Compress fingers toward each other, drawing slightly toward nipple but not sliding skin
- Release pressure, relax hand

Repeat several times. Don't expect anything immediately. Add massage whenever you like. Shift hand to a different position to move milk from other ducts.

Colostrum: collect drops on plastic spoon, tip into baby's mouth or collect with dropper.

Milk: Express into pump funnel or large bowl.

See video at newborns.stanford.edu/Breastfeeding/HandExpression .html.

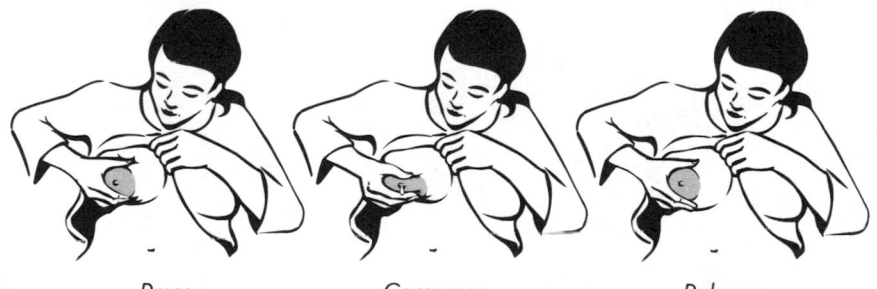

Press.   Compress.   Release.

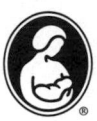

Our Baby Is Here!

———————————————————————

was born on

———————————————————————

weighing

———————————————————————

Please knock *quietly. If we don't answer the door,*
we hope you'll understand.
We're getting to know our baby, and we may be pretty busy right now.

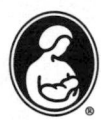

We'd Love Your Help!

Life is very busy for us right now, and it would mean a lot if you could choose one item from this list to help us with:

Groceries: _____

_____

_____

_____

Meals: _____

_____

_____

_____

Errands: _____

_____

_____

_____

Chores: _____

_____

_____

_____

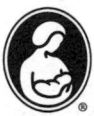

Fussy Baby Ideas

Contact, carry, walk, and talk are age-old baby soothers. Here are some variations on those from mothers who've been there:

- Magic Baby Hold
- Low lights and soothing motions, if the baby isn't totally wound up.
- A shared bath with low lights (best if you have someone there who can console the baby while you get the bath ready). For a baby who isn't in total distress.
- A little jounce rather than swaying. Put a little bump in your walk.
- Dancing together vigorously, especially once you find his favorite music.
- Running water, radio static, or a vacuum or washer as white noise.
- Change of scenery—a different room, a different angle, outdoors.
- Shopping! A car ride and other people/sights may break the spell.
- Bouncing on an exercise ball or birthing ball while you hold her.
- A walk outdoors, if weather permits, with your baby in a sling. Often soothes the baby and you get some exercise! The baby can even nurse discreetly in the sling while you walk.
- Nursing the baby *again*. Hunger isn't always the initial problem, but nursing almost always ends up being the solution; nursing is soothing to your baby.

What works for you?

_____

_____

_____

_____

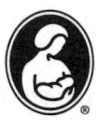

What About Partners?

The mother breastfeeds, and the baby doesn't need you to feed him.
So what can you do?
Anything else!

You are The Safe Person Who Is Not Mama. Nursing and Mama are the center of your baby's world right now, but his world keeps getting bigger, and you are the first person he adds.

You are Different. Your shape, voice, hands, and smell are different. You hold your baby differently. You teach him that different can be good. When your baby is frazzled, you may be just the difference that he needs.

Some things you can do:

- Wear your baby in a sling or other carrier and go for a walk.
- Go out and about; babies are social people.
- Read to your baby—he'll love hearing your voice.
- Change his diaper—even if he hates diaper changes now, he'll love them very soon.
- Take a nap with him on your chest.
- Talk to him about things around the house.
- Take a bath together.
- Take him to his mother whenever he needs her.
- Sleep with him safely (see Chapter 12).
- Use the Magic Baby Hold: with your baby's back against your front, bring your left arm over his left shoulder (one arm on either side of yours), and hold his right thigh.
- Jiggle and sway. Babies tend to like side-to-side motion.

Your first job is to *support* breastfeeding, not *compete* with it. A "relief bottle" may seem helpful, but it's more likely to cause breastfeeding problems and health risks for your baby. Instead:

- Protect your partner from criticism.
- Keep her fed.
- Help her get good help if she needs it (llli.org and ilca.org are good places to start).
- Care for her so that she can care for your child.

Your two separate roles work together to form a strong, secure safety net for the World's Best Baby.

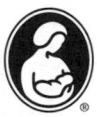

Your Grandchild Is Breastfed?

Here's what's new about breastfeeding a baby:

New research has shown that breastfeeding is important for the baby's health and development and for the mother's health, both now and in the future. It's even good for the environment.

Research has found that breastfeeding works best when the baby is fed in response to hunger cues, not on a schedule. That's usually quite frequently, especially in the beginning. Fortunately, you can't feed too often.

Sore nipples aren't an expected part of breastfeeding; they are a sign that something isn't quite right. With some expert help, the mother should soon be breastfeeding comfortably.

Most medical experts, including the American Academy of Pediatrics and the World Health Organization, recommend that babies be breastfed exclusively—no formula or solid foods—for six months or so, and continue breastfeeding with solid foods added to their diet into these toddler years—even two years or more.

Much of this may be different from what you learned when you had your own babies.

But guess what hasn't changed?

New mothers still need lots of help, lots of support, and lots of loving family members around to prepare meals or throw in a load of laundry. They need people to be patient with them as they figure out both breastfeeding and motherhood. And babies still need their grandparents to love them. Your practical help and support are a golden investment in your grandchild's future, and in your lives together.

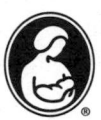

Breastfeeding: It's Just Good Sense

You knew breastfeeding was better. That's why you started. Here's why it's worth getting problems solved.

Breastfeeding
Is a relationship
Is immediate, simple, nearly free
Provides a normal start in life
Promotes normal jaw development
Is the normal follow-up to birth for the mother
Provides mothering hormones
Lets the baby control his own appetite
Saves money for the family

Human Milk
Has many hundreds of known and unknown ingredients, including interferon and white blood cells, antibacterial and antiviral agents, intestinal soothers, growth hormones, and everything else a baby is known to need
Changes to meet the baby's changing needs
Is non-allergenic
Is the human infant's only normal food
Promotes normal brain development

Is always clean
Promotes normal health in infancy and beyond
Smells fine going in and coming out
Is the normal start for the World's Best Baby

Formula-feeding
Is a feeding method
Needs equipment, preparation, money, extra medical care
Is artificial and has risks
Increases need for orthodontia
Is linked to certain women's cancers
Provides no mothering hormones
Can lead to overfeeding and obesity
Makes money for industry

Formula
has far, far fewer ingredients, but includes tropical oils, no anti-infectives, intestinal irritants, poorly absorbed nutrients, known and unknown microdeficiencies

Changes only with manufacturing and preparation errors, which are common

Contanis either of two common allergens—cow milk or soybeans

Isn't what babies are built to handle

Is linked to lower IQ scores

Is easily and frequently contaminated

Is linked to increases in many illnesses and diseases, including SIDS, pneumonia, breast cancer, vision deficits, obesity, diabetes

Smells pretty bad

Is vastly inferior to your milk

If you're not enjoying breastfeeding, get help!
This is too important to both of you to risk losing it.

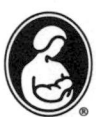

What Mothers Need to Know Before They're Mothers

Words of Wisdom from Real Mothers at a La Leche League Meeting

Newborns don't look like magazine babies.

There are no right answers.

People say things, but they aren't always trying to be judgmental when they say them.

A dirty house builds extra immunities.

Sometimes motherhood stinks.

Should is a poison word that argues against reality.

It's important to see other babies so you know what's really normal.

Sometimes the books are just wrong.

Listen to yourself.

Listen to your baby. Respect him and his intuition. He will tell you what he needs.

Find someone who will listen to you.

You will never achieve an ideal state of motherhood.

Wait long enough and it will change, and the questions and answers will be different.

Pick your battles.

A dog is an excellent floor cleaner.

Respond to questions with "Why do you ask?"

Receiving blankets have all kinds of uses—a surface for public diaper changes, an extra wrap in a car seat, catching spit-up.

Hold off buying things until you know whether you're ever going to use them—like a crib or changing table. Don't get caught up in the consumerism of new parenthood.

The ideal adult-to-baby ratio is about three to one the first week. But if all you have is one mother and one baby, you'll manage.

When people offer help, say yes.

Join a playgroup. It's not for the child, it's for the mother.

After a week or so, get out of the house. The crying doesn't bother other people as much as you think it does, and even the grocery store can seem like a wonderful adventure.

Step outside when you can, throw your shoulders back, take a deep breath, and look up for at least a few seconds.

Don't be surprised at how totally bizarre you feel the first week. It's normal to feel really weird.

You can only do what you can do.

Let go of your expectations and let what is be.

Just because it's fun doesn't mean it's not important.

Babies Don't Keep

The cleaning and scrubbing
Can wait 'til tomorrow,
For babies grow up,
I've learned to my sorrow.

So quiet down, cobwebs.
Dust, go to sleep.
I'm nursing my baby,
And babies don't keep.

Adapted from "Song for a Fifth Child," by Ruth Hulbert Hamilton

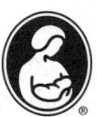

Medications and Breastfeeding

Do you need to wean to take a medication? *Almost certainly not!* The drug is rarely as risky as formula would be. A single bottle of formula increases the risk of many childhood and adult illnesses and diseases, and disrupts the baby's intestines for up to a month. *"Playing it safe" almost always means continued breastfeeding, not weaning.* Here are some of the reasons:

- *Even if a mother's blood level for a given drug is high, it's still very dilute* for her breastfeeding baby to swallow in her milk, digest, and put into *his* bloodstream.
- *Age matters.* Some drugs that might be a concern for premature infants are not a concern for full-term babies. The older the baby, the less the concern. Some mothers are mistakenly told to wean for a drug that may be given directly to babies or small children.
- *When in doubt,* check the baby's blood or just watch for changes like diarrhea or fussiness.
- *Temporary weaning*—and pumping, and bottle-feeding an unhappy baby—*is a huge physical and emotional stress* during an already stressful time.
- *Breastfeeding is not a faucet.* Turning it off abruptly can mean turning it off permanently. Talk about risks!
- *Further risk reduction*: Nursing before taking the dose, waiting five "half-lives," finding a safer drug or treatment, even nursing part-time—all far better choices than even temporary weaning.
- *Drug companies tend to recommend weaning to avoid litigation. The actual research rarely supports weaning.*

For more information, check Thomas Hale's book *Medications and Mothers' Milk* or:

- LactMed, the U.S. National Institutes of Health's *Drugs and Lactation Database* (toxnet.nlm.nih.gov/cgi-bin/sis/htmlgen?LACT)
- Dr. Hale's website (neonatal.ttuhsc.edu/lact)
- The UK National Health Service *Quick Reference Guide for Drugs in Breast Milk* (ukmicentral.nhs.uk/drugpreg/qrg_p1.htm)

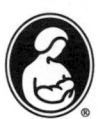

A Few Online Breastfeeding Resources for Mothers

La Leche League International	llli.org
Adoptive breastfeeding resource	fourfriends.com/abrw
American Academy of Pediatrics Breastfeeding Policy Statement	aappolicy.aappublications.org/cgi/content/full/pediatrics;115/2/496
Breastfeeding after breast and nipple surgery	bfar.org
Breastfeeding—general information	kellymom.com
Common Sense breastfeeding (Diane Wiessinger)	normalfed.com
Depression in new mothers	granitescientfic.com
ILCA (International Lactation Consultant Association)	ilca.org
Jack Newman, MD, co-author of *The Ultimate Breastfeeding Book of Answers*	drjacknewman.com
Low milk supply issues	lowmilksupply.org
Oral issues (tongue-tie, dental caries, etc.)	brianpalmerdds.com
Plus-size nursing bra and clothing resources	vireday.com/plus/PlusMat_Nursing.html
Research-based hospital protocols—Academy of Breastfeeding Medicine	bfmed.org
Sleeping safely—and together (Notre Dame Mother-Baby Behavioral Sleep Lab)	nd.edu/~jmckenn1/lab
Thomas Hale (*Medications and Mothers' Milk*)	neonatal.ttuhsc.edu/lact
The United States Breastfeeding Committee	usbreastfeeding.org

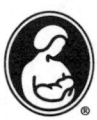

Dealing with Plugs and Blebs

Nursing ideas

- Nurse as often as possible, keeping the affected breast as soft as possible.
- Lay your baby on his back on a folded blanket, head off the edge, face toward the ceiling. Lean over him on elbows and knees, and nurse with breast dangling.

Manual ideas

- Use hand expression and gentle nipple manipulation to work the bleb out.
- After showering or soaking, gently rub surface of nipple to release the bleb.
- Using sterilized needle, gently lift and open skin over bleb; use sterile tweezers if needed. Apply topical antibiotic several times a day, for several days.
- Apply pressure behind the nipple, along with gentle massage and manipulation.

Soaking ideas

- Olive oil on a cotton ball over your nipple inside a bra.
- Vinegar on a breast pad.
- Epsom salts (2 teaspoons in a cup of warm water) four times per day.

Breast ideas

- Stop wearing a bra, or stop wearing an underwire.
- See physiotherapist for ultrasound treatment of the breast.
- Use personal massager, electric razor, electric toothbrush, or lean against washer on spin cycle.
- Lay cabbage leaves over any area of engorgement.

Diet ideas
- Increase fluids.
- Take two tablespoons of lecithin daily (available at health, drug, and vitamin stores).
- Avoid some or all dairy products, sugar, peanuts, chocolate, fats (especially saturated fats), caffeine, antiperspirants, and decaffeinated products.
- Increase immune system boosters like vitamins D and C.

Other ideas
- Ask your doctor about taking an anti-inflammatory medicine.
- Stress? Anemia? Herpes simplex.
- Call an LLL Leader or breastfeeding helper. Why go it alone?

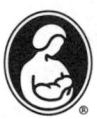

Mastitis, and What You Can Do if You Get It

Mastitis means an inflammation in your breast. It's sometimes due to an infection, but may not be. Signs include:

- A warm or hot, sensitive (sometimes painful) area on one breast (rarely both) that may look red or have reddish streaks
- Sometimes fever and/or chills and/or generalized aching, as though you have the flu.

How did you get it? Often nobody knows. Maybe cracked or damaged nipples that let germs in, plugged ducts, ineffective or infrequent nursing (or pumping), pressure from a bra or baby carrier, being overtired and run-down ("holiday mastitis").

What can you do? You may want to talk to your doctor about a prescription for antibiotics. It may not be an infection, so you could try other treatments first.

- Empty Breast, Lots of Rest. That means (a) frequently nursing, pumping, or hand-expressing to keep the milk moving and (b) spending as much time as possible in bed or lying down, resting or sleeping.
- Cold packs (such as frozen peas wrapped in a cloth) or other sources of cold on the inflamed area, twenty minutes on, twenty minutes off, or a heating pad, whichever feels better.
- Over-the-counter anti-inflammatory medication that your doctor approves.

No worse after 24 hours? You can repeat for another 24. No better? Think about antibiotics.

For more suggestions, see the Academy of Breastfeeding Medicine's mastitis protocol at bfmed.org/Resources/Protocols.aspx.

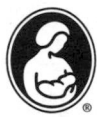

Gaining, Gulping, Grimacing?

Is your baby thriving . . . but nursing is a struggle? Do these sound familiar?

1. My baby chokes and gulps and splutters when she nurses.
2. My breasts always feel full, and/or they spray when my milk releases.
3. My baby "wrestles" with my breast, pulling off, crying, tugging, arching.
4. My baby has *lots* of wet and poopy diapers.
5. My baby is colicky, or gassy, or spits up frequently.
6. My baby sometimes—or always—has frothy or greenish stools. Some diapers may have a little blood.
7. My baby is gaining rapidly, or grew fast at first with weight gain dropping as fussiness increased.
8. My baby rarely falls asleep at my breast; nursing is an athletic event.
9. My baby will nurse only for food, not for comfort.
10. My baby grimaces when she nurses.
11. My baby often seems to have uncomfortable intestines.
12. I try to make a point of nursing on both breasts each time.
13. If it's been less than two hours, I look for some cause for fussiness other than hunger.

Those can mean a baby who's getting "too much soup, not enough cheesecake." The milk that builds up in our breasts between feedings tends to be a lower-fat milk, changing gradually from "soup" to "cheesecake" through the feeding. If we have too much milk, she may not get through all the soup at one sitting. If we switch breasts partway through the nursing "to make sure she takes the other side," or if we try to space our nursings to two hours or more, that can mean the baby plows through a whole lot of soup and never gets much cheesecake. She grows fine. But without the extra fat, milk travels fast through her intestines, doesn't break down fully, and can ferment in her large intestine, causing gas, discomfort, and frothy green stools.

And then there's the fire hose effect. All that milk can squirt into your baby's mouth, making her feel she must swallow or drown. Not much fun. You may find your baby is happier and more settled if you let her "get to the bottom of the barrel," where the cheesecake is, by doing two things:

- Offer to nurse whenever she shows interest, even after just a few minutes. Shorter intervals mean the higher fat milk is still there.
- If she's happy on one side, leave her there. If that side isn't nice and soft afterward, use it again next time. Using one side for a couple hours may be all it takes. Some need to spend four to six hours on one side before using the other. Use your instinct more than the clock. The over fullness on the other side cuts back production, which is what you want. If you're *too* overfull, nurse or express just enough for comfort, then go back to the side you're trying to soften.

These sound like rules, but they're just temporary reminders to help you get past two ideas that may have started the problem—making a point of switching sides, and delaying feedings.

As your supply settles down, you may worry that you've "lost your milk." No more heavy, leaking breasts or choking. If your baby is still getting lots of wet and poopy diapers, and looks relaxed and comfortable during and after nursing, these are signs of good milk supply. If she wants to increase it, all she has to do is nurse more often, or start taking both sides sometimes. Trust her, and trust your body.

You should begin to see a happier baby and easier feedings within a few days. If not, check with an LLL Leader or visit llli.org for more ideas.

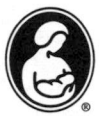

Pumping Chart

Circle Each Hour in Which You've Pumped

Double-pump about 15 minutes at first; adjust as you learn your breasts.

Pump at least once a night.

If you have a non-nursing baby, 10 expressions per day is excellent. Many mothers aim for 8. Try not to fall below 8 in the early weeks. After the first two weeks, 6 is a bare minimum.

For best volume, be sure to follow each pumping session with some hand expression!

Date   **Goal**   **Total**

____ Midnight 1 2 3 4 5 6 7 8 9 10 11 Noon 1 2 3 4 5 6 7 8 9 10 11 ____ ____

____ Midnight 1 2 3 4 5 6 7 8 9 10 11 Noon 1 2 3 4 5 6 7 8 9 10 11 ____ ____

____ Midnight 1 2 3 4 5 6 7 8 9 10 11 Noon 1 2 3 4 5 6 7 8 9 10 11 ____ ____

____ Midnight 1 2 3 4 5 6 7 8 9 10 11 Noon 1 2 3 4 5 6 7 8 9 10 11 ____ ____

____ Midnight 1 2 3 4 5 6 7 8 9 10 11 Noon 1 2 3 4 5 6 7 8 9 10 11 ____ ____

____ Midnight 1 2 3 4 5 6 7 8 9 10 11 Noon 1 2 3 4 5 6 7 8 9 10 11 ____ ____

____ Midnight 1 2 3 4 5 6 7 8 9 10 11 Noon 1 2 3 4 5 6 7 8 9 10 11 ____ ____

____ Midnight 1 2 3 4 5 6 7 8 9 10 11 Noon 1 2 3 4 5 6 7 8 9 10 11 ____ ____

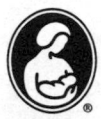

Storing Milk for Your Healthy Full-Term Infant

Where	Temperature	Time	Comments
Room temperature	66° to 78°F (19° to 26°C)	4–8 hours	Containers should be covered and kept as cool as possible; covering the container with a damp towel may keep milk cooler.
Insulated cooler bag	5° to 39°F (-15° to 4°C)	24 hours	Keep ice packs in constant contact with milk containers; limit opening cooler bag.
Refrigerator	39°F (4°C)	3–8 days	Collect in a very clean way to minimize spoilage. Store milk in the back of the main body of the refrigerator.
Freezer compartment of refrigerator	5°F (-15°C)	2 weeks	Store milk away from sides and toward the back of the freezer, where temperature is most constant. Milk stored for longer than these ranges is usually safe, but some of the fats in the milk break down over time.
Freezer compartment of refrigerator with separate doors	0°F (-18°C)	3–6 months	
Deep freezer	-4°F (-20°C)	6–12 months	

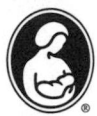

Bottle-Feeding a Breastfed Baby: Ideas for Day Care and Others

- Human milk is safe and sturdy. Don't feel you need to take special precautions with it.
- Feed the baby when he shows hunger cues, not on a schedule.
- Hold the baby snugly. Keep him fairly upright to give him control.
- Hold bottle almost vertically against his lips at the start, as you would hold your finger to say "Shh." When he reaches with his lips, tip the bottle horizontally into his opening mouth. Let him draw it in himself, so his lips close on the fat part of the bottle nipple, *not* just the skinny part.
- Keep him fairly upright, so that the bottle is nearly horizontal when it's in his mouth. The milk won't pour into him automatically, and he'll have much more control. You may hear him sucking some air, but it will just come out his nose.
- If he gets tense or gulps, tilt baby and bottle slightly forward so the milk drains away. He will soon learn to pause on his own.
- Let him pause and take breaks when he wants to.
- When you think he is *nearly* full, twist and remove the bottle. Immediately offer the bottle again to see if he wants more. If he takes it, offer another ten sucks or so, remove, and offer again. Finally he'll just keep his lips closed. This reduces the risk of overfeeding. If he routinely doesn't finish the bottle, put less in it.
- If there's milk left over, don't throw it out! It will keep just fine in the refrigerator until the next feeding.
- If his mother is coming soon, try to distract him, or give him just a small amount. She'll be ready to nurse, and she'll want him to be ready, too.

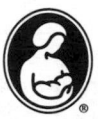

Safe Handling and Storage of Your Milk

Expressing your milk

- Wash your hands before expressing or handling your milk.
- Any clean container works. To avoid known toxins, use glass or look for the number 5 recycling symbol and/or the letters PP on the bottom of the container.
- Put date and name on the bag or bottle *before filling*.

Storing your milk

- Refrigerate or chill your milk right after expressing if it won't be used in the next few hours.
- If milk separates, swirl (don't shake) to redistribute cream before feeding.
- Combine several pumpings in one container by adding cold to cold.
- Milk expands as it freezes, so leave space at the top if you plan to freeze.
- Fill each container with only 2 ounces (60 ml) to minimize waste.
- Unneeded milk can be frozen for use later as needed.
- Store in the back of the freezer away from sides, where temperature is most steady.
- If storing milk in bags, double-bag them or store in sealed container to avoid freezer burn.
- Horizontal bags may save space.
- Use the oldest frozen milk first to keep it from getting too old.

Thawing your milk

- Thaw frozen milk in refrigerator or a bowl of warm water or under warm faucet.
- Don't heat the milk directly on the stove, don't use a microwave.
- Some babies are happy to drink cold milk.
- Thawed can be refrigerated for up to twenty-four hours. Then use, refreeze, or discard.

Acknowledgments

We three writers thank La Leche League International for inviting us to write this new edition of the book that inspired all of us in our early years of mothering. The La Leche League founders, who are the original authors of the book, provided invaluable insights, and we thank them for their careful reading. Barbara Emanuel and LaJuana Oswalt, LLLI Executive management team, have been there every step of the way, coordinating the work we did, along with that of reviewers, researchers, photographers, illustrators, agents, and publishers.

We thank Marnie Cochran, our wonderfully supportive editor at Ballantine Books, whose vision for the book and passion for breastfeeding were inspiring to us. We are grateful for the encouragement, support, and tireless efforts of our agent, Maura Kye-Casella of Don Congdon Associates. We also thank La Leche League International's agent, Stephanie Kip Rostan of Levine|Greenberg Literary Agency, who shepherded the project so adroitly. We thank the LLLI Research Team, coordinated by Marcia Lutostanski: Karen Butler, Helen Butler, Pat Martens, Maria Grant, Cindy Harmon-Jones, Cathy Liles, and Jeanne Mitchell, and LLLI co-chairs Rosemary Gordon and Shirley Phillips for their input and guidance on this important project, Loretta McCallister, and Ron Larracas for project support.

We also thank the lactation experts who contributed their knowledge and insights: Jan Barger, Barbara Behrmann, Diana Cassar-Uhl, Cheryl Chapman, Suzanne Colson, Jean Cotterman, Diane DiSandro, Larry Gartner, Catherine Watson Genna, Rebecca Glover, Kay Hoover, Dee Kassing, Kathy Kendall-Tackett, Katy Lebbing, Lisa Marasco, Jim McKenna, Anne Marie Miller, Nancy Mohrbacher, Jane Morton, Chris Mulford, Jim Murphy, Jack Newman, Nicola O'Byrne,

Amy Peterson, Gill Rapley, Bob Sears, Martha Sears, Tina Smillie, Linda Smith, Betty Sterken, Marsha Walker, and Margaret Wills.

Special thanks for their photographic contributions—David Stark, Neal Rohrer, and Susan Ogden.

Most of all, we thank our tireless brainstorming team and other mothers who became the heart of this book through their wisdom, experiences, and stories, including Jan Barger, Jane Bradshaw, Elisa Brook, Emma Brook, Isabella Brook, Jan Ellen Brown, Kathleen Bruce, Vered Bukai, Cathy Carothers, Diana Cassar-Uhl, Terry Cater-Cyker, Jean Cotterman, Jill Dye, Melissa Ferguson, Chana Fitton, Cathy Genna, Roberta Graham de Escobedo, Cynthia Gration, Lynnette Hafken, Donna Henderson, Kaileigh Hennessey, Sarah Hung, Gloria Jackson, Emily Perl Kingsley, Lynett Koetz, Lisa Rotondi Krempasky, Laura LaRocca, Samantha Leeson, Sherrie Littlefield, Lisa Mandell, Kira Martin, Jeanette McCulloch, Denise Murphy, James Murphy, Nicola O'Byrne, Susan L. Ogden, Nan Perigo, Esmaralda Pitman, Heidi Poliafico, Scott Pryor, Kelly Quinn, Amy Rand, Molly Remer, Bonnie Roberts, Lesley Robinson, Kathleen Salisbury, Jazz Salwen-Grabowski, Enya Santiago, Susan Schade, Lisa Settje, Terriann Shell, Mellanie Sheppard, Newt Sherwin, Linda Smith, Barbara Sturmfels, Lynn Thye, Laura Ulrich, Marianne Vakiener, Kasey Wiessinger, Laura Wiessinger, Margaret Wills, and others who wished to remain anonymous.

This project began over a long weekend in Niagara-on-the-Lake, Ontario, where we first learned how much fun we have working together. But we owe a very special thank-you to La Leche League International co-founder Marian Tompson, who joined us at Diane's cabin in the Adirondack Mountains and set the tone for the book, with dawn wisdoms on the porch and evening memories by the fire. To commemorate the occasion, she signed her name on a hidden place somewhere in the cabin. We'll never tell where!

From Diane Wiessinger: The ripples flow both ways: If my daughters-in-law Laura and Kasey have received anything from me, it's been returned many-fold, in their graceful, intuitive birthing and parenting of my grandchildren, Elizabeth and Max. I couldn't have Laura and Kasey without sons Scott and Eric, who are learning what they taught me: that family is the richest part of life. But this book would have been just plain impossible without the endlessly patient backup of my wonderful husband, John. I love you all! And of course I thank my co-authors: a big thick book and friendship at the finish! I had no idea how life-altering it would be when I set foot in my first La Leche League meeting, four-month-old nursling in arms.

From Diana West: I give my most profound gratitude to my cherished family—my sons, Alex, Ben, and Quinn, and husband, Brad—who are sweetly patient while I work on my books, always supportive of my work to help breast-feeding mothers, and whom I love so very, very much. I also thank La Leche League from the bottom of my heart. You taught me how to mother my children in a way that has created a deep and delightful bond, how to really listen to my friends, and how to discover my own talents and contribute them to the world. I wouldn't be the mother, friend, and professional I am today if you hadn't welcomed me so supportively into the Sisterhood of Mothers when my first baby was born. Finally, I thank my dearest co-authors—two wonderful women and friends with whom it has been a joy and an honor to share the journey of this very special book.

From Teresa Pitman: As always, I am very thankful to my children, Matthew, Lisa, Dan, and Jeremy, who were (and are) the best possible teachers any mother could have. I am equally grateful for the newer additions to my family: my wonderful daughter-in-law, Esmaralda, and my grandchildren Sebastian, Callista, Xavier, and Keagan (who arrived while I was working on this book. Don't worry, I managed to turn off my computer long enough to be present for his beautiful birth at home, like his older siblings). In addition, I have the deepest appreciation for my LLL "family," including my current and past co-Leaders and the many Leaders from around the world who have helped and encouraged me in my work and my life over the years. I count Diana and Diane as part of my family now, too: they are both brilliant, talented, and incredibly hardworking, and have been just amazing to work with.

Selected References

ONE Nesting

5 **there is almost nothing you can do for your child in his whole life that will affect him both emotionally and physically as profoundly as breastfeeding**

Gartner, L.M. et al. 2005. Breastfeeding and the use of human milk; American Academy of Pediatrics Section on Breastfeeding. *Pediatrics* 115(2):496–506.

Ip, S. et al. 2007. Breastfeeding and maternal and infant health outcomes in developed countries. *Evidence Rep Tec Assess (Full Rep.)* 153:1–186.

Kramer, M.S. et al. 2001. Promotion of breastfeeding Intervention Trial (PROBIT): a randomized trial in the Republic of Belarus. *JAMA* 285(4):413–420.

Lönnerdal, B. 2003. Nutritional and physiologic significance of human milk proteins. *Am J Clin Nutr* 77(6):1537S–1543S.

Stuebe, A.M. and E.B. Schwarz. 2010. The risks and benefits of infant feeding practices for women and their children. *J Perinatology* 30(3)155–162.

Turck, D. 2005. Comité de nutrition de la Société française de pédiatrie [Breast feeding: health benefits for child and mother] [Article in French] *Arch Pediatr* 12 Suppl 3:S145–65. (Epub 2005 Nov 21.)

5 **your milk has every vitamin, mineral, and other nutritional element that your baby's body needs**

James, D.C. and R. Lessen. 2009. Position of the American Dietetic Association: promoting and supporting breastfeeding. *J Am Diet Assoc* 109(11):1926–42.

6 **[milk] changes subtly through the meal, day, and year, to match subtle changes in his requirements**

Hale, T.W. and P.E. Hartmann, eds. *Textbook of Human Lactation.* Amarillo, TX: Hale Publishing.

Lawrence, R.A. and R.M. Lawrence. 2005. *Breastfeeding: A Guide for the Medical Profession, 6th edition.* Philadelphia, PA: Elsevier Mosby.

6 **living cells that are unique to your milk**

Goldman, A.S. et al. 1990. Anti-inflammatory systems in human milk. *Adv Exp Med Biol* 262:69–76.

6   **interferon and interleukins are powerful anti-infectives**

Buescher, E.S. 2001. Anti-inflammatory characteristics of human milk: how, where, why. *Adv Exp Med Biol* 501:207–22.

Chien, P.F. and P.W. Howie. 2001. Breast milk and the risk of opportunistic infection in infancy. *Adv Nutr Res* 10:69–104.

Hamosh, M. 2001. Bioactive factors in human milk. *Pediatr Clin North Am* 48(1): 69–86.

6   **your milk can even treat eye infections**

Cugali, N. and D.S. Moore. 1984. Current considerations in neonatal conjunctivitis. *J Nur Midwifery* 29(3):197–204.

6   **ear infections**

Sabirov, A. et al. 2009. Breast-feeding is associated with a reduced frequency of acute otitis media and high serum antibody levels against NTHi and outer membrane protein vaccine antigen candidate P6. *Pediatr Res* 66(5):565.

6   **intestinal upsets**

Dujits, L. et al. 2009. Breastfeeding protects against infectious diseases during infancy in industrialized countries. A systematic review. *Matern Child Nutr* 5(3):199–210.

6   **respiratory problems**

Ogbuanu, I.U. et al. 2009. Effect of breastfeeding duration on lung function at age 10 years: a prospective birth cohort study. *Thorax* 64(1):62–66.

6   **allergies**

Muche-Borowski, C. et al. 2009. Allergy prevention. *J Dtsch Dermatolog Ges* 106(39): 625–631.

6   **dental problems**

Leite-Cavalcanti, A. et al. 2007. Breast-feeding, bottle-feeding, sucking habits and mal-occlusion in Brazilian preschool children. *Rev Salud Publica* 9(2):194–204.

6   **vision**

Agostini, C. and M. Giovannini. 2001. Cognitive and visual development: influence of differences in breast and formula fed infants. *Nutr Health* 15(3–4):183.

6   **his immune system's response to vaccinations is less effective**

Dorea, J.G. 2009. Breastfeeding is an essential complement to vaccination. *Acta Paediatr* 98(8):1244–1250.

6   **the risk of SIDS**

McVea, K.L. et al. 2000. The role of breastfeeding in sudden infant death syndrome. *J Hum Lact* 16(1):13–20.

Venemann, M.M. et al. 2009. Does breastfeeding reduce the risk of sudden infant death syndrome? *Pediatrics* 123(3): e406–e410.

6   **infant death from many other causes is higher**

Chen, A. and W.J. Rogan. 2004. Breastfeeding and the risk of postneonatal death in the United States. *Pediatrics* 113(5):e435–e439.

6   **greater risk of Crohn's disease, ulcerative colitis**

Barclay, A.R. 2009. Systematic review: the role of breastfeeding in the development of pediatric inflammatory bowel disease. *J Pediatr* 155(3):421–426.

6   **heart disease**

Parikh, N.H. et al. 2009. Breastfeeding in infancy and adult cardiovascular disease risk factors. *Am J Med* 122(7):656–663.

6   **certain cancers**

Bener, A. et al. 2008. Does prolonged breastfeeding reduce the risk for childhood leukemia and lymphomas? *Minerva Pediatr* 60(2):155–161.

6   **[if formula-fed] he responds to stress more negatively**

Montgomery, S.M., A. Ehlin, and A. Sacker. 2006. Breastfeeding and resilience against psychological stress. *Arch Dis Child* 91(12):990–994.

6   **obesity**

O'Tierney, P.F. et al. 2009. Duration of breast-feeding and adiposity in adult life. *J Nutr* 139(2):422S–425S.

6   **type 2 diabetes**

Pettit, D.J. et al. 1997. Breastfeeding and the incidence of non-insulin-dependent diabetes mellitus in Pima Indians. *Lancet* 350:166–168.

6   **osteoporosis**

Jones, G. et al. 2000. Breastfeeding in early life and bone mass in prepubertal children: a longitudinal study. *Osteoporosis Int* 11(2):146–152.

6   **IQ studies**

Kramer, M.S. 2008. Breastfeeding and child cognitive development: new evidence from a large randomized trial. *Arch Gen Psychiatry* 65(5):578–584.

6   *pancreatic secretory trypsin inhibitor*

Marchbank, T. et al. 2009. Pancreatic secretory trypsin inhibitor is a major motogenic and protective factor in human breast milk. *Am J Physiol Gastrointest Liver Physiol* 296(4):G697–703.

7   **colostrum is a laxative**

Lawrence, R.A. and R.M. Lawrence. 2005. *Breastfeeding: A Guide for the Medical Profession, 6th edition,* 114. Philadelphia, PA: Elsevier Mosby.

7   **human growth factor continues to develop those intestines, bones, and other organs. Insulin for digestion, long-chain fatty acids for a healthy heart, lactose for brain development—it's all there**

Lawrence, R.A. and R.M. Lawrence. 2005. *Breastfeeding: A Guide for the Medical Profession, 6th edition.* Philadelphia, PA: Elsevier Mosby.

7   **the child who breastfeeds for less than a year is much more likely to need orthodontia later on**

Page, D.C. 2001. Breastfeeding in early functional jaw orthopedics. *Funct Orthod* 18(3):24–27.

8 **when your newborn takes your breast soon after delivery, your uterus contracts and bleeding slows**

Sobhy, S.I. and N.A. Mohame. 2004. The effect of early initiation of breast feeding on the amount of vaginal blood loss during the fourth stage of labor. *J Egypt Public Health Assoc* 79(1–2):1–12.

8 **your periods most likely won't come back for *at least* six months. Your chances of getting pregnant again will be extremely low**

Aryal, T.R. 2007. Differentials of post-partum amenorrhea: a survival analysis. *J Nepal Med Assoc* 46(166):66–73.

8 **breastfeeding helps many (not all) women lose weight readily**

Harder, T. et al. 2005. Duration of breastfeeding and risk of overweight: a meta-analysis. *Am J Epidemiol* 162(5):397–403.

8 **women who haven't breastfed are at greater risk for metabolic syndrome**

Gunderson, E.P. et al. 2007. Lactation and changes in maternal metabolic risk factors. *Obstet Gynecol* 109(3):729–738.

Lawlor, D.A. et al. 2005. Infant feeding and components of the metabolic syndrome: findings from the European Youth Heart Study. *Arch Dis Child* 90:582–588.

Ram, K.T. et al. 2008. Duration of lactation is associated with lower prevalence of the metabolic syndrome in midlife—SWAN, the study of women's health across the nation. *Am J Obstet Gynecol* 198(3):268.e1–6.

Stuebe, A.M. et al. 2005. Duration of lactation and incidence of type 2 diabetes. *JAMA* 294(20):2601–2610.

Stuebe, A.M. and J.W. Rich-Edwards. 2009. The reset hypothesis: lactation and maternal metabolism. *Am J Perinatol* 26(1):81–88.

8 **heart disease**

Schwarz, E.B. et al. 2009. Duration of lactation and risk factors for maternal cardiovascular disease. *Obstet Gynecol* 113(5):974–978.

8 **if you already have insulin-dependent diabetes, you're likely to need less insulin while you're a nursing mother**

Coastal Bend Breastfeeding Coalition. 2009. *Diabetes and breastfeeding—why breastfeed?* <http://www.momsmilk.org/article_diabetes_breastfeeding.html>.

National Collaborating Centre for Women's and Children's Health. 2008. *NICE Clinical Guideline 63: Diabetes in pregnancy. Management of diabetes and its complications from preconception to the postnatal period.* 2008. <http://www.nice.org.uk/CG063>.

Riviello, C. et al. 2009. Breastfeeding and the basal insulin requirement in type I diabetic women. *Endocr Pract* 15(3):187–193.

8 **breastfeeding is also an insurance policy against breast, uterine, and cervical cancer**

Collaborative Group on Hormonal Factors in Breast Cancer. 2002. Breast cancer and breastfeeding: collaborative reanalysis of individual data from 47 epidemiological studies in 30 countries, including 50302 women with breast cancer and 96973 women without the disease. *Lancet* 360(9328):187–195.

Danforth, K.N. et al. 2007. Breastfeeding and risk of ovarian cancer in two prospective cohorts. *Cancer Causes Control* 18(5):517–523.

8 **osteoporosis and fractures are also more common in women who didn't breastfeed**

Cumming, R.G. and R.J. Klineberg. 1993. Breastfeeding and other reproductive factors and the risk of hip fractures in elderly women. *Int J Epidemiol* 22:684–691.

Lopez, J.M. et al. 1996. Bone turnover and density in healthy women during breastfeeding and after weaning. *Osteoporos Int* 6:153–159.

Paton, L.M. et al. 2003. Pregnancy and lactation have no long-term deleterious effect on measures of bone mineral in healthy women: a twin study. *Am J Clin Nutr* 77:707–714.

8 **a formula-feeding mother's blood pressure is likely to be higher**

Jonas, W. et al. 2008. Short- and long-term decrease of blood pressure in women during breastfeeding. *Breastfeeding Med* 3(2):103–109.

8 **mental health**

Mezzacappa, E.S. 2004. Breastfeeding and maternal stress response and health. *Nutr Rev* Jul; 62(7 Pt 1):261–268.

Mezzacappa, E.S. and E.S. Katlin. 2002. Breast-feeding is associated with reduced perceived stress and negative mood in mothers. *Health Psychol* 21(2):187–193.

8 **risk of developing such autoimmune diseases as rheumatoid arthritis**

Brun, J.G. et al. 1995. Breast feeding, other reproductive factors and rheumatoid arthritis. A prospective study. *Br J Rheumatol* 34(6):542–546.

Jacobsson, L.T. et al. 2003. Perinatal characteristics and risk of rheumatoid arthritis. *BMJ* 326(7398):1068–1069.

Pikwer, M. et al. 2009. Breast feeding, but not use of oral contraceptives, is associated with a reduced risk of rheumatoid arthritis. *Ann Rheum Dis* 68(4):526–530.

11 **the breastfeeding experience can also help heal many emotional wounds, from a difficult or traumatic birth to an abusive past**

Coles, J. 2009. Qualitative study of breastfeeding after childhood sexual assault. *J Hum Lact* 25(3):317–324.

16 **evidence that [hand-expressing colostrum prenatally] may also boost your future supply**

Butler, K. and S. Upstone. 2008. *Antenatal Expression of Colostrum*. LLLGB.

Cox, S. 2006. Expressing and storing colostrum antenatally for use in the newborn period. *Breastfeeding Review* 14(3):11–16.

Oscroft, R. 2001. Antenatal expression of colostrum. *Pract Midwife* 4(4):32–35.

19 **babies who aren't "worn" by adults for much of the day fuss more than those who are**

Hunziker, U.A. and R.G. Barr. 1986. Increased carrying reduces infant crying: a randomized controlled trial. *Pediatrics* 77(5):641–648.

23 **your supply won't increase much from about one month on**

Neville, M.C. et al. 1991. Studies in human lactation: milk volume and nutrient composition during weaning and lactogenesis. *Am J Clin Nutr* 54:81–92.

TWO Building Your Network

28 **being part of a supportive community is more important than you might think**

Pitman, T. 2000. Finding your tribe. *Mothering* 102:72–77.

THREE Birth!

43 *the average first labor starts at forty-one weeks or so*

Mittendorf, R. et al. 1990. The length of uncomplicated human gestation. *Obstet Gynecol* 75(6):929–932.

43 **attempts to induce labor with Pitocin (artificial oxytocin, the hormone that causes contractions) often "fail"**

Bidgood, K.A. and P.J. Steer. 1987. A randomized control study of oxytocin augmentation of labour. 2. Uterine activity. *Br J Obstet Gynaecol* 94(6):518–522.

Steer, P.J. et al. 1985. The effect of oxytocin infusion on uterine activity level in slow labour. *Br J Obstet Gynaecol* 92:1120–1126.

43 **added fluids may increase breast engorgement**

Academy of Breastfeeding Medicine Protocol Committee. Berens, P. 2009. ABM clinical protocol #20: Engorgement. *Breastfeed Med* 4(2):111–113.

Cotterman, K.J. 2004. Reverse Pressure Softening: a simple tool to prepare areola for easier latching during engorgement. *J Hum Lact* 20(2): 227–237.

Martens, P.J. and L. Romphf. 2007. Factors associated with newborn in-hospital weight loss: comparisons by feeding method, demographics, and birthing procedures. *J Hum Lact* 23(3):233–241.

43 **eating and drinking as much as you want to in labor**

O'Sullivan, G. et al. 2009. Effect of food intake during labour on obstetric outcome: randomised controlled trial. *BMJ* 338:b784.

44 **catecholamines—fight-or-flight hormones**

Selin, L. et al. 2008. Dystocia in labour—risk factors, management and outcome: a retrospective observational study in a Swedish setting. *Acta Obstet Gynecol Scand* 87(2):216–221.

Simkin, P. 1986. Stress, pain, and catecholamines in labor: a review. *Birth* 13(4): 227–233.

44 **a labor support person, sometimes called a doula**

Hodnett, E.D. et al. 2007. Continuous support for women during childbirth. *Cochrane Database Syst Rev* 18(3):CD003766.

Langer, A. et al. 1998. Effects of psychosocial support during labour and childbirth on breastfeeding, medical interventions, and mothers' wellbeing in a Mexican public hospital: a randomised clinical trial. *Br J Obstet Gynaecol* 105(10):1056–1063.

45   **having to lie still or lie on your back during labor has been shown to lengthen labor**

Albers, L.L. et al. 1997. The relationship of ambulation in labor to operative delivery. *J Nurse Midwifery* 42(1):4–8.

Lawrence, A. et al. 2009. Maternal positions and mobility during first stage labour. *Cochrane Database Syst Rev* 15(2):CD003934.

Varrassi, G. et al. 1989. Effects of physical activity on maternal plasma beta-endorphin levels and perception of labor pain. *Am J Obstet Gynecol* 160(3):707–712.

45   **releases endorphins, the same pain-relieving hormones**

Pancheri, P. et al. 1985. ACTH, beta-endorphin and met-enkephalin: peripheral modifications during the stress of human labor. *Psychoneuroendocrinology* 10(3):289–301.

Smith, R. et al. 1990. Mood changes, obstetric experience and alterations in plasma cortisol, beta-endorphin and corticotrophin releasing hormone during pregnancy and the puerperium. *J Psychosom Res* 34(1):53–69.

Zanardo, V. et al. 2001. Beta endorphin concentrations in human milk. *J Pediatr Gastroenterol Nutr* 33(2):160–164.

45   **epidural**

De Barros Duarte, L. et al. 2007. Placental transfer of bupivacaine enantiomers in normal pregnant women receiving epidural anesthesia for Cesarean section. *Eur J Clin Pharmacol* 63(5):523–526.

O'Hana, H.P. et al. 2008. The effect of epidural analgesia on labor progress and outcome in nulliparous women. *J Matern Fetal Neonatal Med* 21(8):517–521.

Smith, L.J. 2007. Impact of birthing practices on the breastfeeding dyad. *J Midwifery Womens Health* 52(6):621–630.

Smith, L.J. 2008. Why Johnny can't suck: impact of birth practices on infant suck. In *Supporting Sucking Skills in Breastfeeding Infants*. Genna, C.W., ed. Sudbury, MA: Jones and Bartlett.

Thorp, J.A. et al. 1994. Epidural analgesia in labor and Cesarean delivery for dystocia. *Obstet Gynecol Surv* 49(5):362–369.

Yancey, M.K. et al. 2001. Labor epidural analgesia and intrapartum maternal hyperthermia. *Obstet Gynecol* 98(5 Pt 1):763–770.

46   **waiting until her body wants to start pushing means...less risk of tearing or needing help**

Sampselle, C.M. and S. Hines. 1999. Spontaneous pushing during birth: relationship to perineal outcomes. *J Nurse Midwifery* 44(1): 36–39.

Yilirim, G. and N.K. Beji. 2008. Effects of pushing techniques in birth on mother and fetus: a randomized study. *Birth* 35(1): 25–30.

46   **some mammal mothers won't know their babies belong to them if their "stretch receptors" have been numbed**

Blauvelt, H. 1956. Neonate-mother relationship in goat and man. In *Group Processes*. Schaffner, B. ed., 94–140. New York: Josiah Macy Jr. Foundations.

47   **episiotomy...increases the risk of more serious tears**

Nager, M.D. and J.P. Helliwell. 2001. Episiotomy increases perineal laceration length in primiparous women. *Am J Obstet Gynecol* 185(2):444–450.

47   **waiting until the cord stops pulsing**

Van Rheenen, P. and B.J. Brabin. 2004. Late umbilical cord-clamping as an intervention for reducing iron deficiency anaemia in term infants in developing and industrialised countries: a systematic review. *Ann Trop Paediatr* 24(1):3–16.

47   **a new rush of oxytocin**

Feldman, R. et al. 2007. Evidence for a neuroendocrinological foundation of human affiliation: plasma oxytocin levels across pregnancy and the postpartum period predict mother-infant bonding. *Psycholo Sci* 18(11):965–970.

48   **skin contact with his mother**

Bergman, N.J. et al. 2004. Randomized controlled trial of skin-to-skin contact from birth versus conventional incubator for physiological stabilization in 1200- to 2199-gram newborns. *Acta Paediatr* 93(6):779–785.

Moore, E.R. et al. 2007. Early skin-to-skin contact for mothers and their healthy newborn infants. *Cochrane Database Syst Rev* 18(3):CD003519.

49   **if you have twins, the temperature on each breast rises and falls to warm or cool them independently**

Ludington-Hoe, S.M. et al. 2006. Breast and infant temperatures with twins during shared kangaroo care. *J Obstet Gynecol Neonatal Nurs* 35(2):223–231.

49   **still smelling of amniotic fluid**

Schaal, B. et al. 1998. Olfactory function in the human fetus: evidence from selective neonatal responsiveness to the odor of amniotic fluid. *Behav Neurosci* 112(6):1438–1449.

49   **causes yet another whoosh of oxytocin**

Marshall, W.M. et al. 1992. Hot flushes during breastfeeding? *Fertil Steril* 57(6): 1349–1350.

49   **provides a protective, anti-infective coating for his brand-new intestinal tract**

Hanson, L.A. 2004. *Immunobiology of Human Milk*. Amarillo, TX: Pharmasoft Publishing.

51   **home birth is just as safe as hospital birth for low-risk pregnancies**

Fullerton, J.T. et al. 2007. Outcomes of planned home birth: an integrative review. *J Midwifery Womens Health* 52(4):323–333.

Johnson, K. and B.A. Daviss. 2005. Outcomes of planned home births with certified professional midwives: large prospective study in North America. *BMJ* 330(7505):1416.

Symon, A. et al. 2009. Outcomes for births booked under an independent midwife and births in NHS maternity units: matched comparison study. *BMJ* 338:b2060.

54   **avoid routine external fetal monitoring**

Wood, S.H. 2003. Should women be given a choice about fetal assessment in labor? *J Matern Child Nurs* 28(5):292–298.

55   **common interventions**

Chalmers, B. et al. 2009. Maternity Experiences Study Group of the Canadian Perinatal Surveillance System; Public Health Agency of Canada. Use of routine interventions in vaginal labor and birth: findings from the Maternity Experiences Survey. *Birth* 36(1):13–25.

Childbirth Connection. 2002. *Listening to Mothers I Report.* <http://www.childbirthconnection.org/article.asp?ck=10068>.

Medoff-Cooper, B. et al. 2005. The AWHONN near-term infant initiative: a conceptual framework for optimizing health for near-term infants. *J Obstet Gynecol Neonatal Nurs* 34(6):666–671.

Thacker, S.B. et al. 2006. Continuous electronic heart rate monitoring for fetal assessment during labor. *Cochrane Database Syst Rev* 3:CD000063.

55 **the World Health Organization recommends limiting medical inductions to those that are truly necessary, fewer than 10 percent of all births**

Chalmers, B. et al. 2001. WHO principles of perinatal care: the essential antenatal, perinatal, and postpartum care course. *Birth* 28(3):202–207.

55 **ask that misoprostol (Cytotec) *not* be used**

Cecatti, J.G. et al. 2006. Effectiveness and safety of a new vaginal misoprostol product specifically labeled for cervical ripening and labor induction. *Acta Obstet Gynecol Scand* 85(6):706–711.

Wagner, M. 2008. *Born in the USA: How a Broken Maternity System Must Be Fixed to Put Women and Children First.* Los Angeles: University of California Press.

Weaver, S.P. et al. 2006. Vaginal misoprostol for cervical ripening in term pregnancy. *Am Fam Physician* 73(3):511–512.

57 **reduce your risk of a C-section**

Althabe, F. and J.F. Belizán. 2006. Caesarean section: the paradox. *Lancet* 368(9546): 1472–1473.

FOUR Latching and Attaching

63 **an approach that takes advantage of the natural instincts you both have**

Colson, S. 2007. Biological nurturing (1): a non-prescriptive recipe for breastfeeding. *Pract Midwife* 10(9):42–48.

Colson, S. 2007. Biological nurturing (2): the physiology of lactation revisited. *Pract Midwife* 10(10):14–19.

Colson, S.D. et al. 2008. Optimal positions for the release of primitive reflexes stimulating breastfeeding. *Early Hum Dev* 84(7):441–449.

68 **What Babies Need**

Glover, R. and D. Wiessinger. 2008. The infant-maternal breastfeeding conversation: helping when they lose the thread. In *Supporting Sucking Skills in Breastfeeding Infants.* Genna, C.W. ed., 97–129. Sudbury, MA: Jones and Bartlett.

Smith, L.J. 2008. Why Johnny can't suck: impact of birth practices on infant suck. In *Supporting Sucking Skills in Breastfeeding Infants.* Genna, C.W. ed., 58–59. Sudbury, MA: Jones and Bartlett.

Wolf, J. 2003. Low breastfeeding rates and public health in the United States. *Am J Public Health* 93(12):2000–2010.

FIVE The First Few Days: Hello, Baby...

87 **your bare or diaper-only baby on your bare skin**

Ludington-Hoe, S.M. et al. 2000. Kangaroo care compared to incubators in maintaining body warmth in preterm infants. *Biol Res Nurs* 2(1):60–73.

Moore, E.R. et al. 2007. Early skin-to-skin contact for mothers and their healthy newborn infants. *Cochrane Database Syst Rev* (3):CD003519.

Riordan, J. and K. Hoover. 2010. Perinatal and intrapartum care. In *Breastfeeding and Human Lactation, 4th edition*. Riordan, J. and K. Wambach, ed., 218, 220–221, 244. Sudbury, MA: Jones and Bartlett.

90 **how long, which side, and how often**

Kent, J. et al. 2006. Volume and frequency of breastfeedings and fat content of breast milk throughout the day. *Pediatrics* 117(3):e387–e395.

Riordan, J. 2010. Anatomy and physiology of lactation. In *Breastfeeding and Human Lactation, 4th edition*. Riordan, J. and K. Wambach, ed., 79–116. Sudbury, MA: Jones and Bartlett.

Smith, L.J. and J. Riordan. 2010. Postpartum care. In *Breastfeeding and Human Lactation, 4th edition*. Riordan, J. and K. Wambach, ed., 272. Sudbury, MA: Jones and Bartlett.

92 **sharing sleep safely in the hospital**

McKenna, J.J. and L.T. Gettler. 2007. Mother-infant cosleeping with breastfeeding in the Western industrialized context. In *Textbook of Human Lactation*. Hale, T.W. and P.E. Hartmann, ed. Amarillo, TX: Hale Publishing.

93 **giving your baby formula, for any reason, in these first days is not something to be taken lightly**

Riordan, J. 2010. The biological specificity of breastmilk. In *Breastfeeding and Human Lactation, 4th edition*. Riordan, J. and K. Wambach, ed., 133, 139. Sudbury, MA: Jones and Bartlett.

Walker, M. 1993. A fresh look at the risks of artificial infant feeding. *J Hum Lact* 9(2):97–107.

95 **babies shouldn't lose any more than 7 percent of their body weight before they start gaining**

Martens, P.J. and L. Romphf. 2007. Factors associated with newborn in-hospital weight loss: comparisons by feeding method, demographics, and birthing procedures. *J Hum Lact* 23(3):233–241.

99 **swaddling is popular at the moment, but there's research that raises alarms**

Bystrova, K. et al. 2009. Skin-to-skin contact may reduce negative consequences of "the stress of being born": a study on temperature in newborn infants, subjected to different ward routines in St. Petersburg. *Acta Paediatr* 92(3):320–326.

Bystrova, K. et al. 2009. Early contact versus separation: effects on mother-infant interaction one year later. *Birth* 36(2):97–109.

Van Sleuwen, B.E. et al. 2007. Swaddling: a systematic review. *Pediatrics* 120(4): e1097–e1106.

six The First Two Weeks: Milk!

105 **baby latches and begins sucking**

Genna, C.W. and L. Sandora. 2008. Breastfeeding: normal sucking and swallowing. In *Supporting Sucking Skills in Breastfeeding Infants*. Genna, C.W., ed., 3809. Sudbury, MA: Jones and Bartlett.

107 **level of *cholecystokinin* (CCK) has risen**

Uvnäs-Moberg, K. et al. 1993. Plasma cholecystokinin concentrations after breast feeding in healthy 4 day old infants. *Arch Dis Child* 68(1 Spec No):46–48.

107 **nursings often cluster together**

Kent, J.C. 2007. How breastfeeding works. *J Midwifery Womens Health* Nov-Dec; 52(6):564–570.

Kent, J. et al. 2006. Volume and frequency of breastfeedings and fat content of breast milk throughout the day. *Pediatrics* 117(3):e387–e395.

Renfrew, M.J. et al. 2000. Feeding schedules in hospitals for newborn infants. *Cochrane Database Syst Rev* (2):CD000090.

108 **the number of wet and poopy diapers should increase day by day**

Nommsen-Rivers, L.A. et al. 2008. Newborn wet and soiled diaper counts and timing of onset of lactation as indicators of breastfeeding adequacy. *J Hum Lact* 24(1):27–33.

110 **look for a return to birth weight by two weeks. An average gain after that is roughly 1 ounce (30 g) a day, but your baby may gain somewhat more or less**

Crossland, D.S. et al. 2008. Weight change in the term baby in the first 2 weeks of life. *Acta Paediatr* 97(4):425–429.

Martens, P.J. and L. Romphf. 2007. Factors associated with newborn in-hospital weight loss: comparisons by feeding method, demographics, and birthing procedures. *J Hum Lact* 23(3):233–241.

112 **the more milk that is removed during this time, the higher your long-term milk supply will be**

Daly, S.E. and P.E. Hartmann. 1995. Infant demand and milk supply. Part 1: infant demand and milk production in lactating women. *J Hum Lact* 11(1):21–26.

Daly, S.E. and P.E. Hartmann. 1995. Infant demand and milk supply. Part 2: the short-term control of milk synthesis in lactating women. *J Hum Lact* 11(1):27–37.

West, D. and L. Marasco. 2009. *The Breastfeeding Mother's Guide to Making More Milk*. New York: McGraw-Hill.

112 **breast compressions**

Newman, J. and T. Pitman. 2006. *The Ultimate Breastfeeding Book of Answers*. New York: Three Rivers Press.

113 **guidelines you can give them for food**

Bronner, Y.L. 2010. Maternal nutrition during lactation. In *Breastfeeding and Human Lactation, 4th edition*. Riordan, J. and K. Wambach, ed., 498. Sudbury, MA: Jones and Bartlett.

114 **safe co-sleeping**

McKenna, J.J. 2007. *Sleeping with Your Baby: A Parent's Guide to Cosleeping.* Washington DC: Platypus Media.

McKenna, J.J. et al. 2007. Mother-infant cosleeping, breastfeeding and sudden infant death syndrome: what biological anthropology has discovered about normal infant sleep and pediatric sleep medicine. *Yearbook Phys Anthropol* 50:133–161.

116   **baby blues**

Kendall-Tackett, K. 2005. *Depression in New Mothers: Causes, Consequences, and Treatment Alternatives,* 4. Binghamton, NY: Haworth Maltreatment and Trauma Press.

118   **hard-to-settle baby**

Barr, R.G. et al. 1989. Feeding and temperament as determinants of early infant crying/fussing behavior. *Pediatrics* 84(3):514–521.

Jones, S. 1992. *Crying Baby, Sleepless Nights: Why Your Baby Is Crying and What You Can Do About It,* 73. Boston: Harvard Common Press.

124   **you don't need more fluids than you want in order to make milk, and your supply won't decrease if you're mildly dehydrated**

Dusdieker, L. et al. 1985. Effect of supplemental fluids on human milk production. *J Pediatr* 106(2):207–211.

Olsen, A. 1939. Nursing under conditions of thirst or excessive ingestion of fluids. *Acta Obstet et Gynecol* 10(4):312–343.

125   **your baby will learn the family menu through breastfeeding**

Mennella, J.A. 1995. Mother's milk: a medium for early flavor experiences. *J Hum Lact* 11(1):39–45.

Mennella, J.A. et al. 2009. Early milk feeding influences taste acceptance and liking during infancy. *Am J Clin Nutr* 90(3):780S–788S.

Sullivan, S and L. Birch. 1994. Infant dietary experience and acceptance of solid foods. *Pediatrics* 93(2):271–277.

125   **go easy on caffeine**

Berlin, C.M. et al. 1984. Disposition of dietary caffeine in milk, saliva and plasma of lactating women. *Pediatrics* 73(1):59–63.

Ryu, J.E. 1985. Caffeine in human milk and in serum of breast-fed infants. *Dev Pharmacol Ther* 8(6):329–337.

128   **pacifiers are linked to early weaning**

Kramer, M.S. et al. 2001. Pacifier use, early weaning, and cry/fuss behavior: a randomized controlled trial. *JAMA* 18;286(3):322–326.

Righard, L. and M.O. Alade. 1997. Breastfeeding and the use of pacifiers. *Birth* 24(2):116–120.

Victora, C.G. et al. 1997. Pacifier use and short breastfeeding duration. Cause, consequence or coincidence? *Pediatrics* 99(3):445–453.

128   **children who use pacifiers in day care are more prone to thrush and ear infections**

Warren, J.J. et al. 2001. Pacifier use and the occurrence of otitis media in the first year of life. *Pediatr Dent* 23(2):103–107.

128 **[pacifiers] can affect mouth development**

Palmer, B. 1999. Breastfeeding: reducing the risk for obstructive sleep apnea. *Breastfeeding Abstracts* Feb;18(3):19–20.

Viggiano, D. et al. 2005. Breastfeeding, bottlefeeding, and non-nutritive sucking: effects on occlusion in deciduous dentition. *Arch Dis Child* 89(12):1121–1123.

SEVEN Two to Six Weeks: Butterfly Smiles

134 **mothers were often told to feed on a schedule**

Aksit, S. et al. 2002. Effect of sucking characteristics on breast milk creamatocrit. *Paediatr Perinat Epidemiol* 16(4):355–360.

Tyson, J. et al. 1992. Adaptation of feeding to a low fat yield in breast milk. *Pediatrics* 89(2):215–220.

Woolridge, M.W. et al. 1990. Do changes in pattern of breast usage alter the baby's nutrient intake? *Lancet* Aug 18;336(8712):395–397.

136 **breasts feel fairly soft most of the time**

Cregan, M.D. and P.E. Hartmann. 1999. Computerized breast measurement from conception to weaning: clinical implications. *J Hum Lact* 15(2):89–96.

137 **gaining weight appropriately**

Hermanussen, M. et al. 2001. Growth tracks in early childhood. *Acta Paediatr* 90(4):381–386.

World Health Organization. <who.int/childgrowth/standards/en>.

138 **most exclusively breastfed babies take about 25 to 27 ounces (750 to 800 ml) of milk a day**

Butte, N.F. et al. 2000. Energy requirements derived from total energy expenditure and energy deposition during the first 2 y of life. *Am J Clin Nutr* 72(6):1558–1569.

Kent, J. et al. 2006. Volume and frequency of breastfeedings and fat content of breast milk throughout the day. *Pediatrics* 117(3):e387–e395.

141 **babies who aren't held cry significantly more than babies who are**

Sears, W. and M. Sears. 2001. *The Attachment Parenting Book*. Boston: Little, Brown.

147 **women don't have a fight-or-flight response to stress; ours is called "tend and befriend"**

Taylor, S.E. et al. 2000. Biobehavioral responses to stress in females: tend-and-befriend, not fight-or-flight. *Psychol Rev* 107(3):411–429.

EIGHT Six Weeks to Four Months: Hitting Your Stride

151 **crying tends to peak around six to eight weeks**

Hiscock, H. and B.I. Jordan. 2004. Problem crying in infancy. *Med J Aust* 181(9):507–512.

Hunziker, U.A. and R.G. Barr. 1986. Increased carrying reduces infant crying: a randomized controlled trial. *Pediatrics* 77(5):641–648.

Jones, S. 1992. *Crying Baby, Sleepless Nights: Why Your Baby Is Crying and What You Can Do About It.* Boston: Harvard Common Press.

154   **around six weeks or so, though, some babies stop having the several bowel movements each day that are expected up until this point**

Mohrbacher, N. and J. Stock. 2003. *The Breastfeeding Answer Book, 3rd edition.* Schaumburg, IL: La Leche League International.

155   **most studies have found no significant difference in the volume, taste, or composition of milk after exercise**

Wallace, J.P. et al. 1992. Infant acceptance of postexercise breast milk. *Pediatrics* 89 (6 Pt 2):1245–1247.

156   **working out can improve your mood, give you more energy, and help you sleep better at night**

Da Costa, D. 2009. A randomized clinical trial of exercise to alleviate postpartum depressed mood. *J Psychosom Obstet Gynaecol* 30(3):191–200.

Dritsa, M. et al. 2008. Effects of a home-based exercise intervention on fatigue in postpartum depressed women: results of a randomized controlled trial. *Ann Behav Med* 35(2):179–187.

156   **aim for losing no more than about 1 pound (0.5 kg) a week**

Bronner, Y.L. 2010. Maternal nutrition during lactation. In *Breastfeeding and Human Lactation, 4th edition.* Riordan, J. and K. Wambach, ed. Sudbury, MA: Jones and Bartlett.

Dusdieker, L.B. et al. 1994. Is milk production impaired by dieting during lactation? *Am J Clin Nutr* 59(4):833–840.

Institute of Medicine, Food and Nutrition Board, National Research Council. 2005. *Dietary Reference Intakes for Energy, Carbohydrates, Fiber, Fat, Fatty Acids, Cholesterol, Protein, and Amino Acids.* Washington, DC: National Academy Press.

Specker, B.L. 1994. Nutritional concerns of lactating women consuming vegetarian diets. *Am J Clin Nutr* 59(5 Suppl):1182S–1186S.

158   **vitamin D**

Lips, P. 2006. Vitamin D physiology. *Prog Biophys Mol Biol* 92(1):4–8.

159   **extra iron**

Griffin, I.J. and S.A. Abrams. 2001. Iron and breastfeeding. *Pediatr Clin North Am* Apr;48(2):401–413.

Yang, Z. et al. 2009. Prevalence and predictors of iron deficiency in fully breastfed infants at 6 mo of age: comparison of data from 6 studies. *Am J Clin Nutr* 89(5):1433–1440.

163   **fussy and demanding**

Sears, W. and M. Sears. 2002. *The Fussy Baby Book: How to Bring Out the Best in Your High-Need Child, revised edition.* Schaumburg IL: La Leche League International.

165   **sleeping through the night can slow his rate of growth and risks early weaning**

Ball, H.L. et al. 2006. Randomised trial of infant sleep location on the postnatal ward. *Arch Dis Child* 91(12):1005–1010.

Doan, T. et al. 2007. Breast-feeding increases sleep duration of new parents. *J Perinat Neonatal Nurs* 21(3):200–206.

169   **Lactational Amenorrhea Method**

Infact Canada. 1996. Breastfeeding and child spacing: LAM: lactational amenorrhea method. <http://www.infactcanada.ca/bfchild.htm>.

Kippley, S. 2008. *The Seven Standards of Ecological Breastfeeding.* Self-published.

NINE Four to Nine Months: In the Zone

175   **World Health Organization (WHO) weight gain charts reflect these normal changes**

World Health Organization. <who.int/childgrowth/standards/en/>.

179   **when solids start**

Rapley, G. and T. Murkett. 2008. *Baby-Led Weaning: Helping Your Baby to Love Good Food.* London: Vermilion.

182   **human milk itself rarely contributes to decay and actually has tooth-strengthening properties**

Mohebbi, S.Z. et al. 2008. Feeding habits as determinants of early childhood caries in a population where prolonged breastfeeding is the norm. *Community Dent Oral Epidemiol* 36(4):363–369.

Palmer, B. 2000. Infant dental decay: is it related to breastfeeding? <http://www .brianpalmerdds.com/pdf/caries.pdf>.

Slavkin, H.C. 1999. Streptococcus mutans, early childhood caries and new opportunities. *J Am Dental Assoc* 130(12):1787–1792.

Torney, P.H. 1992. *Prolonged, on-demand breastfeeding and dental caries—an investigation.* M.Dent.Sc. thesis, University of Dublin, Ireland.

184   **return to fertility**

Infact Canada. 1996. Breastfeeding and child spacing: LAM: lactational amenorrhea method. <infactcanada.ca/bfchild.htm>.

Kennedy, K.I. 2010. Fertility, sexuality, and contraception during lactation. In *Breastfeeding and Human Lactation, 4th edition.* Riordan, J. and K. Wambach, ed., 707–709. Sudbury, MA: Jones and Bartlett.

186   **breastfeeding ultimately protects against adult obesity**

Arenz, S. and R. Von Kries. 2009. Protective effect of breast-feeding against obesity in childhood: can a meta-analysis of published observational studies help to validate the hypothesis? *Adv Exp Med Biol* 639:145–52.

Arenz, S. et al. 2004. Breast-feeding and childhood obesity—a systematic review. *Int J Obes Relat Metab Disord* 28(10):1247–1256.

Harder, T. et al. 2005. Duration of breastfeeding and risk of overweight: a meta-analysis. *Am J Epidemiol* 162(5):397–403.

TEN Nine to Eighteen Months: On the Move

192   **reduce the risk of allergies**

Fiocchi, A. et al. 2006. Food allergy and the introduction of solid foods to infants: a consensus document. Adverse Reactions to Foods Committee, American College of Allergy, Asthma and Immunology. *Ann Allergy Asthma Immunol* 97(1):10–20.

Halken, S. 2004. Prevention of allergic disease in childhood: clinical and epidemiological aspects of primary and secondary allergy prevention. *Pediatr Allergy Immunol* 15 Suppl 16:4–5, 9–32.

Trotters Independent Publishing Services Ltd. 2008. Cup feeding revisited <tipslimited.com/cupfeeding.htm#bacterial>.

UNICEF. 2003. Governmental changes recommendation to 6 months' exclusive breastfeeding. <babyfriendly.org.uk/items/item_detail.asp?item=93>.

192 **families with a predisposition for diabetes do best by waiting until a year to introduce cow milk**

Savilahti, E. and K.M. Saarinen. 2009. Early infant feeding and type 1 diabetes. *Eur J Nutr* 48(4):243–249.

Vaarala, O. et al. 1999. Cow's milk formula feeding induces primary immunization to insulin in infants at genetic risk for type 1 diabetes. *Diabetes* 48(7):1389–1394.

193 **a daily dose of 500 to 1,000 mg of a calcium and magnesium supplement from the middle of your cycle through the first three days of your period may help minimize any drop in supply**

West, D. and L. Marasco. 2009. *The Breastfeeding Mother's Guide to Making More Milk,* 138. New York: McGraw-Hill.

ELEVEN Nursing Toddlers and Beyond: Moving On

202 **normal "weaning window"**

Dettwyler, K.A. 1995. A time to wean: the hominid blueprint for the natural age of weaning in modern human populations. In *Breastfeeding: Biocultural Perspectives.* Stuart-Macadam, P. and K.A. Dettwyler, ed., 39–73. New York: Aldine De Gruyter.

204 **the World Health Organization . . . recommends that children be breastfed for *at least* two years**

World Health Organization. 2003. *Global Strategy for Infant and Young Child Feeding.* <who.int/nutrition/publications/gs_infant_feeding_text_eng.pdf>.

TWELVE Sleeping Like a Baby

222 **a baby relies totally on his mother to keep him stable and secure**

Van der Horst, F.C. and R. Van der Veer. 2008. Loneliness in infancy: Harry Harlow, John Bowlby and issues of separation. *Integr Psychol Behav Sci* 42(4):325–335.

224 **co-sleeping**

Academy of Breastfeeding Medicine Protocol Committee. 2008. ABM clinical protocol #6: guideline on co-sleeping and breastfeeding. *Breastfeeding Medicine* 3(1):38–43.

Ball, H.L. 2006. Parent-infant bed-sharing behaviour: effects of feeding type, and presence of father. *Human Nature* 17(3):301–318.

Doan, T. et al. 2007. Breast-feeding increases sleep duration of new parents. *J Perinat Neonatal Nurs* 21(3):200–206.

Hauck, F.R. et al. 2008. Infant sleeping arrangements and practices during the first year of life. *Pediatrics* 122(suppl 2):S113–S120.

Horsley, T. et al. 2007. Benefits and harms associated with the practice of bed-sharing: a systematic review. *Arch Pediatr Adolesc Med* 161(3):237–245.

Kahn, A. et al. 2000. Factors influencing the determination of arousal thresholds in infants—a review. *Sleep Med* 1(4):273–278.

McKenna, J.J. 2007. *Sleeping with Your Baby: A Parent's Guide to Cosleeping.* Washington, DC: Platypus Media.

McKenna, J.J. et al. 1997. Bedsharing promotes breastfeeding. *Pediatrics* 100(2): 214–219.

Wailoo, M. et al. 2004. Infants bed-sharing with mothers. *Arch Dis Child* 89(12): 1082–1083.

228 **SIDS (crib death) and co-sleeping**

American Academy of Pediatrics. 2005. Task Force on Sudden Infant Death Syndrome policy statement: the changing concept of sudden infant death syndrome: diagnostic coding shifts, controversies regarding the sleeping environment, and new variables to consider in reducing risk. *Pediatrics* 116(5):1245–1255.

Arnestad, A.M. et al. 2001. Changes in the epidemiological pattern of sudden infant death syndrome in southeast Norway, 1984–1998: implications for future prevention and research. *Arch Dis Child* 85(2):108–115.

Blair, P.S. et al. 2006. Major epidemiological changes in sudden infant death syndrome: a 20-year population-based study in the UK. *Lancet* 367(9507):314–319.

Hauck, F.R. et al. 2005. Do pacifiers reduce the risk of sudden infant death syndrome? A meta-analysis. *Pediatrics* 116(5):e716–e723.

Li, D.K. et al. 2006. Use of a dummy (pacifier) during sleep and risk of sudden infant death syndrome (SIDS): population based case-control study. *BMJ* 332(7532):18–22.

McKenna, J.J. and T. McDade. 2005. Why babies should never sleep alone: a review of the co-sleeping controversy in relation to SIDS, bedsharing and breast feeding. *Paediatr Respir Rev* 6(2):134–152.

Mosko, S. et al. 1997. Maternal proximity and infant CO_2 environment during bedsharing and possible implications for SIDS research. *Am J Phys Anthropol* 103(3):315–328.

Mosko, S. et al. 1997. Infant arousals during mother-infant bed-sharing: implications for infant sleep and sudden infant death syndrome research. *Pediatrics* 100(5):841–849.

231 **letting your baby fall asleep at the breast**

Uvnäs-Moberg, K. et al. 1993. Plasma cholecystokinin concentrations after breast feeding in healthy 4 day old infants. *Arch Dis Child* 68(1 Spec No):46–48.

241 **adding solid foods doesn't help babies sleep more**

Keane, V. et al. 1988. Do solids help baby sleep through the night? *Am J Dis Child* 142:404–405.

Macknin, M.L. et al. 1989. Infant sleep and bedtime cereal. *Am J Dis Child* 143(9):1066–1068.

241 **no evidence that nighttime nursing causes cavities**

Matee M.I. et al. 1992. Mutans streptococci and lactobacilli in breast-fed children with rampant caries. *Caries Res* 26(3):183–187.

Mattos-Granera, R.O. et al. 1998. Association between caries prevalence and clinical, microbiological and dietary variables in 1.0 to 2.5-Year-Old Brazilian children. *Caries Res* 32(5):319–323.

Palmer, B. 2000. Infant dental decay: is it related to breastfeeding? <http://www.brianpalmerdds.com/pdf/caries.pdf>.

Slavkin, H.C. 1999. Streptococcus mutans, early childhood caries and new opportunities. *J Am Dental Assoc* 130(12):1787–1792.

Torney, P.H. 1992. *Prolonged, on-demand breastfeeding and dental caries—an investigation.* M.Dent.Sc. thesis.

THIRTEEN The Scoop on Solids

246 **introduction of complementary feedings before six months of age generally does not increase total caloric intake or rate of growth**

Birch, L.L. et al. 1991. The variability of young children's energy intake. *N Engl J Med* 324(4):232–235.

Butte, N.F. et al. 1991. Energy requirements of breast-fed infants. *J Am Coll Nutr* 10(3):190–195.

Butte, N.F. et al. 2000. Energy requirements derived from total energy expenditure and energy deposition during the first 2 y of life. *Am J Clin Nutr* 72(6):1558–1569.

Canadian Paediatric Society. 2005. Exclusive breastfeeding should continue to six months. *Paediatr Child Health* 10(3):148.

Dewey, K.G. 2001. Nutrition, growth, and complementary feeding of the breastfed infant. *Pediatr Clin North Am* 48(1):87–104.

Fox, M.K. et al. 2006. Sources of energy and nutrients in the diets of infants and toddlers. *J Am Diet Assoc* 106(1 Suppl 1):S28–S42.

Gartner, L.M. et al. 2005. Breastfeeding and the use of human milk; American Academy of Pediatrics Section on Breastfeeding. *Pediatrics* 115(2):496–506.

González, C. 2005. *My Child Won't Eat.* Schaumburg, IL: La Leche League International.

Naylor, A.J. and A.L. Morrow, ed. 2001. *Developmental Readiness of Normal Full Term Infants to Progress from Exclusive Breastfeeding to the Introduction of Complementary Foods: Reviews of the Relevant Literature Concerning Infant Immunologic, Gastrointestinal, Oral Motor and Maternal Reproductive and Lactational Development.* Washington, DC: Linkages Project of the Academy of Educational Development.

United Kingdom Scientific Advisory Committee on Nutrition (Subgroup on Maternal and Child Nutrition). 2003. <sach.gov.uk/pdfs/smcn_03_08.pdf>.

World Health Organization. 2003. *Global Strategy for Infant and Young Child Feeding* <http://whqlibdoc.who.int/publications/2003/9241562218.pdf>.

249 **around six months...substances can slip through the intestinal walls into the bloodstream**

Saarinen, U. and M. Kajosaari. 1995. Breastfeeding as a prophylaxis against atopic disease: prospective follow-up study until 17 years old. *Lancet* 346(8982):1065–1069.

249   **digestive enzymes are up and running at around six months**

Lebenthal, E. 1985. Impact of digestion and absorption in the weaning period on infant feeding practices. *Pediatrics* 75(1):207–213.

251   **waiting until she does it herself**

Rapley, G. and T. Murkett. 2008. *Baby-Led Weaning: Helping Your Baby to Love Good Food.* London: Vermilion.

254   **"Servings" may be tiny**

Fox, M.K. et al. 2006. Average portions of foods commonly eaten by infants and toddlers in the United States. *J Am Diet Assoc* 106(1 Suppl 1):S66–S76.

Mrdjenovic, G. and D.A. Levitsky. 2005. Children eat what they are served: the imprecise regulation of energy intake. *Appetite* 44(3):273–282.

Rolls, B.J. et al. 2000. Serving portion size influences 5-year-old but not 3-year old children's food intakes. *J Am Diet Assoc* 100:232–234.

258   **gluten (present in wheat, rye, and barley) must be introduced between four and seven months of age to avoid having problems**

Chertok, I.R. 2007. The importance of exclusive breastfeeding in infants at risk for celiac disease. *MCN Am J Matern Child Nurs* 32(1):50–54.

Norris, J.M. et al. 2005. Risk of celiac disease autoimmunity and timing of gluten introduction in the diet of infants at increased risk of disease. *JAMA* 293(19):2343–2351.

259   **a family dinner is linked to improved children's grades, reduced risk of obesity, and even reduced risk of substance abuse in the years ahead**

Eisenberg, M. et al. 2004. Correlations between family meals and psychosocial well-being among adolescents. *Arch Pediatr Adolesc Med* 158:792–796.

FOURTEEN   When You Can't Be with Your Baby

266   **having a longer leave *after* the baby is born increases breastfeeding success... women who start their leave a few weeks *before* the baby's birth are less likely to have a Cesarean section**

Guendelman, S. et al. 2009. Maternity leave in the ninth month of pregnancy and birth outcomes among working women. *Womens Health Issues* 19(1):30–37.

267   **gives you a chance to pick up some of the germs and bacteria in the center, so that you can start producing antibodies**

Lee, M.B. and J.D. Greig. 2008. A review of enteric outbreaks in child care centers: effective infection control recommendations. *J Environ Health* 71(3):24–32, 46.

Riordan, J. 2010. The biological specificity of breastmilk. In *Breastfeeding and Human Lactation, 4th edition.* Riordan, J. and K. Wambach ed., 140–144. Sudbury, MA: Jones and Bartlett.

273   **breastfeeding mothers—and other employees—feel more positive about companies that support them in continuing to breastfeed**

Glass, J. and L. Riley. 1998. Family responsive policies and employee retention following childbirth. *Social Forces* 76:1401–1436.

Guendelman, S. et al. 2009. Juggling work and breastfeeding: effects of maternity leave and occupational characteristics. *Pediatrics* 123(1):e38–e46.

Hakim, C. et al. 2008. *Little Britons: Financing Childcare Choice*. London: Policy Exchange.

Johnston, M.L. and N. Esposito. 2007. Barriers and facilitators for breastfeeding among working women in the United States. *J Obstet Gynecol Neonatal Nurs* 36(1):9–20.

Neifert, M. 2000. Supporting breastfeeding mothers as they return to work. *Amer Acad Pediatrics*. <healthychildcare.org/pdf/BFarticle.pdf>.

280 **a baby who is separated from his mother for the hours that full-time outside work requires has elevated cortisol levels**

Ainsworth, M.D.S. 1985. Attachments across the life span. *Bull NY Acad Med* 61(9): 792–812.

Bowlby, R. 2007. Babies and toddlers in non-parental daycare can avoid stress and anxiety if they develop a lasting secondary attachment bond with one carer who is consistently accessible to them. *Attach Hum Dev* 9(4):307–319.

Cao, Y. et al. 2009. Are breast-fed infants more resilient? Feeding method and cortisol in infants. *J Pediatr* 154(3):452–454.

Geoffroy, M.C. et al. 2006. Daycare attendance, stress, and mental health. *Can J Psychiatry* 51(9):607–615. Erratum in: *Can J Psychiatry* Oct;51(11):726.

Ouellet-Morin, I. et al. 2009. Diurnal cortisol secretion at home and in child care: a prospective study of 2-year-old toddlers. *J Child Psychol Psychiatry* Oct 5 (Epub ahead of print).

Vermeer, H. and M. Van IJzendoorn. 2006. Children's elevated cortisol levels at daycare: a review and meta-analysis. *Early Child Res Q* 21(3):390–401.

Waynforth, D. 2007. The influence of parent-infant cosleeping, nursing, and childcare on cortisol and SIgA immunity in a sample of British children. *Dev Psychobiol* 49(6):640–648.

FIFTEEN Milk to Go

292 **expressing milk**

Becker, G.E. et al. 2008. Methods of milk expression for lactating women. *Cochrane Database Syst Rev* 2008(4):CD006170.

Brown, S.L. et al. 2005. Breast pump adverse events: reports to the Food and Drug Administration. *J Hum Lact* 21(2):169–174.

Ohyama, M., H. Watabe, et al. 2010. Manual expression and electric breast pumping in the first 48 hours after delivery. *Pediatr Iot* 52(1):39–43.

Walker, M. 2010. Breastpumps and other technologies. In *Breastfeeding and Human Lactation, 4th edition*. Riordan, J. and K. Wambach, ed., 403. Sudbury, MA: Jones and Bartlett.

Wilson-Clay, B. and K. Hoover. 2008. *The Breastfeeding Atlas, 4th edition*. Austin, TX: LactNews Press.

297 **breast flanges**

Jones, E. and S. Hilton. 2009. Correctly fitting breast shields are the key to lactation success for pump dependent mothers following preterm delivery. *J Neonatal Nurs* 15(1):14–17.

298 **put in eight to twelve pumping sessions each day**

Cregan, M.D. et al. 2002. Milk prolactin, feed volume and duration between feeds in women breastfeeding their full-term infants over a 24 h period. *Exp Physiol* 87(2):207–214.

Kent, J. et al. 2006. Volume and frequency of breastfeedings and fat content of breast milk throughout the day. *Pediatrics* 117(3):e387–e395.

Lawrence, R. and R. Lawrence. 2005. *Breastfeeding: A Guide for the Medical Profession, 6th edition*, 1018–1020. St. Louis: Mosby.

Riordan, J. 2010. Anatomy and physiology of lactation. In *Breastfeeding and Human Lactation, 4th edition*. Riordan, J. and K. Wambach, ed., 88–90. Sudbury, MA: Jones and Bartlett.

305 **storing your expressed milk**

Adeola, K.F. and O.O. Adunni. 1998. Effect of storage temperature on microbial quality of infant milk. *J Trop Pediatr* 44(1):54–55.

Barger, J. and P. Bull. 1987. Comparison of the bacterial composition of breast milk stored at room temperature and stored in the refrigerator. *Int J Childbirth Ed* 2:29–30.

Cook, P. 2006. *Handling and Storage of Expressed Breast Milk*. London: Food Standards Agency.

Hamosh, M. et al. 1996. Breastfeeding and the working mother: effect of time and temperature of short term storage on proteolysis, lipolysis, and bacterial growth in milk. *Pediatrics* 97(4):493–498.

Hands, A. 2003. Safe storage of expressed breast milk in the home. *MIDIRS Midwifery Digest* 13(3):378–385.

Hanna, N. et al. 2004. Effect of storage on breast milk antioxidant activity. *Arch Dis Child Fetal Neonatal Ed* 89(6):518–520.

Igumbor, E.O. et al. 2000. Storage of breast milk: effect of temperature and storage duration on microbial growth. *Cent Afr J Med* 46(9): 247–251.

Jones, F. and M.R. Tully. 2006. *Best Practice for Expressing, Storing and Handling Human Milk in Hospitals, Homes and Child Care Settings, 2nd edition*. Raleigh, NC: Human Milk Banking Association of North America.

Mannel, R. et al. 2007. *Core Curriculum for Lactation Consultant Practice, 2nd edition*, 534–535. Sudbury, MA: Jones and Bartlett.

Martinez-Costa, C. et al. 2007. Effects of refrigeration on the bactericidal activity of human milk: a preliminary study. *J Pediatr Gastroenterol Nutr* 45(2):275–277.

Ogundele, M.O. 2000. Techniques for the storage of human breast milk: implications for anti-microbial functions and safety of stored milk. *Eur J Pediatr* 159(11):793–797.

Ogundele, M.O. 2002. Effects of storage on the physicochemical and antibacterial properties of human milk. *Br J Biomed Sci* 59(4):205–211.

Pardou, A. et al. 1994. Human milk banking: influence of storage processes and of bacterial contamination on some milk constituents. *Biol Neonate* 65(5):302–309.

Pittard, W.B. III et al. 1985. Bacteriostatic qualities of human milk. *J Pediatr* 107(2):240–243.

Silvestre, D. et al. 2006. Bactericidal activity of human milk: stability during storage. *Br J Biomed Sci* 63(2):59–62.

Williams-Arnold, L.D. 2000. *Human Milk Storage for Healthy Infants and Children*. Sandwich, MA: Health Education Associates.

305 **use containers that are not made with the endocrine disruptor bisphenol-A (BPA)**

National Toxicology Program. 2008. *Draft NTP Brief on Bisphenol A. CAS No. 80–05–7*. National Institute of Environmental Health Sciences, National Institutes of Health. Washington, DC: U.S. Department of Health and Human Services.

307 *don't* **use a microwave [to heat your milk]**

Quan, R. et al. 1992. Effects of microwave radiation on anti-infective factors in human milk. *Pediatrics* 89(4 Pt 1):667–669.

Sigman, M. et al. 1989. Effects of microwaving human milk: changes in IgA content and bacterial count. *J Am Diet Assoc* 89(5):690–692.

SIXTEEN Everybody Weans

314 **when should [Ending breastfeeding] end**

Dettwyler, K.A. 2003. A time to wean: the hominid blueprint for the natural age of weaning in modern human populations. In *Breastfeeding: Biocultural Perspectives*. Stuart-Macadam, P. and K.A. Dettwyler, ed., 39–73. New York: Aldine De Gruyter.

Flower, H. 2003. *Adventures in Tandem Nursing*. Schaumburg, IL: La Leche League International.

Habicht, J.P. 2004. WHO Expert Consultation. Expert consultation on the optimal duration of exclusive breastfeeding: the process, recommendations, and challenges for the future. *Adv Exp Med Biol* 554:79–87.

Kramer, M.S. and R. Kakuma. 2004. The optimal duration of exclusive breastfeeding: a systematic review. *Adv Exp Med Biol* 554:63–77.

Mean, M, and N. Newton. 1967. Cultural patterns of perinatal behavior. In *Childbearing: Its Social and Psychological Aspects*. Richardon, S.A. and A.F. Guttmacher, ed. Baltimore: Williams & Wilkins.

UNICEF. 2009. *The Baby-Friendly Hospital Initiative: Ten Steps to Successful Breastfeeding*. <http://www.unicef.org/nutrition/index_24806.html>.

316 **the longer you breastfeed the better it is for both of you**

Bachrach, V.R. et al. 2003. Breastfeeding and the risk of hospitalization for respiratory disease in infancy: a meta-analysis. *Arch Pediatr Adolesc Med* 157(3):237–243.

Chantry, C.J. et al. 2006. Full breastfeeding duration and associated decrease in respiratory tract infection in US children. *Pediatrics* 117(2):425–432.

Collaborative Group on Hormonal Factors in Breast Cancer. 2002. Breast cancer and breastfeeding: collaborative reanalysis of individual data from 47 epidemiological studies in 30 countries, including 50302 women with breast cancer and 96973 women without the disease. *Lancet* 360(9328):187–195.

Daniels, M.C. and L.S. Adair. 2005. Breast-feeding influences cognitive development in Filipino children. *J Nutr* 135(11):2589–2595.

Helewa, M. et al. 2002. Breast cancer, pregnancy, and breastfeeding. *J Obstet Gynaecol Can* 24(2):164–180.

Ip, S. et al. 2007. Breastfeeding and maternal and infant health outcomes in developed countries. *Evidence Report/Technology Assessment No 153. AHRQ Publication No. 07-E007.* Rockville, MD: Agency for Health Care Research and Quality.

Kokkonen, J. et al. 2004. Gastrointestinal complaints and diagnosis in children: a population-based study. *Acta Paediatr* 93(7):880–886.

Kramer, M.S. et al. 2008. Breastfeeding and child cognitive development: new evidence from a large randomized trial. *Arch Gen Psychiatry* 65(5):578–584.

Lee, S.Y. et al. 2003. Effect of lifetime lactation on breast cancer risk: a Korean women's cohort study. *Int J Cancer* 105(3):390–393.

Montgomery, S.M. et al. 2006. Breast feeding and resilience against psychosocial stress. *Arch Dis Child* 91(12):990–994.

Oddy, W.H. et al. 2004. The relation of breastfeeding and body mass index to asthma and atopy in children: a prospective cohort study to age 6 years. *Am J Public Health* 94(9):1531–1537.

UNICEF et al. 2002. *Facts for Life, 3rd edition.* New York: UNICEF.

321 **pregnancy rarely *requires* that you wean**

Newton, N. and M. Theotokjatos. 1979. Breastfeeding during pregnancy in 503 women: does a psychobiological weaning mechanism exist in humans? *Emotion Reprod* 20B:845–849.

West, D. and L. Marasco. 2009. *The Breastfeeding Mother's Guide to Making More Milk,* 167–192. New York: McGraw-Hill.

Zhu, B.P. et al. 2001. Effect of the interval between pregnancies on perinatal outcomes among white and black women. *Am J Obstet Gynecol* 185(6):1403–1410.

322 **one situation that can affect your fertility even when you're having regular periods is a short *luteal phase***

Karamardian L.M. and D.A. Grimes. 1992. Luteal phase deficiency: effect of treatment on pregnancy rates. *Am J Obstet Gynecol* Nov;167(5):1391–1398.

McNeilly, A.S. et al. 2008. Fertility after childbirth: adequacy of post-partum luteal phases. *Clin Endocrin* 17(6):609–615.

323 **there's no need to stop breastfeeding (or to pump and throw your milk away) if you have general anesthesia**

Montgomery, A. et al. 2006. The Academy of Breastfeeding Medicine Protocol Committee. ABM clinical protocol #15: Analgesia and anesthesia for the breastfeeding mother. *Breastfeeding Medicine* 1(4):271–277.

323 **there are *very few* medications that don't work with breastfeeding**

Hale, T.W. 2008. *Medications and Mothers' Milk, 13th edition.* Amarillo, TX: Hale Publishing.

326 **"Triple Nipple Syndrome": breast, pacifier, and bottle**

Latham, M.C. et al. 1986. Infant feeding in urban Kenya: a pattern of early triple nipple feeding. *J Trop Pediatr* 32(6):276–280.

326 **if a baby has learned that a breast is just food and a pacifier or a bottle is for comfort, he can decide that it's not worth the bother of negotiating for the breast**

Neifert, M. et al. 1995. Nipple confusion: toward a formal definition. *J Pediatr* 126(6):S125–S129.

Peterson, A., and M. Harmer. 2010. *Balancing Breast and Bottle: Reaching Your Breastfeeding Goals.* Amarillo, TX: Hale Publishing.

Viggiano, D. et al. 2005. Breastfeeding, bottlefeeding, and non-nutritive sucking: effects on occlusion in deciduous dentition. *Arch Dis Child* 89(12):1121–1123.

336 **early night weaning is a risk factor**

McKenna, J.J. 2007. *Sleeping with Your Baby: A Parent's Guide to Cosleeping,* 38–145. Washington, DC: Platypus Media.

Pantley, E. 2005. *The No-Cry Sleep Solution for Toddlers and Pre-schoolers,* 3–16, 141–144. New York: McGraw-Hill.

SEVENTEEN Alternate Routes

340 **some women pump exclusively**

Mohrbacher, N. 1996. Mothers who chose to pump instead of breastfeeding. *Circle of Caring* 9(2):1.

343 **[breastfeeding] a premature baby**

Cregan, M. et al. 2002. Initiation of lactation in women after preterm birth. *Acta Obstet Gynecol Scand* 81(9):870–877.

Henderson, J.J. et al. 2008. Effect of preterm birth and antenatal corticosteroid treatment on lactogenesis II in women. *Pediatrics* 121(1):e92–e100.

Hill, P.D. et al. 2001. Initiation and frequency of pumping and milk production in mothers of non-nursing preterm infants. *J Hum Lact* 17(1):9–13.

Hurst, N.M. and P.P. Meier. 2010. Breastfeeding the preterm infant. In *Breastfeeding and Human Lactation, 4th edition.* Riordan, J. and K. Wambach, ed. 444–447. Sudbury, MA: Jones and Bartlett.

McGuire, W. and M.Y. Anthony. 2003. Donor human milk versus formula for preventing necrotising enterocolitis in preterm infants: systematic review. *Arch Dis Child Fetal Neonatal Ed* 88(1):F11-F14.

Morton, J. et al. 2009. Combining hand techniques with electric pumping increases milk production in mothers of preterm infants. *J Perinatol* 29(11):757–764.

Schanler, R.J. et al. 1999. Feeding strategies for premature infants: beneficial outcomes of feeding fortified human milk versus preterm formula. *Pediatrics* 103(6 Pt 1):1150–1157.

Schanler, R.J. et al. 2005. Randomized trial of donor human milk versus preterm formula as substitutes for mothers' own milk in the feeding of extremely premature infants. *Pediatrics* 116(2):400–406.

345 **the value of Kangaroo Care**

Bergman, N.J. et al. 2004. Randomized controlled trial of skin-to-skin contact from birth versus conventional incubator for physiological stabilization in 1200- to 2199-gram newborns. *Acta Paediatr* 93:779–785.

Charpak, N. et al. 2005. Influence of feeding patterns and other factors on early somatic growth of healthy, preterm infants in home-based kangaroo mother care: A cohort study. *Pediatr Gastroenterol Nutr* 41(4):430–437.

Conde-Agudelo, A. et al. 2003. Kangaroo mother care to reduce morbidity and mortality in low birthweight infants. *Cochrane Database Syst Rev* 2003(2):CD002771.

Dodd, V. 2005. Implications of kangaroo care for growth and development in preterm infants. *J Obstet Gynecol Neonatal Nurs* 34(2):218–232.

Ellett, M. et al. 2004. Feasibility of using kangaroo (skin-to-skin) care with colicky infants. *Gastroenterol Nursing* 27(1):9–15.

Feldman, R. et al. 2002. Comparison of skin-to-skin (kangaroo) and traditional care: parenting outcomes and preterm development. *Pediatrics* 110(1):16–26.

Johnston, C. et al. 2003. Kangaroo care is effective in diminishing pain response in preterm neonates. *Arch Pediatr Adolesc Med* 157(11):1084–1088.

Kirsten, G. et al. 2001. Part 2: The management of breastfeeding. Kangaroo mother care in the nursery. *Pediatric Clin N Am* Apr;48(2):443–452.

Ludington-Hoe, S. et al. 2005. Skin-to-skin contact (kangaroo care) analgesia for preterm infant heel stick. *AACN Clinical Issues* 16(3):373–387.

McCain, G. et al. 2005. Heart rate variability responses of a preterm infant to kangaroo care. *J Obstet Gynecol Neonatal Nurs* 34(6):689–694.

Penalva, O. and J. Schwartzman. 2006. Descriptive study of the clinical and nutritional profile and follow-up of premature babies in a Kangaroo Mother Care Program. *J Pediatr* 82(1):33–39.

Worku, B. and A. Kassie. 2005. Kangaroo Mother Care: a randomized controlled trial on effectiveness of early Kangaroo Mother Care of the low birthweight infants in Addis Ababa, Ethiopia. *J Trop Pediatr* 51(2):93–97.

350 **help your near-term baby breastfeed**

Walker, M. 2008. Breastfeeding the late preterm infant. *J Obstet Gynecol Neonatal Nurs* Nov-Dec;37(6):692–701.

351 **breastfeeding twins, triplets, or more**

Flidel-Rimon, O. and E.S. Shinwell. 2006. Breast feeding twins and high multiples. *Arch Dis Child Fetal Neonatal Ed* 91(5):F377–F380.

Gromada, K. and A. Spangler. 1998. Breastfeeding twins and higher-order multiples. *J Obstet Gynecol Neonatal Nurs* 27(4):441–449.

Leonard, L.G. 2002. Breastfeeding higher order multiples: enhancing support during the postpartum hospitalization period. *J Hum Lact* 18(4):386–392.

Leonard, L.G. 2003. Breastfeeding rights of multiple birth families and guidelines for health professionals. *Twin Res* 6(1):34–45.

354 **relactation**

Agarwal, A. and A. Jain. 2009. Early successful relactation in a case of prolonged lactation failure. *Indian J Pediatr* Nov 20 (Epub ahead of print).

Alves, J.G. 1999. Relactation improves nutritional status in hospitalized infants. *J Trop Pediatr* 45(2):120–121.

Banapurmath, S. et al. 2003. Initiation of lactation and establishing relactation in outpatients. *Indian Pediatr* 40(4):343–347.

Butler, K. 2009. Relactation. *LLLGB Feedback*. Autumn:19–21.

De, N.C. et al. 2002. Initiating the process of relactation: an Institute based study. *Indian Pediatr* 39(2):173–178.

Menon, J. and L. Mathews. 2002. Relactation in mothers of high risk infants. *Indian Pediatr* 39(10):983–984.

358 **bringing in a milk supply without having been pregnant**

Auerbach, K.G. and J. Avery. 1981. Induced lactation: a study of adoptive nursing by 240 women. *Am J Dis Child* 135(4):340–343.

Banapurmath, S. et al. 2003. Initiation of lactation and establishing relactation in outpatients. *Indian Pediatr* 40(4):343–347.

Biervliet, F.P. et al. 2001. Induction of lactation in the intended mother of a surrogate pregnancy: case report. *Hum Reprod* 16(3):581–583.

Bryant, C.A. 2006. Nursing the adopted infant. *J Am Board Fam Med* 19(4):374–379.

Cheales-Siebenaler, N. 1999. Induced lactation in an adoptive mother. *J Hum Lact* 15(1):41–43.

Goldfarb, L. and J. Newman. 2002. *The Protocols for Induced Lactation: A Guide for Maximizing Breastmilk Production*. <asklenore.info/breastfeeding/induced_lactation/protocols_intro.html>.

362 **a mother who has diabetes and breastfeeds**

Hartmann, P. and M. Cregan. 2001. Lactogenesis and the effects of insulin-dependent diabetes mellitus and prematurity. *J Nutr* 131(11):3016S–3020S.

National Collaborating Centre for Women's and Children's Health. 2008. *NICE Clinical Guideline 63: Diabetes in Pregnancy: Management of Diabetes and Its Complications from Preconception to the Postnatal Period*. <nice.org.uk/CG063>.

Owen, C.G. et al. 2006. Does breastfeeding influence risk of type 2 diabetes in later life? A quantitative analysis of published evidence. *Am J Clin Nutr* 84(5):1043–1054.

Taylor, J.S. et al. 2005. A systematic review of the literature associating breastfeeding with type 2 diabetes and gestational diabetes. *J Am Coll Nutr* 24(5):320–326.

363 **the risk of an infant contracting HIV from an infected mother is much higher if the baby is both breastfed *and* receives formula supplementation than if he is exclusively breastfed or exclusively formula-fed**

Morrison, P. 2008. Taking another look at global policy on HIV and infant feeding. AnotherLook. <anotherlook.org>.

Shearer, W.J. 2008. Breastfeeding and HIV infection. *Pediatr* 121(5):1046–1047.

WHO; UNICEF; UNAIDS; UNFPA. 2007. *HIV Transmission Through Breastfeeding: A Review of Available Evidence—An Update from 2001 to 2007.* <who.int/nutrition/topics/ Paper_5_Infant_Feeding_bangkok.pdf>.

WHO; UNICEF; UNAIDS; UNFPA. 2007. *HIV and Infant Feeding: Update 2007.* <who .int/child_adolescent_health/documents/9789241595964/en/index.html>.

364 **how much these tests affect breastfeeding and your ability to make milk depends on what's done and what stage of lactation you're in**

ACR Committee on Drugs and Contrast Media. 2001. Administration of contrast medium to breastfeeding mothers. *ACR Bulletin* 57(10):12–13.

Helewa, M. et al. 2002. Breast cancer, pregnancy, and breastfeeding. *J Obstet Gynaecol Can* Feb;24(2):164–180.

Higgins, S. and B. Haffty. 1994. Pregnancy and lactation after breast-conserving therapy for early stage breast cancer. *Cancer* Apr 15;73(8):2175–2180.

Newman, J. 2007. Breastfeeding and radiologic procedures. *Canadian Family Physician* 53:630–631.

Tralins, A.H. 1995. Lactation after conservative breast surgery combined with radiation therapy. *Am J Clin Oncol* Feb;18(1):40–43.

367 **all previous breast and nipple surgeries, including breast reductions, breast augmentations, and nipple inversion release surgeries, can affect future milk production**

Ahmed, A. and P. Kolhe. 2000. Comparison of nipple and areolar sensation after breast reduction by free nipple graft and inferior pedicle techniques. *Br J Plast Surg* 53(2):126–129.

Chiummariello, S. et al. 2008. Breastfeeding after reduction mammaplasty using different techniques. *Aesth Plast Surg* 32(2):294–297.

Cruz, N. and L. Korchin. 2007. Lactational performance after breast reduction with different pedicles. *Plast Reconstr Surg* 120(1):35–40.

Hurst, N.M. 1996. Lactation after augmentation mammaplasty. *Obstet Gynecol* 87(1):30–34.

Kakagia, D. et al. 2005. Breastfeeding after reduction mammaplasty: a comparison of 3 techniques. *Ann Plast Surg* 55(4):343–345.

Michalopoulos, K. 2007. The effects of breast augmentation surgery on future ability to lactate. *Breast J* 13(1):62–67.

Modfid, M.M. et al. 2006. Nipple-areola complex sensitivity after primary breast augmentation: a comparison of periareolar and inframammary incision approaches. *Plast Reconstr Surg* 117(6):1694–1698.

Nommsen-Rivers, L. 2003. Cosmetic breast surgery—is breastfeeding at risk? *J Hum Lact* 19(1):7–8.

West, D. 2001. *Defining Your Own Success: Breastfeeding After Breast Reduction Surgery.* Schaumburg, IL: La Leche League International.

Widdice, L. 1993. The effects of breast reduction and breast augmentation surgery on lactation: an annotated bibliography. *J Hum Lact* 9(3):161–167.

368 the baby born with a disability or medical problem needs the stimulation, attention, and closeness that naturally happen with breastfeeding even more than a healthy baby does

Genna, C.W. et al. 2008. Neurological issues and breastfeeding. In *Supporting Sucking Skills in Breastfeeding Infants*. Genna, C.W., ed., 253–303. Sudbury, MA: Jones and Bartlett.

Lactation Consultant Series Two, Unit 9. Schaumburg, IL: La Leche League International.

Page-Goertz, S. and J. Riordan. 2010. The ill child: breastfeeding implications. In *Breastfeeding and Human Lactation, 4th edition*. Riordan, J. and K. Wambach, ed., 639–640, 650, 652, 654–655. Sudbury, MA: Jones and Bartlett.

369 immunological properties in your milk are very important if you have a baby with Down syndrome

Cooley, W. 1993. Supporting the family of the newborn with Down syndrome. *Compreh Therapy* 19(3):111–115.

Mizuno, K. and A. Ueda. 2001. Development of sucking behavior in infants with Down's syndrome. *Acta Paediatr* 90:1384–1388.

Pisacane, A. 2003. Down syndrome and breastfeeding. *Acta Paediatr* 92(12): 1479–1481.

Saenz, R.B. 2004. *Helping a Mother Breastfeed Her Baby with Down Syndrome*. Schaumburg, IL: La Leche League International.

370 a baby with an opening in his palate has difficulty creating suction, which makes it difficult to remove milk effectively no matter how he is fed

Cohen, M. et al. 1992. Immediate unrestricted feeding of infants following cleft lip and palate repair. *J Craniofac Surg* 3(1):30–32.

Denk, M.J. 1998. Topics in pediatric plastic surgery. *Ped Clin No Amer* 45(6): 1479–1506.

Mcheik, J. et al. 2006. Early repair for infants with cleft lip and nose. *Int J Pediatr Otorhinolaryng* 70(10):1785–1790.

Sandberg, D.J. et al. 2002. Neonatal cleft lip and cleft palate repair. *AORN J* 75(3):490–498.

371 breastfeeding your baby with *cystic fibrosis*, *celiac disease*, or other malabsorption problems can protect him from respiratory infections and help him gain weight more normally

Duncan, L.L. and S.B. Elder. 1997. Breastfeeding the infant with PKU. *J Hum Lact* 13(3):231–235.

Gaskin, K. and Waters, D. 1994. Nutritional management of infants with cystic fibrosis. *J Paediatr Child Health* 30:1–2.

Greve, L. et al. 1994. Breast-feeding in the management of the newborn with phenylketonuria: a practical approach to dietary therapy. *J Am Diet Assoc* 94:305–309.

Holliday, K. et al. 1991. Growth of human milk-fed and formula-fed infants with cystic fibrosis. *J Pediatr* 118:77–79.

Luder, E. et al. 1990. Current recommendations for breastfeeding in cystic fibrosis centers. *Am J Dis Child* 144:1153–1156.

McCabe, L. 1989. The management of breast feeding among infants with phenylketonuria. *J Inher Metab Dis* 12:467–474.

Motzfeldt, L. et al. 1999. Breastfeeding in phenylketonuria. *Acta Paediatr Suppl* 88(432):25–27.

Rooney, K. 1988. Breastfeeding a baby with cystic fibrosis. *New Beginnings* 4:43–44.

Riva, E. et al. 1996. Early breastfeeding is linked to higher intelligence quotient scores in dietary treated phenylketonuric children. *Acta Paediatr* 85:56–58.

EIGHTEEN   Tech Support

375   **[alcohol is] generally safe in moderation**

Cobo, E. 1973. Effect of different doses of ethanol on the milk-ejecting reflex in lactating women. *Am J Obstet Gynecol* 115(6):817–821.

Coiro, V. et al. 1992. Inhibition by ethanol of the oxytocin response to breast stimulation in normal women and the role of endogenous opioids. *Acta Endocrinol (Copenh)* 126(3):213–216.

Koren, G. 2002. Drinking alcohol while breastfeeding: will it harm my baby? *Canadian Family Physician* 48:39–41.

Little, R.E. et al. 2002. ALSPAC Study Team. Alcohol, breastfeeding, and development at 18 months. *Pediatrics* 109(5):E72–2.

Mennella, J.A. 1997. The human infant's suckling responses to the flavor of alcohol in mother's milk. *Alcoholism Clin Exper Res* 21:581–585.

Mennella, J.A. 2001. Alcohol's effect on lactation. *Alcohol Res Health* 25(3):230–234.

Mennella, J.A. and G.K. Beauchamp. 1991. The transfer of alcohol to human milk: effects on flavor and the infant's behavior. *N Engl J Med* 325: 981–985.

Mennella, J.A. and G.K. Beauchamp. 1993. Beer, breast feeding and folklore. *Dev Psychobiol* 26: 459–466.

376   **you can definitely breastfeed after bariatric surgery**

Celiker, M.Y. and A. Chawla. 2009. Congenital B_{12} deficiency following maternal gastric bypass. *J Perinatol* 29(9):640–642.

Grange, D.K. and J.L. Finlay. 1994. Nutritional vitamin B_{12} deficiency in a breastfed infant following maternal gastric bypass. *Pediatr Hematol Oncol* 11(3):311–318.

Kombol, P. 2008. International Lactation Consultant Association. ILCA's Inside Track: a resource for breastfeeding mothers. Breastfeeding after weight loss surgery. *J Hum Lact* 24(3):341–342.

Martens, W.S. II et al. 1990. Failure of a nursing infant to thrive after the mother's gastric bypass for morbid obesity. *Pediatrics* 86(5):777–778.

Wardinsky, T.D. et al. 1995. Vitamin B_{12} deficiency associated with low breast-milk vitamin B$_{12}$ concentration in an infant following maternal gastric bypass surgery. *Arch Pediatr Adolesc Med* 149(11):1281–1284.

377 **Blebs**

Huml S. 1999. Sore nipples. A new look at an old problem through the eyes of a dermatologist. *Pract Midwife* 2(2):28–31.

378 **Blood in Your Milk**

Virdi, V.S. et al. 2001. Rusty-pipe syndrome. *Indian Pediatr* 38(8):931–932.

380 **An abscess requires prompt medical care**

Agrawal, A. and M. Kissin. 2007. Breast abscess. *Br J Hosp Med (Lond)* 68(11): M198–M199.

Betzold, C.M. 2007. An update on the recognition and management of lactational breast inflammation. *J Midwifery Womens Health* 52(6):595–605.

Martin, J.G. 2009. Breast abscess in lactation. *J Midwifery Womens Health* 54(2): 150–151.

Wilson-Clay, B. 2008. Case report of methicillin-resistant *Staphylococcus aureus* (MRSA) mastitis with abscess formation in a breastfeeding woman. *J Hum Lact* 24(3):326–329.

380 **lumps that come and go are not a cause for any concern. If there's a particular lump that is persistently there, it may require some investigation.**

Bevin, T.H. and C.K. Pearson. 1993. Breastfeeding difficulties and a breast abscess associated with a galactocele: a case report. *J Hum Lact* 9(3):177–178.

Petok, E.S. 1995. Breast cancer and breastfeeding: five cases. *J Hum Lact* 11(3): 205–209.

Whang, I.Y. et al. 2007. Galactocele as a changing axillary lump in a pregnant woman. *Arch Gynecol Obstet* 276(4):379–382.

381 **Insufficient glandular tissue, or *breast hypoplasia*...can...have less milk-making tissue**

Huggins, K., E. Petok, and O. Mireles. 2000. Markers of lactation insufficiency: a study of 34 mothers. In *Current Issues in Clinical Lactation*, K. Auerbach, ed., 25–35. Sudbury, MA: Jones and Bartlett.

Knight, C.H. and A. Sorensen. 2001. Windows in early mammary development: critical or not? *Reproduction* 122(3):337–345.

383 **Colic**

Hewston, R. et al. 2007. Researching colic: a crying matter. Part 1: causes and risk factors. *Pract Midwife* 10(10):20–23.

Hewston, R. et al. 2007. Researching colic: a crying matter. Part 2: treatments. *Pract Midwife* 10(11):30–33.

Metcalf, T. et al. 1994. Simethicone in the treatment of infantile colic. *Pediatrics* 94: 29–34.

385 **Eating Disorders**

Bowles, B.C. and B.P. Williamson. 1990. Pregnancy and lactation following anorexia and bulimia. *J Obstet Gynecol Neonatal Nurs* 19(3):243–248.

Micali, N. et al. 2009. Infant feeding and weight in the first year of life in babies of women with eating disorders. *J Pediatr* 154(1):e55–e60.

Weekly, S.J. 1992. Diets and eating disorders: implications for the breastfeeding mother. *NAACOGS Clin Issu Perinat Womens Health Nurs* 3(4):695–700.

385 Engorgement

Academy of Breastfeeding Medicine Protocol Committee. Berens P. 2009. ABM clinical protocol #20: Engorgement. *Breastfeed Med* 4(2):111–113.

Arora, S. et al. 2008. A comparison of cabbage leaves vs. hot and cold compresses in the treatment of breast engorgement. *Indian J Community Med* 33(3):160–162.

Cotterman, K.J. 2004. Reverse pressure softening: a simple tool to prepare areola for easier latch during engorgement. *J Hum Lact* 20(2):227–237.

Roberts, K.L. 1995. A comparison of chilled cabbage leaves and chilled gelpaks in reducing breast engorgement. *J Hum Lact* 11(1):17–20.

Snowden, H.M. et al. 2001. Treatments for breast engorgement during lactation. *Cochrane Database Syst Rev* (2):CD000046.

392 if possible, talk with the anesthesiologist about the drugs that will be used. In almost all cases, breastfeeding is fine as soon as you're alert enough to hold your baby.

Academy of Breastfeeding Medicine Protocol Committee. Montgomery, A. et al. 2006. ABM clinical protocol #15: analgesia and anesthesia for the breastfeeding mother. *Breastfeeding Medicine* 1(4):271–277.

Hale, T.W. 1999. Anesthetic medications in breastfeeding mothers. *J Hum Lact* 15(3):185–194.

Hale, T.W. 2008. *Medications and Mothers' Milk, 13th edition.* Amarillo, TX: Hale Publishing.

Hale, T.W. 2010. Drug therapy and breastfeeding. In *Breastfeeding and Human Lactation, 4th edition.* Riordan, J. and K. Wambach, ed., 188–189. Sudbury, MA: Jones and Bartlett.

393 Hypoglycemia

Committee on Fetus and Newborn, American Academy of Pediatrics. 1993. Routine evaluation of blood pressure, hematocrit and glucose in newborns. *Pediatr* 92(3):474–476.

Cornblath, M. et al. 1990. Hypoglycemia in infancy: the need for a rational definition. *Pediatr* 85(5):834–837.

Cornblath, M. 1993. In *Metabolism and Endocrinology, Primary Care of the Newborn. Johns Hopkins Children's Center.* Seidel, Rosenstein and Pathak, ed. St. Louis, MO: Mosby YearBook.

Cornblath, M. and R. Schwartz. 1993. Hypoglycemia in the neonate. *J Pediatr Endocrinol* 6(2):113–129.

Hawdon, J.W. et al. 1992. Patterns of metabolic adaptation for preterm and term neonates in the first postnatal week. *Arch Dis Child* 67:357–365.

Hawdon, J.W. et al. 1994. Prevention and management of neonatal hypoglycemia. *Arch Dis Child* 70:F60–F65.

394 **Hypothermia**

See Kangaroo Care references in Chapter 17.

395 **Jaundice**

American Academy of Pediatrics Subcommittee on Hyperbilirubinemia. 2004. Management of hyperbilirubinemia in the newborn infant 35 or more weeks of gestation. *Pediatrics* 114(1):297–316.

Buiter, H.D. et al. 2008. Neonatal jaundice and stool production in breast- or formula-fed term infants. *Eur J Pediatr* 167(5):501–507.

Gourley, G. et al. 1999. Neonatal jaundice and diet. *Arch Pediatr Adolesc Med* 153:184–188.

ILCA Professional Development Committee. 2007. ILCA's Inside Track: my baby is jaundiced—what's that? *J Hum Lact* 23(2):199–200.

Mishra, S. et al. 2008. Jaundice in the newborn. *Indian J Pediatr* 75(2):157–63.

396 **there are ways to help...the milk supply**

Butler, K. 2009. *My Baby Needs More Milk.* LLLGB.

Crossland, D.S. et al. 2008. Weight change in the term baby in the first 2 weeks of life. *Acta Paediatr* 97(4):425–429.

Maisels, M.J. et al. 1994. The effect of breastfeeding frequency on serum bilirubin levels. *Am J Obstet Gynecol* 170:880–883.

West, D. and L. Marasco. 2009. *The Breastfeeding Mother's Guide to Making More Milk*, 15–37, 103–118. New York: McGraw-Hill.

397 **A galactagogue...may add to the boost that good milk removal provides**

Academy of Breastfeeding Medicine. 2004. *Protocol #9: Use of Galactagogues in Initiating or Augmenting Maternal Milk Supply.* <http://www.bfmed.org/Resources/Protocols.aspx>.

Anderson, P.O. and V. Valdés. 2007. A critical review of pharmaceutical galactagogues. *Breastfeed Med* 2(4):229–242.

Anfinson, T. 2002. Akathisia, panic, agoraphobia, and major depression following brief exposure to metoclopramide. *Psychopharmacol Bul* 36(1):82–93.

Da Silva, O. et al. 2001. Effect of domperidone on milk production in mothers of premature newborns: a randomized, double-blind, placebo-controlled trial. *CMAJ* 164(1):17–21.

Dalvi, S.S. 1990. Effect of Asparagus racemosus (Shatavari) on gastric emptying time in normal healthy volunteers. *J Postgrad Med* 36(2):91–94.

Ehrenkrantz, R. and B. Ackerman. 1986. Metoclopramide effect on faltering milk production by mothers of premature infants. *Pediatric* 78(4):614–620.

Feillet, N. et al. 1996. Metaclopramide and depression: apropos of a case of a pregnant woman. [French] *Therapie* 51(5):600–601.

Gabay, M.P. 2002. Galactagogues: medications that induce lactation. *J Hum Lact* 18(3):274–279.

Goyal, R.K. et al. 2003. Asparagus racemosus—an update. *Indian J Med Sci* 57(9):408–414.

Humphrey, S. 2003. *The Nursing Mother's Herbal*. Minneapolis: Fairview Press.

Humphrey, S. and D. McKenna. 1997. Herbs and breastfeeding. *Breastfeeding Abstracts* 17(2):11–12.

Kauppila, A. et al. 1981. Metoclopramide increases prolactin release and milk secretion in puerperium without stimulating the secretion of thyrotropin and thyroid hormones. *J Clin Endocrinol Metab* 52(3):436–439.

Nice, F. et al. 2000. Herbals and breastfeeding: which herbals are safe to take while breastfeeding. *Birth Issues* 9(3).

Patel, A. and U. Kanitkar. 1969. Asparagus racemosus wild-form bordi, as a galactagogue, in buffaloes. *Indian Vet J* 46(8):718–721.

Petraglia, F. et al. 1985. Domperidone in defective and insufficient lactation. *Eur J Obstet Gynecol Reprod Biol* 19(5):281–287.

Prakash, A. and A. Wagstaff. 1998. Domperidone. A review of its use in diabetic gastropathy. *Drugs* 56(3):429–445.

Reddymasu, S. et al. 2007. Domperidone: review of pharmacology and clinical applications in gastroenterology. *Am J Gastroenterol* 102(9):2036–2045.

Sabnis, P. et al. 1968. Effects of alcoholic extracts of Asparagus racemosus on mammary glands of rats. *Indian J Exp Biol* 6(1):55–57.

Sharma, S. et al. 1996. Randomized controlled trial of Asparagus racemosus (Shatavari) as a lactogogue in lactational inadequacy. *Indian Pediatr* 33(8):675–677.

Soykan, I. et al. 1997. The effect of chronic oral domperidone therapy on gastrointestinal symptoms, gastric emptying, and quality of life in patients with gastroparesis. *Am J Gastroenterol* 92(6):976–980.

Swafford, S. and P. Berens. 2000. Effect of fenugreek on breast milk volume. *ABM News & Views* 6(3):21.

398 Mastitis

Academy of Breastfeeding Medicine Protocol Committee. 2008. ABM clinical protocol #4: Mastitis. *Breastfeed Med* 3(3):177–180.

Spencer, J.P. 2008. Management of mastitis in breastfeeding women. *Am Fam Physician* 78(6):727–731.

400 Medications and Breastfeeding

American Academy of Pediatrics Committee on Drugs. 2001. The transfer of drugs and other chemicals into human milk. *Pediatrics* 108(3):776–789.

Hale, T.W. 2008. *Medications and Mothers' Milk, 13th edition*. Amarillo, TX: Hale Publishing.

404 *inverted nipples*

Arsenault, G. 1997. Using a disposable syringe to treat inverted nipples. *Can Fam Physician* 43:1517–1518.

Dewey, K.G. et al. 2003. Risk factors for suboptimal infant breastfeeding behavior, delayed onset of lactation, and excess neonatal weight loss. *Pediatrics* 112(3 Pt 1):607–619.

Patel, Y. 2008. Inverted nipples: correction using a simple disposable syringe. *East Afr Med J* 85(1):51–52.

Vazirinejad, R. et al. 2009. The effect of maternal breast variations on neonatal weight gain in the first seven days of life. *Int Breastfeed J* 18(4):13.

Vogel, A. et al. 1999. Factors associated with the duration of breastfeeding. *Acta Paediatr* 88(12):1320–1326.

404 nipple shields

Bodley, V. and D. Powers. 1996. Long-term nipple shield use—a positive perspective. *J Hum Lact* 12(4):301–304.

Chertok, I.R. 2009. Reexamination of ultra-thin nipple shield use, infant growth and maternal satisfaction. *J Clin Nurs* 18(21):2949–2955.

Chertok, I.R. et al. 2006. A pilot study of maternal and term infant outcomes associated with ultrathin nipple shield use. *J Obstet Gynecol Neonatal Nurs* 35(2):265–272.

Clum, D. and J. Primomo. 1996. Use of a silicone nipple shield with premature infants. *J Hum Lact* 12(4):287–290.

Elliott, C. 1996. Using a silicone nipple shield to assist a baby unable to latch. *J Hum Lact* 12(4):309–313.

Meier, P.P. et al. 2000. Nipple shields for preterm infants: effect on milk transfer and duration of breastfeeding. *J Hum Lact* 16(2):106–114.

Powers, D. and V.B. Tapia. 2004. Women's experiences using a nipple shield. *J Hum Lact* 20(3):327–334.

Wilson-Clay, B. 1996. Clinical use of silicone nipple shields. *J Hum Lact* 12(4):279–285.

Woodworth, M. and E. Frank. 1996. Transitioning to the breast at six weeks: use of a nipple shield. *J Hum Lact* 12(4):305–307.

408 oversupply

Butler, K. and S. Upstone. 2009. *Too Much Milk*. LLLGB.

Livingstone, V. 1997. The maternal hyperlactation syndrome. *Medicine North America* 20(2):42–46.

Smillie, C.M. et al. 2005. Hyperlactation: how left-brained rules for breastfeeding can wreak havoc with a natural process. *Newborn Infant Nurs Rev* 5(1):49–58.

Van Veldhuizen-Staas, C. 2007. Overabundant milk supply: an alternate way to intervene by full drainage and block feeding. *Int Breastfeed J* 2(11).

Wilson-Clay, B. 2006. Milk oversupply. *J Hum Lact* 22(2):218–220.

412 nipple piercings don't usually affect milk production

Angel, E. 2009. *The Piercing Bible: The Definitive Guide to Safe Body Piercing*. Berkeley, CA: Celestial Arts.

414 Postpartum Depression

Kendall-Tackett, K. 2005. *Depression in New Mothers: Causes, Consequences, and Treatment Alternatives*. Binghamton, NY: Haworth Maltreatment and Trauma Press.

417 *research does not support thickened feeds* [for reflux]

Horvath, A. et al. 2008. The effect of thickened-feed interventions on gastroesophageal reflux in infants: systematic review and meta-analysis of randomized, controlled trials. *Pedatrics* 122(6):e1268–e1277.

417 **Sore Nipples**

Glover, R. and D. Wiessinger. 2008. The infant-maternal breastfeeding conversation: helping when they lose the thread. In *Supporting Sucking Skills in Breastfeeding Infants.* Genna, C.W., ed., 122–123. Sudbury, MA: Jones and Bartlett.

McClellan, H. et al. 2008. Infants of mothers with persistent nipple pain exert strong sucking vacuums. *Acta Paediatr* 97(9):1205–1209.

Smillie, C.M. 2008. How infants learn to feed: a neurobehavioural model. In *Supporting Sucking Skills in Breastfeeding Infants.* Genna, C.W., ed., 79–86. Sudbury, MA: Jones and Bartlett.

Smith, L.J. 2008. Why Johnny can't suck: impact of birth practices on infant suck. In *Supporting Sucking Skills in Breastfeeding Infants.* Genna, C.W., ed., 57–78. Sudbury, MA: Jones and Bartlett.

Wiessinger, D. 2004. The world of latch-on: one Leader's journey. *Leaven* 40(1):3–6.

420 **Supplementation**

Hunt, S. 2002. Breastfed babies: to supplement or not to supplement? *Pract Midwife* 5(6):20–21.

Kassing, D. 2002. Bottle-feeding as a tool to reinforce breastfeeding. *J Hum Lact* 18(1):56–60.

Li, R. et al. 2008. Association of breastfeeding intensity and bottle-emptying behaviors at early infancy with infants' risk for excess weight at late infancy. *Pediatrics* 122 (Suppl 2):S77–S84.

Rechtman, D.J. et al. 2006. Effect of environmental conditions on unpasteurized donor human milk. *Breastfeeding Medicine* 1(1):24–26.

Robke, F.J. 2008. Effects of nursing bottle misuse on oral health. Prevalence of caries, tooth malalignments and malocclusions in North-German preschool children. *J Orofac Orthop* 69(1):5–19.

427 **for the mother who smokes, breastfeeding is still a safer choice than formula**

Amir, L.H. 2001. Maternal smoking and reduced duration of breastfeeding: a review of possible mechanisms. *Early Hum Dev* 64(1):45–67.

Haug, K. et al. 1998. Secular trends in breastfeeding and parental smoking. *Acta Paediatr* 187(10):1023–1027.

Ilett, K.F. et al. 2003. Use of nicotine patches in breastfeeding mothers: transfer of nicotine and cotinine into human milk. *Clin Pharmacol Ther* 74(6):516–524.

Mennella, J.A. et al. 2007. Breastfeeding and smoking: short-term effects on infant feeding and sleep. *Pediatrics* 120(3):497–502.

Nafstad, P. et al. 1996. Breastfeeding, maternal smoking and lower respiratory tract infections. *Eur Respir J* 9(12):2623–2629.

Ratner, P.A. et al. 1999. Smoking relapse and early weaning among postpartum women: is there an association? *Birth* 26(2):76–82.

Steldinger, R. et al. 1988. Half lives of nicotine in milk of smoking mothers: implications for nursing. *J Perinat Med* 16(3):261–262.

428 **Tongue-tie**

Ballard, J.L. et al. 2002. Ankyloglossia: assessment, incidence, and effect of frenuloplasty on the breastfeeding dyad. *Pediatrics* 110(5):e63.

Başaklar, A.C. 2008. Ankyloglossia and effects on breast-feeding, speech problems and mechanical/social issues in children. *B-ENT* 4(2):81–85.

Chu, M.W. and D.C. Bloom. 2009. Posterior ankyloglossia: a case report. *Int J Pediatr Otorhinolaryngol* 73(6):881–883.

Coryllos, E.V. et al. 2008. Minimally invasive treatment for posterior tongue-tie (the hidden tongue-tie). In *Supporting Sucking Skills in Breastfeeding Infants*. Genna, C.W., ed., 227–234. Sudbury, MA: Jones and Bartlett.

Dollberg, S. et al. 2006. Immediate nipple pain relief after frenotomy in breast-fed infants with ankyloglossia: a randomized, prospective study. *J Pediatr Surg* 41(9):1598–1600.

Geddes, D.T. et al. 2008. Frenulotomy for breastfeeding infants with ankyloglossia: effect on milk removal and sucking mechanism as imaged by ultrasound. *Pediatrics* 122(1):e188–e194.

Geddes, D.T. et al. 2009. Sucking characteristics of successfully breastfeeding infants with ankyloglossia: a case series. *Acta Paediatr* (Epub ahead of print).

Genna, C.W. 2008. Influence of anatomic and structural issues on sucking skills. In *Supporting Sucking Skills in Breastfeeding Infants*. Genna, C.W., ed., 181–203 Sudbury, MA: Jones and Bartlett.

Genna, C.W. and L. Sandora. 2008. Breastfeeding: normal sucking and swallowing. In *Supporting Sucking Skills in Breastfeeding Infants*. Genna, C.W., ed., 1–42. Sudbury, MA: Jones and Bartlett.

Karabulut, R. et al. 2006. Ankyloglossia in breastfeeding infants: the effect of frenotomy on maternal nipple pain and latch. *Breastfeed Med* 1(4):216–224.

Lalakea, M.L. and A.H. Messner. 2003. Ankyloglossia: does it matter? *Pediatr Clin North Am* 50(2):381–397.

Messner, A.H. et al. 2000. Ankyloglossia: incidence and associated feeding difficulties. *Arch Otolaryngol Head Neck Surg* 126(1):36–39.

430 **Vasospasm**

Holmen, O.L. and B. Backe. 2009. An underdiagnosed cause of nipple pain presented on a camera phone. *BMJ* 339:b2553; 631–2.

Morino, C. and S.M. Winn. 2007. Raynaud's phenomenon of the nipples: An elusive diagnosis. *J Hum Lact* 23(2); 191–3.

433 **Yeast Infections**

Brent, N.B. 2001. Thrush in the breastfeeding dyad: results of a survey on diagnosis and treatment. *Clin Pediatr (Phila)* 40(9): 503–506.

da Costa Zöllner, M.S.A. and A.O. Jorge. 2003. Candida spp. occurrence in oral cavities of breast feeding infants and in their mothers' mouths and breasts. *Pesqui Odontol Bras* 17(2):151–155.

Francis-Morrill, J. et al. 2003. Detecting *Candida albicans* in human milk. *J Clin Microbiol* 41(1):475–478.

Francis-Morrill, J. et al. 2004. Diagnostic value of signs and symptoms of mammary candidosis among lactating women. *J Hum Lact* 20(3):288–94.

Francis-Morrill, J. et al. 2005. Risk factors for mammary candidosis among lactating women. *J Obstet Gynecol Neonatal Nurs* 34(1):37–45.

Graves, S. et al. 2003. Painful nipples in nursing mothers: fungal or staphylococcal? A preliminary study. *Aust Fam Physician* 32(7):570–571.

Hale, T.W. et al. 2009. The absence of *Candida albicans* in milk samples of women with clinical symptoms of ductal candidiasis. *Breastfeed Med* 4(2):57–61.

Panjaitan, M. et al. 2008. Polymerase chain reaction in detection of *Candida albicans* for confirmation of clinical diagnosis of nipple thrush. *Breastfeeding Med* 3(3):185–187.

Wiener, S. 2006. Diagnosis and management of Candida of the nipple and breast. *J Midwifery Womens Health* 51(2):125–128.

Picture Credits

Index

Would You Like to Know More?

La Leche League International is a source of information, support, and encouragement. La Leche League Groups meet all over the world to share breastfeeding and mothering experiences. To become a member of LLLI, your local Group, or to find a Leader in your community, visit the LLLI website at llli.org.

La Leche League International offers many resources in addition to this edition of *The Womanly Art of Breastfeeding:*

Local Resources

- Accredited La Leche League Leaders in sixty-eight countries
- Gatherings of mothers, babies, and La Leche League Leaders for information and support
- Phone and online help from accredited La Leche League International Leaders

Online Support and Information

- Mother-to-mother forums
- Help forms (mothers enter questions online and receive personalized answers from La Leche League Leaders via e-mail)
- Breastfeeding answers on a variety of topics of interest—general breastfeeding, maternal breastfeeding, infant/child breastfeeding, families, and more

Online support can be accessed by clicking the "Resources" link on our website home page at llli.org.

Publications

- Books on a variety of subjects such as breastfeeding, parenting, nutrition, children's books, and professional texts
- Information sheets—breastfeeding tips, is my baby getting enough milk, establishing your milk supply—for a full listing visit our website store. llli.org
- Online e-magazines

Our printed publications are available in our online store at store.llli.org or directly from our home page via the navigational tab. Additional publications are offered to members by various LLL entities around the world. These can be found by visiting the local websites linked on the llli.org home page.